The
Hospital Autopsy
A Manual of Fundamental Autopsy Practice

The
Hospital Autopsy
A Manual of Fundamental Autopsy Practice

THIRD EDITION

Julian L Burton MBChB (Hons) MEd FHEA
Senior Teaching Fellow and Senate Award Fellow (Learning and Teaching) at the University of Sheffield, Sheffield
and
Coronial Pathologist at the Medico-Legal Centre, Sheffield

Guy Rutty MD MBBS FRCPath DipRCPath(Forensic) FFFLM FFSSoc
Professor of Forensic Pathology, Chief Forensic Pathologist, East Midlands Forensic Pathology Unit, University of Leicester
and
Home Office Registered Forensic Pathologist, Leicester, UK

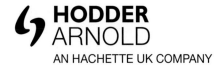
HODDER
ARNOLD
AN HACHETTE UK COMPANY

First published in Great Britain in 2001 by
Arnold a member of the Hodder Headline Group;
This third edition published in 2010 by Hodder Arnold, an imprint of Hodder Education, an Hachette UK company, 338 Euston Road, London NW1 3BH

http://www.hoddereducation.com

Hachette's policy is to use papers that are natural, renewable and recyclable products and made from wood grown in sustainable forests. The logging and manufacturing processes are expected to conform to the environmental regulations of the country of origin.

Whilst the advice and information in this book are believed to be true and accurate at the date of going to press, neither the author nor the publisher can accept any legal responsibility or liability for any errors or omissions that may be made. In particular (but without limiting the generality of the preceding disclaimer) every effort has been made to check drug dosages; however it is still possible that errors have been missed. Furthermore, dosage schedules are constantly being revised and new side-effects recognized. For these reasons the reader is strongly urged to consult the drug companies' printed instructions before administering any of the drugs recommended in this book.

British Library Cataloguing in Publication Data
A catalogue record for this book is available from the British Library

Library of Congress Cataloging-in-Publication Data
A catalog record for this book is available from the Library of Congress

ISBN   978 0 340 96514 6
1 2 3 4 5 6 7 8 9 10

Publisher: Caroline Makepeace
Commissioning Editor: Philip Shaw
Production Editor: Amy Mulick and Joanna Silman
Production Controller: Kate Harris
Cover Designer: Laura DeGrasse
Indexer: Laurence Errington

Typeset in 10 on 13pt Minion by Phoenix Photosetting, Chatham, Kent
Printed and bound in Italy

What do you think about this book? Or any other Hodder Arnold title?
Please visit our website: www.hoddereducation.com

CONTENTS

CONTRIBUTORS

Caroline Browne
Head of Regulation
Human Tissue Authority, London

Julian L Burton MBChB (Hons), MEd, FHEA
Senior Teaching Fellow and Senate Award Fellow
(Learning and Teaching) at the University of
Sheffield; and Coronial Pathologist at the
Medico-Legal Centre, Sheffield

Marta C Cohen MD
Consultant Paediatric Histopathologist
Histopathology Department Sheffield Children
NHS Foundation Trust. Honorary Senior Lecturer.
University of Sheffield, Sheffield

Steven Donlon MRSPH (Cert/Dip) FAAPT CFM
MBAHiD MCIFA
Mortuary Services Manager, Crosshouse Hospital,
Kilmornock, Ayrshire

Christopher P Dorries OBE
HM Coroner, The Medico-Legal Centre, Sheffield

Alexander RW Forrest BSc, MBChB, LLM, MCB, FRCP,
FRCPath, CSci, CChem, FRSC, FFSSoc, FFFLM, DObstRCOG
Honary Professor of Forensic Chemistry
Centre for Analytical Sciences, Department of
Chemistry, University of Sheffield,
Sheffield

David J Harvey MBChB, BSc (Hons), MRCP
Microbiology Department, Sheffield Teaching
Hospitals NHS Foundation Trust, Sheffield

Amanda J Jeffery MBChB, FRCPath(Forensic), MFFLM
Senior Lecturer in Forensic Pathology and Home
Office Registered Forensic Pathologist
East Midlands Forensic Pathology Unit, University
of Leicester, Leicester

James Lowe BMedSci, BMBS, DM, FRCPath
Professor of Neuropathology, University of
Nottingham Medical School and Honorary
Consultant Histopathologist to Queen's Medical
Centre, Nottingham

Sebastian Lucas BMBCh, FRCP, FRCPath
Department of Histopathology, King's College
London School of Medicine, St Thomas' Hospital,
London

G Harry Millward-Sadler BSc(Hons), MBChB, FRCPath
Honorary Consultant and Senior Lecturer
Southampton University Hospitals;
Central Pathology Assessor for Maternal Deaths
CMACE (was CEMACH)

Richard SH Pumphrey FRCPath
Honorary Consultant Clinical Immunologist
Central Manchester University Hospitals NHS
Foundation Trust, Manchester

Vimal Raj MBBS, FRCR, PGDMLS, EDM
Specialist Registrar in Radiology
University Hospitals of Leicester NHS Trust,
Leicester

Elisabeth J Ridgway MBBS, BSc (Hons), MD, FRCPath
Microbiology Department, Sheffield Teaching
Hospitals NHS Foundation Trust, Sheffield

Ian SD Roberts MBChB, FRCPath
Department of Cellular Pathology, John Radcliffe
Hospital, Oxford

Guy N Rutty MD, MBBS, FRCPath, DipRCPath(Forensic),
FFFLM, FFSSoc
Chief Forensic Pathologist
East Midlands Forensic Pathology Unit, University
of Leicester; and Home Office Registered Forensic
Pathologist, Leicester

Jane E Rutty MSc, BSc(Hons), DPSN, RGN, FHEA
Principal Lecturer (Nursing)
School of Nursing and Midwifery, Faculty of Health
and Life Sciences, De Montfort University, Leicester

James Underwood MD, FRCPath, FRCP, FMedSci
Emeritus Professor of Pathology
University of Sheffield, Sheffield

PREFACE TO THE THIRD EDITION

We are delighted to present the third edition of this established book, which again brings together the experience and guidance of recognised experts in autopsy practice and related subjects from across the United Kingdom into an illustrated, authoritative textbook.

Since the publication of the second edition, the hospital autopsy rate has continued to decline to such an extent that in many centres autopsies that are not performed on the instruction of a medicolegal authority have become a rarity. This has necessitated the addition of a subtitle to the title of this edition of the book to denote that this book now aims to provide information to a wider range of pathologists engaged in autopsy practice. This includes those examinations undertaken at the request of a medico-legal authority but who do not need the expertise of a forensic pathologist, and those performed with the consent of the relatives of the deceased.

In this third edition all of the chapters have been updated – in most cases by the original authors – to take account of advances that have taken place in the nine years since the second edition. It reflects the comments we gratefully received on the second edition, the increasing body of knowledge required of pathologists engaged in autopsy practice, and the increasing difficulty with which junior pathologists can come by the requisite experience to complete their training. We have also taken into account the changing world of autopsy practice with the increased use of so called minimally invasive or near virtual autopsies using radiological imaging modalities. Bearing all this in mind we have included six new chapters on the role of the autopsy in medical education, religious attitudes to the autopsy, autopsies of patients with high-risk infections, peri-operative and post-operative deaths, the radiological autopsy and the unascertained autopsy. We have further increased the number of photographs and illustrations in the book, almost all of which now appear in full colour.

In the United Kingdom, autopsy practice has been influenced by a number of publications, most notably the Guidelines on Autopsy Practice by the Royal College of Pathologists, and by amendments to the Coroners' Rules, the new Human Tissue Act, reports from the National Confidential Enquiry into Patient Outcome and Death and the formation of the Human Tissue Authority. The relevant parts of these documents and guidelines have been incorporated, where appropriate, into the chapters of the book. In light of these, we remain convinced that there is a need not for more autopsies, but for autopsies performed to a higher standard. There remains no single 'right way' to undertake an autopsy but the methods set out here are, we hope, a useful guide. We hope that the third edition of *The Hospital Autopsy* will continue the tradition of its predecessors: i.e. to inform junior and senior pathologists alike of best practices in both the basic techniques of the autopsy and the ancillary specialist techniques that are occasionally required.

Dr Julian L Burton and Professor Guy N Rutty 2010

Dr JL Burton is a coronial pathologist at the Medico-Legal Centre in Sheffield. His is active in autopsy practice and his practice focuses on sudden unexpected deaths in the community including those from natural causes, road traffic collisions, drug overdoses, industrial deaths and suicides. He has experience of postoperative death autopsies and an interest in autopsies performed on decomposed bodies. Dr Burton is also medical educationalist with a research interest in the role of the autopsy in undergraduate and postgraduate medical education.

Professor GN Rutty holds the Foundation Chair of Forensic Pathology, University of Leicester, UK where he is Chief Forensic Pathologist to the East Midlands Forensic Pathology Unit. He is a Home Office Registered Forensic Pathologist. He is the Chair of the Forensic Pathology Sub-Committee of the Royal College of Pathologists, and a member of the Home Office Policy Advisory Board for Forensic Pathology. He is active in autopsy practice, teaching and research with a pedigree of autopsy related publications. His current principle area of research relates to the use of radiological imaging in autopsy practice, mass fatality investigation and identification.

ACKNOWLEDGEMENTS

We would like to thank the following people who helped us during the preparation of this book:

- Drs Simon Cross and Dennis Cotton for the inspiration to write the first edition and then allowing us to take forward the concept into the second and third editions.
- The anatomical pathology technologists at The Medico-Legal Centre in Sheffield for their help and support.
- Joanna Silman of Hodder Arnold who motivated and supported us throughout the production of this book.
- Mr Carl Vivian of the University of Leicester Audio Visual Services for assisting with some of the images in the book.
- The Medical Illustration Unit of the University Hospitals of Leicester for one of the drawings used in the book.
- The relatives who gave permission for photographs to appear in the editions. Where permissions are not required the book adheres to current GMC guidelines related to images acquired at autopsy examination.

Chapter 1

THE HISTORY OF THE AUTOPSY

Julian L Burton

The greater the opportunity that hospitals give us for observing rare diseases – and this applies even more to the commoner diseases – the more often am I obliged to bewail the lot of the ancient physicians, who lacked hospitals … But, if after hospitals began to exist, it had been permitted to investigate diseases not only in sick persons but also in those who had died after every sickness, the advances that the medical profession would have made in the subsequent ten centuries can easily be estimated by considering the advances that have been made since both kinds of examination began to be permitted, about the beginning of the 16th century.

Morgagni (1761)

Introduction

The term 'autopsy' means 'to see for oneself' and is synonymous with the terms 'post-mortem', 'post-mortem examination' and 'necropsy'. None of these terms has a specific meaning that allows the extent or precise nature of the investigation to be inferred from their use. In modern practice, an autopsy is usually taken to indicate a detailed examination that includes the external examination of the corpse, and the evisceration and subsequent careful dissection of the contents of the cranial, thoracic, abdominal and pelvic cavities. Nonetheless, examinations restricted to a particular body cavity (either by the relatives' wishes or because of some infectious hazard), or to the sampling of the organs in the unopened body with a biopsy needle, are also regarded as autopsy examinations. In some countries, such as Scotland, where a 'view and grant' system of death certification exists, the term 'post-mortem examination' may refer only to the external examination, with no effort being made to examine the internal organs. So-called 'scan and grant' virtual autopsies, in which bodies are subjected to imaging rather than dissection, have also emerged in recent years (Rutty, 2007).

We can consider that there are two principal types of autopsy: hospital examinations, performed on the request of a clinician with the consent of the next of kin, and medicolegal autopsies. The latter can be subcategorised into those where there is a criminal or civil interest (forensic autopsies) and those where death is presumed to be due to natural causes (non-forensic medicolegal autopsies).

The variations in the scope of the examination implied by these terms must be remembered in any historical account of the autopsy. Furthermore, other terms have historically been used to describe what we now call 'autopsy'. Among these, the term 'dissection' is now taken to refer solely to the process of cutting apart or separating tissues and organs from one another for further study. 'Anatomisation' is a term that has fallen into disuse, but carries the connotation of a degree of dissection that sounds extreme.

Throughout recorded history, humans have felt both revulsion and fascination at the prospect of examination of the human body after death. These attitudes have been inextricably linked with the prevailing religious and political climates of the time, and, further, reflect the epistemological advances in our understanding of medicine and disease. As the nineteenth century French philosopher Auguste Comte (1798–1875) argued, the human mind has progressed from a theological stage, through a metaphysical stage, to a final positive stage. In the theological stage, primitive attempts are made to explain behaviour in terms of spiritual or supernatural entities. The metaphysical stage is a modification of this and explains behaviour in terms of abstractions, essences or forces. The positive stage dispenses with these concepts and turns to observation and reason as a means of understanding behaviour (Cohen and Manion, 1998). Such 'positivism' is the underlying principle of the modern scientific method. Thus, the purposes for which post-mortem examinations were performed have evolved from the prophetic, through a search for an imbalance of the humours, to a 'scientific' approach to the evaluation of the nature and extent of disease and the cause of death. Modern medicine has an anatomical and physiological attitude underlying most diseases and, even when such causes cannot be proven, we assume that they will someday be elucidated in these terms. Our continuing fascination with the autopsy in the twenty-first century is evidenced by the proliferation of web pages and television programmes discussing autopsies.

What follows is a brief account of the history of the modern autopsy. More detailed discussion is to be found in the excellent commentaries by Porter (1999), Park (1995) and King and Meehan (1973). Any historical account of the subject will lean heavily on their definitive studies.

Antiquity

The ancient Egyptians, whose civilisation rose under the Pharaohs around 3000 BC, practised medicine that had both an empirical and a magico-religious aspect. Human dissection was confined to the process of mummification, in which embalmers attempted to preserve the body intact. The internal organs were removed through small incisions (although the heart, believed to be the seat of the soul, was left *in situ*) and the brain was removed via the nose using hooks. Once removed, the organs were stored in special Canopic jars. While it was acceptable to tamper with the body of the deceased in this manner, the procedure was performed for entirely magico-religious reasons and no attempt was made to understand disease in the living from an examination of the dead.

In the other great civilisation of the time, that of Mesopotamia (the lands between the rivers Tigris and Euphrates), disease was similarly thought to be due to supernatural intervention. Rather than looking to the human corpse for an understanding of disease, omen-based prognostic practices flourished, including the examination of the liver (hepatoscopy) and entrails (haruspicy) of sacrificed animals (Porter, 1999). Hepatoscopy and haruspicy can be traced back to the time of Sargon I of Babylon (*c.* 3500 BC). Disease was regarded in an anamistic fashion – i.e. controlled by gods or spiritual forces, whose intentions could be read in the liver by the haruspex (King and Meehan, 1973).

The Greek civilisation began to emerge around 1000 BC, but little is known of their medicine before 500 BC. Hippocrates (*c.* 460–377 BC), whose work has been deduced from legend, promoted a naturalistic philosophy that disease resulted from 'natural' causes. Early Greek physicians had a sound grasp of surface anatomy, but the cultural mores against human dissection limited their knowledge of internal anatomy to that gleaned from the inspection of wounds and the dissection of animals. The use of animal dissection, promoted by Aristotle (384–322 BC), was subsequently used to ground biomedical knowledge in Alexandrian medicine. Hirophilus (*c.* 330–255 BC), however, is reported to have performed dissections on live humans (probably condemned criminals) and public dissections on human cadavers. It was he who discovered and named the prostate, duodenum (from the Greek for 12 fingers), and the structure that bears his name, the torcular Herophili (the confluence of the intracranial sinuses) (King and Meehan, 1973). That Hirophilus describes the rete mirabile (a network of arteries found at the base of the brain in primates) demonstrates that some of his dissections were also performed in animals; the rete mirabile is not present in humans.

The application of human dissection altered little over the subsequent four centuries. The classical Greeks and their successors were working with an entirely different concept of disease; namely a misbalance of humours. This model gives no particular significance to the physical state of the organs and therefore does not see any particular clinical interest in the autopsy. The work and views of Galen (AD 129–c.216) were to dominate medicine for the next millennium. However, while he prided himself on being an expert clinician, he was also a medical scientist and performed dissections. These were mainly performed on apes, sheep, pigs, goats, and even an elephant's heart. Human dissection was out of the question, though he told of examining two skeletons observed by chance, one washed from a grave by a flood and another of an unburied thief picked clean by carrion birds (King and Meehan, 1973). Given Galen's dominance over the medical establishment, his assertions on human anatomy based on comparative anatomy in apes and other mammals were to remain largely unchallenged for 1400 years (Porter, 1999).

Human dissection in the Dark Ages

With the fall of the Roman Empire, the West began its decline into the Dark Ages. Little of what passed for medical practice between 476 and 1000 in the West is known. Human dissections for scientific purposes in the West are unrecorded in this time.

Thanks to a number of writers in the Greek East, we can be certain that the practice of human dissection did continue and that the history of the autopsy is unbroken from ancient times to the modern day. Both Pseudo-Eustathius (c. 325) and Symeon the Theologian (949–1022) report that autopsies intended to search for disease were performed on the dead bodies of criminals (Bliquez and Kazhdan, 1984; Burton, 2005). It is apparent that the practice

of human vivisection also continued. As Theophanes (752–818) records:

> … an apostate from the Christian faith and leader of the Scameri was captured. They cut off his hands and feet on the Mole of St Thomas, brought in physicians, and dissected him from his pubic region to his chest while he was alive. This they did with a view to understanding the structure of man. In this condition they gave him over to the flames.
>
> (Bliquez and Kazhdan, 1984)

Clearly, the Eastern Church did not have the same mores against human dissection that had plagued the ancient Greeks or that would feature prominently in the West. Moreover, these Byzantine dissections were perhaps the first true autopsies, seeking to understand the nature of disease and not just anatomical structure (Burton, 2005). Such autopsies would not be seen in the West for another 450 years.

The medieval autopsy

In Anglo Saxon England, the Tutonic pagan belief that disease was caused by 'the worm', 'onfliers', 'elf-shot' and contagious magic meant that further investigation of the body was not only fruitless but might also be positively dangerous. The appropriate activity in that context was the proper observance of the ritual of cleansing, disposal and grief with perhaps some vengeance on supposed sources of disease. Elements of these attitudes persist in all cultures, as the expensive procedures of funeral and bereavement rituals attest.

Little is known of autopsy practices in the early Middle Ages. In the early medieval west, dissection of the human cadaver remained closely bound up with the religious beliefs of the time. Dissection for scientific advancement was all but unheard of. Indeed no mention of human dissection for such purposes is to be found in Binski's (1996) account of medieval death, ritual and representation.

In England, Germany and France, human dissection was limited to the process of 'division of the corpse'. In general terms, this practice consisted either of the evisceration of the body in preparation for a state funeral or of a complete dismemberment ('anatomy'). The latter was undertaken largely on the bodies of the saints (Park, 1995; Binski, 1996) and allowed several religious communities to have local access to a part of such an illustrious person. Such relics often consisted of severed body parts and were preserved within the alter or a shrine within the church (Binski, 1996). Division of the corpse was also undertaken to facilitate its transportation for burial when death occurred far from home. Such a practice is clearly exemplified in this account of the division of Henry I of England in 1135:

> Although he had died in Rouen, the king wished to be buried in Reading. Accordingly, he was decapitated, and his brain, eyes, and viscera were removed and buried in Rouen. The rest of his body was cut into pieces, heavily salted, and packed into oxhides against the smell, which, according to the chronicler, had already killed the man responsible for extracting the brain. By the time the funeral procession had reached Caen, the corpse was exuding a liquid so foul that its attendants could not drain it without what Henry of Huntington called 'horror and faintings.'

(Park, 1995)

In contrast, such practices were only rarely adopted in twelfth and thirteenth century Italy. Indeed, division in preparation for burial in Italy was prohibited by Pope Boniface VIII in 1299 and punishable by excommunication – itself a form of social death (Park, 1995).

In thirteenth century England, dissection of the dead to determine the cause of death was largely unknown. Autopsies were not used in early coronial inquests – instead, the jury met with the coroner around the body (Seabourne and Seabourne, 2001). Disease, death and decay were considered to be signs of sin and the will of God. Further, as bubonic plague (and, later, smallpox) ravaged the country there were fears that cadavers were sources of contagion. However, given that the diagnosis of death was often certain, but not always accurate (giving rise to several 'miracles' of resurrection), the absence of autopsy practice was perhaps comforting (Horrox, 1999)!

Italy is the birth-place of the examination of the dead that evolved into the autopsy we are familiar with today. The earliest report of such an autopsy dates from 1286 when a doctor in Cremona undertook an autopsy examination to investigate an epidemic (Park, 1995). The chronicles of Fra Salimbene, a Franciscan friar, tell of a physician who opened a hen and found an abscess at the tip of the heart. He then opened a man who had died of apparently the same disease and found a similar lesion. The autopsy was to soon have a place in medicolegal investigations, and the report of Azzolino, who died in Bologna in 1302 in suspicious circumstances and was autopsied on the order of the court, concludes 'We have assured ourselves of the condition by the evidence of our own senses and by the anatomisation of the parts' (King and Meehan, 1973).

The Renaissance autopsy

The ruling of Pope Boniface VIII was taken by many to include all forms of dissection, but the attitude of the church was to be slowly modified, and, in 1410, Pope Alexander was autopsied by Pietro D'Argelata following his sudden death. A bill was subsequently issued by Pope Sixtus IV (1471–1484) permitting studies on human bodies at Padua and Bologna (in fact the first public human dissection in Bologna occurred around 1315). The bill was confirmed by Clement VII (1523–1534). The performance of forensic autopsies was sanctioned by Emperor Charles V in 1532 with the introduction of the Constituto Criminalis Carolina (Dada and Ansari, 1996). By 1556 the autopsy was fully accepted by the Catholic church (King and Meehan, 1973; Porter, 1999).

It was Andreas Vesalius (1514–1564) who was to not only restore but transcend Galenic anatomy. Born in Brussels and trained in Paris, he moved to Padua in 1537 and rapidly made a name for himself as a skilled dissector. His familiarity with anatomy led him to challenge the accepted Galenic version of human anatomy. In 1539, having acquired a large supply of cadavers from executed criminals, he produced the *De humani corporis fabrica* (On the fabric of the human body), which was finished in 1542. In daring to think that Galen was wrong, Vesalius's work had a profound effect on our understanding of anatomy (Porter, 1999). Vesalius's fame rapidly spread through northern Europe. So it was that, when King Henry II of France suffered a jousting wound in his eye on 30 June 1559, Vesalius was called to attend the King, along with surgeon Ambrose Paré. The King's wound proved fatal. Death occurred 3 days later, and Vesalius and Paré performed the autopsy (Martin, 2001).

Although dissection of the human body undertaken as an anatomical exploration was the subject of much interest, the description of pathological states was, in keeping with the times, somewhat understated. Antonio Benivieni (1443–1502) did much to promote autopsies and pathology, yet his text *De abditis nonnullis ac mirandis morborum et sanatotionum causis* (On some remarkable hidden causes of diseases and of cures), published in 1507, includes the autopsy report of a man who died following protracted vomiting. The entire pathological report reads:

It was found that the opening of his stomach had closed up and it had hardened down to the lowest part with the result that nothing could pass through to the organs beyond, and death inevitably followed.

(King and Meehan, 1973)

Autopsies in the seventeenth and eighteenth centuries

The performance of incomplete dissections, the failure to correlate morphological with clinical findings, and the brevity of reports continued to hamper the autopsy through the sixteenth and seventeenth centuries (Dada and Ansari, 1996). Boerhaave recognised this and in 1724 described in detail the case of a nobleman who died from oesophageal rupture. In particular, he emphasised the importance of the history: 'Everything pertaining to the case must be listed, nor that the least thing neglected which a critical reader might rightly seek to understand the malady.' The case is repeated by King and Meehan (1973).

Preceding the fatal illness, he ate a most injudicious meal: 'veal soup with fragrant herbs; … a little white cabbage boiled with sheep; spinach; and calf sweetbreads lightly roasted (or fried); a little duck, thigh and breast; two larks; a bit of apple compote and bread; and … dessert consisting of pears, grapes, and sweetmeats. With his meal he drank a little beer and a little wine from Moselle. Shortly after he felt that something had 'irritated the opening to his stomach'. After unsuccessful attempts to obtain relief by vomiting, he felt a horrible pain and declared that 'something near the upper part of his stomach was ruptured, torn, or dislocated'. Suffering great agonies, he took a great deal of medication by mouth, including many emetics and much fluid, but all without relief. He passed very little urine despite the great amount of fluid ingested. The sufferings were horrible and he died in agony, while the physicians stood by, helpless and completely baffled.

The autopsy procedure, narrated at great length, fills almost six large pages of closely printed text, far more than the reports of the previous century. The autopsy was carefully performed, the incision beginning at the xiphisternum, down to the pubis, 'and then to the lumbar areas so as to injure nothing and to remove nothing from its position'. The different organs and regions of the abdomen are described cursorily where there was little change, and at length where the appearance was abnormal. No organs were removed. Since the abdominal examination did not explain the clinical findings, 'the true cause of death was believed to lie in the thorax'. Therefore, after the abdominal organs were all restored to their 'natural position', the thorax was carefully opened and found to contain over 10 litres of fluid. The actual rupture of the oesophagus and the adjacent pleura, and the collapse of the lungs, are vividly described, as is the precise method of the examination. Except for a small incision made in the oesophagus, the organs were neither incised nor removed.

The autopsy and the anatomical dissection became sources of human tissue for archiving and display. Frederik Ruysch (1638–1731), working as chief anatomist for the city of Amsterdam, perfected a preservation technique for archiving the brain. The blood vessels were injected with a mixture of wax and red pigment, before immersing the tissues in a transparent alcoholic liquid of his own devising (Gere, 2003). Ruysch's collection of artistic and educational anatomical specimens was purchased in 1717 by Peter the Great for 30 000 guilders (Gere, 2003).

The nineteenth century autopsy

The history of the autopsy examination in its modern form begins in Padua in the mid-eighteenth century with the work of Giovanni Battista Morgagni (1682–1771). Morgagni further emphasised the importance of careful observation and the correlation of clinical and pathological findings suggested by Boerhaave. He was a keen academic. At the age of 16 (in 1698) he was already learned in algebra, archaeology, geometry, astronomy and agriculture, and enrolled as a medical undergraduate at the University of Bologna. As a graduate student he trained under Antonio Valsalva, and at age 29 was appointed as assistant professor of theoretical medicine in Padua. From the outset he was opposed to Galenic principles, favouring instead observation and experimentation. Four years later he held the Chair of Anatomy and devoted the next 55 years to his students, his morphological studies and his family (Hill and Anderson, 1996).

A significant turning point in the history of the autopsy took place at the end of the eighteenth century with the work of Xavier Bichat. Although his career was only short (he died of tuberculosis at the age of 30), Bichat – known as the Father of Histology – revolutionised the autopsy examination, directing attention away from the organs to the tissues. Without the aid of a microscope he distinguished 21 types of tissue, recognising that it was the tissues making up the organs of the body, rather

than the organs themselves, that held the key to understanding disease. A busy clinician, it is said he performed some 600 autopsies in the year of his own death (King and Meehan, 1973; Hill and Anderson, 1996). Without doubt he was convinced of their value:

> You may take notes for 20 years, from morning to night at the bedside of the sick, upon the diseases of the viscera, and all will be to you only a confusion of symptoms, ... a train of incoherent phenomena. Open a few bodies and this obscurity will disappear.

The father of the modern autopsy is widely regarded to be Karl Rokitansky (1804–1878). Working at the Allgemein Krankenhaus in Vienna, he performed over 30 000 autopsies during his career and is thought to have supervised some 70 000 autopsies. In addition, he amassed a collection of tens of thousands of anatomical specimens, collections of skulls and pelvic bones, and treasures including the report on the autopsy of Ludwig van Beethoven. (Beethoven's autopsy was performed by Johann Wagner in 1827, just months before Rokitansky joined the staff.) Rokitansky, and his colleagues Johann Wagner and Lorenz Biermayer, were perhaps the first professors of pathology anywhere. Rokitansky initiated the concept of a thorough and systematic autopsy examination that ensured that every part of the body would be examined in identical fashion, regardless of the clinical history. Ironically, he also set the precedent of the pathologist divorced from clinical practice. In so doing, he may have foreshadowed the decline of the appreciation of the autopsy (Hill and Anderson, 1996).

In England, renewed interest in anatomy and the autopsy at the start of the nineteenth century meant that the demand for cadavers rapidly outstripped the supply afforded by the courts; the bodies of criminals sentenced to death were given to doctors for 'anatomisation'. Grave robbing developed as a profitable enterprise, but relatives and the authorities began to take preventative measures and the practice fell into decline. The practice was in part controlled by legislation (Anatomy Act 1832) that gave the unclaimed bodies of paupers who died in hospitals and workhouses a further punishment for their poverty by turning them over to the anatomists (Rugg, 1999). So-called 'resurrectionists' took to providing corpses for dissection by murder. The most famous of these were William Burke (1792–1829) and William Hare (1792–1870) in Edinburgh, who suffocated their intoxicated victims. Burke sat on the victim's chest, occluding the mouth and nose, while Hare dragged the victim round the room by the feet ('Burking'). Brought to justice in 1829, Hare turned King's evidence and Burke was hanged, his body being publicly anatomised and flayed, and his skin tanned and sold by the strip (Porter, 1999).

Rudolf Virchow (1821–1902), working in Berlin, advanced the autopsy yet further beyond the work of Rokitansky, extending the understanding of disease to the cellular level – a pivotal point in the development of the modern understanding of pathology. His short textbook *A Description and Explanation of the Method of Performing Post-mortem Examinations* (Virchow, 1876) makes fascinating reading.

A relatively modern collection of autopsy reports is Sir William Osler's (1849–1919) autopsy protocols. The surviving three volumes record 428 autopsies in considerable detail although many are rather synoptic. Further autopsy accounts can also be found within his thesis, which is based on 20 autopsies and the preparation of gross and microscopic specimens (Golden, 2007). His published text on 'The Principles of Medicine' is notable in that it can be clearly seen that the autopsy contributed significantly to Osler's understanding of disease (Rodin, 1973). His belief in the value of the autopsy extended even to his own death. 'Archie, you lunatic,' he said to his friend Dr T. Archibald Mallock 3 weeks before he died, 'I've been watching this case for 2 months and I'm sorry I shall not see the postmortem.' (Hill and Anderson, 1996).

The late nineteenth century witnessed the emergence of the minimally invasive autopsy. Howard Kelly proposed a method of 'post mortem examination of the thoracic and abdominal viscera through the vagina, perineum, and rectum and without incision of the abdominal parieties' (Bonello, 2003). This was prompted by a recognition that, even then, physicians struggled to gain consent for autopsies because of concerns that the body would be visibly mutilated. In Kelly's method, an incision was made into the perineum once the legs had been elevated or placed into the lithotomy position. The hand and arm, bared to the shoulder, were then worked into the abdominal cavity to free the viscera with the aid of a scalpel as needed. In this way, the internal organs could be removed for inspection (Bonello, 2003).

Nineteenth century autopsies were not without contention. The physicians present at the autopsy of Napoleon expressed divergent opinions as to the true cause of death. Theories ranging from gastric carcinoma to poisoning with arsenic, antimony or mercurous chloride to quinine overdosage have been suggested. Mari *et al.* (2004) suggest torsades de pointes secondary to chronic arsenic poisoning and a quinine overdose.

The twentieth century autopsy

At the start of the twentieth century the autopsy was considered to be central to medical research, education and professional development (Roulson *et al.*, 2005; Burton and Underwood, 2007). By the 1960s the situation had changed and the autopsy has subsequently undergone a steady decline, which continues to the present day (Start *et al.*, 1993; Burton and Underwood, 2003). This decline has been almost, but not entirely, universal. A number of studies have been able to significantly increase autopsy rates although the rates decline again when the study interventions are discontinued (Burton and Underwood, 2007).

As the role of pathology in medicine became established, autopsies moved out of anatomy theatres and private homes and into hospital and public mortuaries. Autopsies had certainly been performed in the homes of the deceased or in physicians' consulting rooms in the nineteenth century – a firm kitchen table in a well-lit room was recommended for the purpose. The practice was continued, to a diminishing extent and usually by general practitioners, until the 1960s. By an interesting quirk of fate, Sir John Mackenzie was autopsied by John Parkinson (of Wolff–Parkinson–White fame) in 1925 using a set of autopsy instruments that the former had advised the latter to purchase for home autopsies some 12 years prior to his death (Hollman, 2001; Burton, 2005).

There is a certain popular reluctance to permit autopsies on deceased relatives. In practice, however, this is not the limiting factor in the hospital autopsy rate since, for specific survey purposes, a number of published studies have sought and achieved very high autopsy rates (up to 80 per cent) over periods of a year or so. Instead, the limiting factor appears to be the willingness of clinicians to request autopsies. One study found that consent was sought for an autopsy in only 6.2 per cent of natural deaths and 43.4 per cent of these requests were granted (Burton and Underwood, 2003). Thus, the well-documented decline in hospital autopsy rates is presumably because clinicians do not want them. The reasons offered by clinicians for not requesting autopsies are varied and range from a simple distaste for the procedure to a belief that modern investigative techniques are so accurate that the autopsy can add nothing not known in life. That the process of obtaining informed consent is now very time-consuming is also likely to have a negative impact on request rates.

Pathologists have countered this with numerous studies showing that the discrepancy rate between the cause of death offered by clinicians before autopsy and that revealed by the autopsy is from 15 to 30 per cent, even when restricted to major discrepancies. Minor discrepancies and incidental, significant, conditions unsuspected in life provide an added error rate of the same sort of order. Similar findings have been reported from numerous countries and are unaffected by the degree of certainty felt by the clinician regarding the pre-autopsy diagnosis.

In retrospect, these studies may have been counter-productive, since what they are providing is detailed demonstration of error on the part of clinicians and it is naive to suppose that this will provide routine motivation to have more errors demonstrated, since it is clinicians who must request the autopsy. Whether consent will be granted depends greatly on the strength of the requesting clinician's recommendation that an autopsy is needed (Burton

et al., 2004; Burton and Underwood, 2007). Within the current climate of increasing litigation, it is unlikely that individual clinicians can be expected to reverse the trend in the demand for autopsies. (This is further compounded by the growing concern of the general public regarding the removal and retention of organs and tissues at autopsy, particularly from children.) There remain admirable exceptions, and many clinicians continue to value the opportunity to improve their understanding of clinical disease, even at the expense of having to admit that they are sometimes wrong.

Nonetheless, the requests for hospital autopsies continue to decline (Burton and Underwood, 2003) and so, consequently, does the hospital autopsy rate. The implications of this for modern pathological practice and training have yet to be fully realised, although many trainees already find it difficult to obtain sufficient autopsy practice. With the advent of systematised audit demand may increase again, and this is discussed further in Chapter 22.

The twenty-first century autopsy

Although the autopsy declined in the twentieth century, the past two decades have seen remarkable innovations. There has been a continuing rise in the number of autopsy-related publications and new technologies are increasingly being applied.

There has been a surge of interest in the radiological autopsy. While the use of ultrasound (echopsy) and endoscopic techniques are principally research tools, the use of computerised tomography and magnetic resonance imaging is on the increase, and these are discussed in more detail in Chapter 19.

Curiously, the most detailed autopsies ever performed have been carried out on ancient corpses for purely academic reasons and are even published in semi-popular format for the general public. These include the incredibly detailed study of Lindow Man, a corpse dating from before AD 240 and found in a bog in Cheshire in 1984 (Stead et al., 1986). The account includes: forensic analysis; radiocarbon dating; computerised tomography; scanning electron microscopy; thin-layer chromatography; botanical and zoological analysis of his last meal; and the study of pollen in palaeofaeces.

In developing countries and in countries where social and/or religious mores against the autopsy persist, a new technique – the verbal autopsy – is emerging in the literature. These 'autopsies' require no examination of the body and comprise structured interviews conducted some months after death in an attempt to reach a probable cause of death that may inform national mortality data. The technique is of low specificity, although some authors have reported a high sensitivity for cancer diagnoses. These verbal autopsies fall outside the remit of this book and will not be discussed further.

It is clear that the autopsy has a long and at times ignoble history that has seen a marked change in both the form and the function of the procedure. At all times it has been firmly linked to prevailing socio-political and religious societal views. The nature of the autopsy has been reinvented several times, and it is likely that this process will continue so that the examination remains relevant to modern practice and acceptable to contemporary society. Perhaps most pressing will be a need not for more autopsies but for autopsies performed to a higher standard, and this is the subject of the rest of this book.

References

Binski P (1996). *Medieval Death, Ritual and Representation*. London: British Museum Press.

Bliquez LJ, Kazhdan A (1984). Four testimonia to human dissection in Byzantine times. *Bull. Hist. Med.* **58**:554–7.

Bonello JP (2003). Minimally invasive autopsy circa 1882: Howard Kelly's innovative and imaginative series. *Surg Laparos Endosc Percutan Tech* **13**:223–6.

Burton EC, Phillips RS, Covinsky KE *et al.* (2004). The relation of autopsy rate to physicians' beliefs and recommendations regarding autopsy. *Am J Med* **117**:255–61.

Burton JL (2005). A bite into the history of the autopsy: from ancient roots to modern decay. *Forensic Med Sci Pathol* **1**:277–84.

Burton JL, Underwood JCE (2003). Autopsy practice after the 'organ retention scandal': requests, performance and tissue retention. *J Clin Pathol* **56**:537–41.

Burton JL, Underwood JCE (2007). Clinical, educational and epidemiological value of autopsy. *Lancet* **369**: 1471–80.

Cohen R, Manion L. (1998) *Research Methods in Education*, 4th edn. London: Routledge.

Dada MA, Ansari NA (1996). The postmortem examination in diagnosis. *J Clin Pathol* **49**:965–6.

Gere C (2003). A brief history of brain archiving. *J Hist Neurosci* **12**:396–410.

Golden RL (2007). Osler's lost thesis. *J Med Biogr* **15**(suppl 1):71–8.

Hill RB, Anderson RE (1996). The recent history of the autopsy. *Arch Pathol Lab Med* **120**:702–12.

Hollman A (2001). Postmortems on the kitchen table. *Br Med J* **323**:1472–3.

Horrox R (1999). Purgatory, prayer and plaque. In: Jupp PC, Gittings C (eds), *Death in England: An Illustrated History*. Manchester: Manchester University Press.

King LS, Meehan MC (1973). A history of the autopsy: a review. *Am J Pathol* **73**:514–44.

Mari F, Bertol E, Fineschi V, Karch SB (2004). Channelling the Emperor: what really killed Napoleon? *J R Soc Med* **97**:397–9.

Martin G (2001). The death of Henry II of France: a sporting death and post-mortem. *ANZ J Surg* **71**:318–20.

Park K (1995). The life of the corpse: division and dissection in late medieval Europe. *J Hist Med Allied Sci* **50**:111–32.

Porter R (1999). *The Greatest Benefit to Mankind: A Medical History of Humanity from Antiquity to the Present*. London: Fontana.

Rodin AE (1973). Osler's autopsies; their nature and utilization. *Med Hist* **17**:37–48.

Roulson J, Benbow EW, Hasleton PS (2005). Discrepancies between clinical and autopsy diagnosis and the value of post mortem histology; a meta-analysis and review. *Histopathology* **47**:551–9.

Rugg J (1999). From reason to regulation: 1760–1850. In: Jupp PC, Gittings C (eds), *Death in England: An Illustrated History*. Manchester: Manchester University Press.

Rutty GN (2007). Are autopsies necessary? *Rechtsmedizin* **17**:21–8.

Seabourne A, Seabourne G (2001). Suicide or accident: self-killing in medieval England. Series of 198 cases from the Eyre records. *Br J Psychiatry* **178**:42–7.

Start RD, McCulloch TA, Benbow EW, Lauder I, Underwood JCE (1993). Clinical autopsy rates during the 1980s: the continued decline. *J Pathol* **141**:63–6.

Stead IM, Bourke JB, Brothwell D (1986). *Lindow Man: The Body in the Bog*. London: Guild Publishing.

Virchow R (1876). *A Description and Explanation of the Method of Performing Post-mortem Examinations*. London: J&A Churchill.

Chapter 2

THE FUTURE OF THE AUTOPSY

James Underwood

Introduction

Hospital autopsy rates (i.e. autopsies other than those required by law) have been declining since the 1950s, prompting concerns about the impact on clinical audit, medical education and research (Burton and Underwood, 2007). In the UK, even in teaching hospitals, the autopsy rate has plummeted to significantly less than 10 per cent of deaths (Start *et al.*, 1993; Burton and Underwood, 2003) and, in many other hospitals, fewer than 5 per cent. At this rate of decline, clinical autopsies and the pathologists sufficiently experienced to perform them face extinction. The future practice of medicine will be blind to the many adverse consequences of clinical interventions and innovations. Research into cardiac and central nervous system disorders in particular will be severely affected. Scientific validation of public health measures to reduce mortality from common fatal conditions will be compromised (Squier and Ironside, 2006). There will be detrimental effects on clinical audit and medical education (Carr *et al.*, 2004). However, by anticipating the likely adverse impact on medicine, and by proactive measures to reverse the decline, we may be able to avert the death of the clinical autopsy and ensure that information from it continues to sustain high medical standards.

Autopsies required by law have a more secure future because of the continuing reliance on the findings for accurate death certification in cases of sudden or unexpected natural death and for legal purposes in the further investigation of deaths due to unnatural causes. However, even for these cases, some causes of death may be determined by non-invasive post-mortem imaging such as computerised tomography and/or magnetic resonance imaging (MRI), although its reliability is still being validated.

This chapter comments briefly on the current status of the autopsy and then draws attention to some recent advances that could be developed further to enhance the clinical utility and the public acceptability of autopsies.

Reasons for the decline

Declining autopsy rates result from:

- diminishing clinical interest and increasing clinical confidence in ante-mortem diagnosis, so fewer autopsies are requested;
- increasingly complex consent procedures necessitated by more stringent human tissue legislation;
- insufficient priority given to autopsies by pathologists burdened with increasing workloads of surgical resections, biopsies and cytology;
- insufficient exposure to autopsies during medical undergraduate training;
- the low esteem of autopsy-based research.

Clinicians attribute the falling numbers of hospital autopsies to their increasing confidence in the clinical cause of death, despite many studies showing significant discrepancies between the certified cause of death and the actual cause of death as revealed by autopsy (see Chapter 22). Even when confronted with these data, they then question whether knowledge of these discrepancies ever influences clinical management in such a way that the care of future patients is improved. Such evidence is difficult to adduce except in a few specific instances; for example, the investigation of deaths after new surgical procedures can lead to improvements in surgical techniques and in postoperative management and improve the criteria for case selection for surgery.

The clearest manifestation of the low level of clinical interest in the autopsy is the fact that, first, consent from relatives is sought usually by the most junior and inexperienced member of the clinical team and, second, senior clinicians rarely appear in the post-mortem room to witness the findings in their cases. Clinicians also contest that clinical autopsy requests are not received because relatives do not wish to give consent. A study by Burton and Underwood (2003) demonstrated that relatives are frequently not given an opportunity to express or withhold consent. When such opportunities are given, consent is more often given than refused.

Lately, in the UK, there has been considerable adverse media attention to the retention of organs, particularly hearts and brains (paradoxically, the organs most difficult to study during life and yet which, in many societies, have the greatest symbolic and emotional significance). Consequently, new human tissue legislation necessitates more complex arrangements for obtaining relatives' consent. The consent process is now more time-consuming, often necessitating appropriately trained bereavement staff to assist the relatives.

Many pathologists have withdrawn from autopsy practice, sometimes because of the public opprobrium evoked by 'organ retention'. Byard (2005) has hinted that the autopsy's current decline is in part due to pathologists' lack of enthusiasm, which is all too evident to their clinical colleagues. He comments that autopsies 'are sometimes seen as some sort of atavistic medical throwback, to be undertaken only by second-rate academics and those who are unemployable in the real world of 21st century anatomical pathology!'

The future of the autopsy lies in educating students, doctors, health service managers and the public, in modernising the techniques used in the examination of the body after death, in greater flexibility in adapting autopsy techniques to satisfy relatives' concerns, and in improving the communication of the results of autopsies.

Autopsies and medical education

Autopsies are unrivalled as an educational tool for teaching by clinicopathological correlation. The impact of witnessing the morbid anatomical features of disease is potent and enduring. Also, the discovery of clinicopathological discrepancies in the post-mortem room conveys powerfully knowledge of the innate fallibility of medical practice and of the need for clinical audit utilising autopsy data. However, many pathologists – although they themselves were once students – do not appreciate students' psychological reactions to seeing dissected cadavers; this emotional experience may detract from the potential educational benefit. Therefore, pathologists demonstrating post-mortem findings to students should be aware of these reactions, declare that they acknowledge them and take steps to minimise them. When autopsies are used for teaching, Benbow (1990) urges that pathologists should keep the unpleasant aspects of post-mortem demonstrations to a minimum; this can be done, for example, by placing a screen around the cadaver that might otherwise be in the full view of students examining the internal organs, bearing in mind that they may have seen the patient during life. Otherwise, some students may form the irrevocable impression that the autopsy is a disrespectful procedure and shun any further exposure to it, thus ceasing to experience the benefits to medicine.

The declining clinical autopsy rate, combined with recent changes in medical undergraduate curricula, is resulting in many clinical students graduating from some medical schools without ever having witnessed an autopsy. Consequently, in many places, the next generation of doctors will have even less knowledge of the role of the autopsy in verifying the cause of death, in determining the reliability of diagnostic investigations, or in determining the beneficial and adverse effects of treatment (Hooper and Geller, 2007). Nor will these new doctors have had any personal experience of autopsies to enable them to give informed answers to the concerns of relatives whose agreement is being requested. These adverse trends must be reversed by leadership from within the specialty of pathology (Horowitz and Naritoku, 2007).

The educational roles of the autopsy are considered in more detail in Chapter 3.

Non-invasive autopsies

Because of personal, religious or cultural objections to the autopsy by dissection and the stressful nature, even for doctors, of seeking consent at a time of bereavement, non-invasive autopsy by imaging is being evaluated.

In one study, 20 stillborn, miscarried or aborted fetuses were examined by MRI and by subsequent autopsy dissection. Although there was complete agreement between the two procedures in only eight cases, the MRI examination revealed information in four cases that was not evident by autopsy dissection (Brookes et al., 1996). A more recent study comparing MRI and conventional autopsy examination of the central nervous system in 100 fetuses concluded that, despite a high frequency of agreement, essential information would be lost in many cases if MRI were the only investigation, thus compromising the counselling of parents (Cohen et al., 2008).

Similar studies are examining the reliability and effectiveness of MRI in investigating deaths in adults (Dirnhofer et al., 2006), particularly in communities with strong religious or cultural objections to dissection of the body after death. However, it is doubtful whether the MRI autopsy will ever supersede dissection, visual examination of the internal organs and histology of tissue samples, for several reasons.

- MRI does not have the spatial resolution to identify very small but significant lesions.

- MRI cannot sample the body for micro-organisms or toxins.
- There is no histological confirmation of the findings.
- Most MRI machines are used fully for the investigation of living patients, often after a prolonged waiting period.

Nevertheless, there may be some cases in which a very specific problem needs investigating that could be achieved by MRI, after proof of its reliability and subject to other clinical priorities for access to the machine. The radiological autopsy does have a place in medicolegal practice and this is discussed in more detail in Chapter 19.

Limited autopsies

The full autopsy is unrivalled as a method of auditing the reliability of clinical diagnosis; complete dissection of the body ensures that all significant unexpected findings are detected. However, there may be objections to performing a full autopsy: for example, in cases in which there is a hazard of infection not outweighed by the likelihood of significant unexpected findings; or in cases in which the relatives cannot tolerate the prospect of agreeing to a full autopsy, but might allow a less extensive examination.

Thus, a limited autopsy may be problem-oriented by focusing on the organ or body cavity in which there is the greatest clinical interest. Alternatively, an anatomically more widespread examination may be made using endoscopic techniques not requiring the large incisions or removal of organs for which some relatives may withhold their agreement. These techniques are described in Chapter 11 and have recently been reviewed by Rutty (2007). Although there are several individual cases reported in the literature, the most thorough evaluation of the endoscopic, thoracoscopic and laparoscopic autopsies appears to be that reported by Avrahami et al. (1995a) from Israel. They report 100 per cent concordance between endoscopic and full autopsy findings for major traumatic lesions, such as ruptured liver and spleen, but a lower correlation for some other lesions such as retroperitoneal abnormalities. Their experience appears to be derived disproportionately from deaths due to trauma where, in most countries, the legal requirement for a full autopsy by dissection cannot be blocked by relatives' objections. The sensitivity of these techniques seems to be unacceptably low for non-traumatic lesions causing death (Avrahami *et al.*, 1995b).

With needle autopsies, there is no gross information other than from the external examination of the body. However, the technique may enable relatives to agree to a less disfiguring method of autopsy investigation, provided they are aware of the limitations. Needle autopsy, performed under lawful circumstances, also enables very fresh tissue (e.g. for microbiology, genetic studies or autolysis-free histology) to be obtained very soon after death irrespective of whether there is subsequently to be full autopsy. The most recent published study reports that a cause of death could be given in 67 per cent of needle autopsy cases (Huston *et al.*, 1996).

Role of the autopsy in advancing medical knowledge

Our knowledge of diseases of the central nervous system (CNS) and the heart relies greatly on autopsies. Three factors bear on this: first, diseases of the CNS and heart account for the majority of deaths in 'developed' countries; second, these organs are the least amenable to investigation (by biopsy) during life; third, these organs, more than any other, have the greatest symbolic significance and their emotive associations underlie the reluctance of many relatives to agree to their retention at autopsy. Autopsies are still essential for the detailed characterisation of diseases of the CNS and of the heart. Our knowledge of variant Creutzfeldt–Jakob disease relies heavily on the study of post-mortem brain tissue. The autopsy should also be considered in protocols for the verification of cause of death in clinical trials in which death, or its avoidance, is an outcome measure; deaths in clinical trials may be due to the intervention (e.g. unexpected fatal side-effect of the

treatment), to unrelated disease or to the condition at the trial's focus.

Some argue that the autopsy ('seeing for oneself') is obsolete in an era of modern medical imaging and clinical testing of presumed high reliability. Nevertheless, although the frequency of clinical errors revealed by autopsies has declined (Sonderegger-Iseli *et al.*, 2000) – and the decline may well be due to the use of autopsy data in clinical audit – it is still at a level at which the autopsy may well be capable of enabling a further reduction (see Chapter 22).

The molecular autopsy

DNA is robust enough for the reliable genetic analysis of post-mortem tissue, even when it has been processed into paraffin wax blocks and archived for many years. Although RNA is more labile, viral RNA has been recently extracted from lung tissue from those who died in the influenza pandemic of 1918.

The potential of genetic analysis to further investigate autopsy findings is illustrated by a search for the factor V Leiden mutation in tissue from deaths due to pulmonary embolism (Gorman *et al.*, 1999); however, the positive rate in 82 cases was so close to that of the general population that routine testing would not be warranted. Nevertheless, in cases of sudden unexpected death in which an inherited genetic cause may underlie the fatal lesion, it can be worthwhile to use post-mortem samples for molecular analyses where no suitable ante-mortem material is available; the findings could be used to counsel the family of the deceased about their risks and about possible prophylactic measures. This is, of course, important in deaths from potentially heritable cardiac arrhythmia syndromes (Tester and Ackerman, 2007).

The autopsy has an important potential role in assessing the effectiveness and side-effects of gene therapy. Autopsy not only enables the opportunity to assess the extent to which gene therapy has ameliorated the disease for which it is given, but also enables access to a wide range of tissue and cell types in order to investigate the specificity of the localisation of retroviral vectors. This approach in a study of 32 autopsy cases has given important reassurance that the retroviral vector was confined to the site of inoculation (Long *et al.*, 1999).

Improving communication

Surveys of hospital and community doctors generally show that they appreciate receiving autopsy reports and that, in a high proportion of cases, the findings are unexpected and could influence their future clinical practice (Karunaratne and Benbow, 1997). Information from autopsies also has important benefits for bereaved relatives; many bereaved parents find it helpful to have a sensitive and reasonably full explanation for the death of their child in order to help them come to terms with their loss. In a survey of family members of 102 patients who died in a university teaching hospital in the USA, 88 per cent responded that they considered autopsy beneficial, citing as reasons the advancement of medical knowledge, comfort from knowing the actual cause of death and reassurance that the clinical care was appropriate (McPhee *et al.*, 1986). However, many family members complained about the long delay in receiving information about the autopsy findings.

Pathologists have been slow to apply modern image capture and storage techniques to autopsies so as to enable surgeons and physicians with commitments in wards, operating theatres and clinics to view autopsies at a time when living patients are not competing with the dead for their attention. The stored images may also be helpful in institutional risk management and in defending spurious litigation.

Autopsies could regain public and professional support by improving the speed and quality of the reporting process.

Increasing the autopsy consent rate

Some institutions have succeeded in maintaining a high clinical autopsy rate or reversing a declining rate – an even greater challenge. Factors contributing to a sustained high autopsy rate include: the effective organisation, management and integration of all aspects of the autopsy service; timely communication of autopsy findings to clinicians; and use of

autopsy data in institutional risk management (Haque *et al.*, 1996). Other interventions used successfully to reverse declining autopsy rates include emphasising to relatives the quality-control benefits of unexpected findings and training in the seeking of consent. In one Swiss hospital, these strategies increased the autopsy rate from 16 to 30 per cent within 6 months and up to 36 per cent after 1 year; when these interventions were discontinued, the autopsy rate fell to 6 per cent (Lugli *et al.*, 1999). The importance of fully informing relatives of the value of an autopsy and of close collaboration between clinicians and pathologists has been borne out by other studies (Clayton, 1992).

Reviving the autopsy: conclusions

Reviving the autopsy, in terms of both autopsy rates and quality, requires simultaneous attention to many factors:

- better exposure of medical students to autopsies;
- improved mortuary design to create a more attractive environment;
- better training of pathology trainees and a greater commitment from senior staff;
- use of modern image recording and archiving to enable clinicians to see and to discuss the gross findings with the pathologist;
- improved public education about autopsies and their benefits for the health of future patients and of the nation;
- application of modern laboratory methods in the post-mortem detection of genetic and biochemical abnormalities.

There is a huge task to be done in educating the public generally about the examination of the body after death so that, as bereaved relatives, they are better prepared to come to terms with autopsies either when required by law or when requested for clinical reasons. We also need to raise awareness of the importance of being able to keep tissues and, sometimes, whole organs from autopsies. After all, many spouses and close relatives already have discussions about the disposal of their bodies – expressing a preference for burial or cremation or some other lawful process – and this could lead on naturally to declaring preferences about autopsy consent and tissue and organ retention, provided that the relevant information is made available to assist such decisions. In this respect, the production of information leaflets for the public and bereaved relatives is important for the revival of the autopsy. Nevertheless, even now, bereaved relatives are more likely to give autopsy consent more often than they are given the opportunity by clinicians to do so.

However, perhaps it is mistaken to judge the current status of the autopsy on the basis of the number performed. Maybe, as Hall (1999) suggested, we need even fewer autopsies but performed to a much higher standard and directed to answering specific questions. By restricting the autopsy to a postmortem examination intended to answer only the unresolved clinical questions – the problem-oriented autopsy – and to conform to the requirements of the relatives in individual cases in terms of restricting the anatomical extent of the examination, the autopsy may regain some clinical and public support. But this would very seriously compromise the value of the autopsy in clinical audit because the unexpected conditions may be overlooked.

So, in the opinion of this author, the future lies in promoting public support for autopsies, in some cases adapting the autopsy to address specific questions or to the limits imposed by relatives, in making more effective use of information from autopsies, and in ensuring that the next generation of doctors has experienced the powerful educational benefit of examining the body after death. Perhaps, in years to come, some bereaved relatives may question why they have not been offered an opportunity to have the cause of death fully and reliably investigated and thus, by supporting education, research and audit, to cause some good to be derived from their grief – as happens already with organ donation for transplantation.

References

Avrahami R, Watemberg S, Daniels-Philips E, Kahana T, Hiss J (1995a). Endoscopic autopsy. *Am J Forensic Med Pathol* **16**:147–50.

Avrahami R, Watemberg S, Hiss Y, Deutsch AA (1995b). Laparoscopic vs conventional autopsy: a promising perspective. *Arch Surg* **130**:407–9.

Benbow EW (1990). Medical students' views of necropsies. *J Clin Pathol* **43**:969–76.

Brookes JA, Hall-Craggs MA, Sams VR, Lees WR (1996). Non-invasive perinatal necropsy by magnetic resonance imaging. *Lancet* **348**:1139–41.

Burton JL, Underwood J (2003). Autopsy practice after the 'organ retention scandal': requests, performance and tissue retention. *J Clin Pathol* **56**:537–41.

Burton JL, Underwood J (2007). Clinical, educational and epidemiological value of autopsy. *Lancet* **369**:1471–80.

Byard RW (2005). Who's killing the autopsy? A new tool for assessing the causes of falling autopsy rates. *Med J Aust* **183**:654–5.

Carr U, Bowker L, Ball RY (2004). The slow death of the clinical post-mortem examination: implications for clinical audit, diagnostics and medical education. *Clin Med* **4**:417–23.

Clayton SA (1992). Improving the autopsy rate at a university hospital. *Am J Med* **92**:428.

Cohen MC, Paley MN, Griffiths PD, Whitby EH (2008). Less invasive autopsy: benefits and limitations of the use of magnetic resonance imaging in the perinatal postmortem. *Pediatr Dev Pathol* **11**:1–9.

Dirnhofer R, Jackowski C, Vock P, Potter K, Thali MJ (2006). VirTopsy: minimally invasive, imaging-guided virtual autopsy. *Radiographics* **26**:1305–33.

Gorman TE, Arcot AN, Baker P, Prior TW, Brandt JT (1999). Prevalence of the factor V Leiden mutation among autopsy patients with pulmonary thromboembolic disease using an improved method for factor V Leiden detection. *Am J Clin Pathol* **111**:413–17.

Hall PA (1999). Do we really need a higher necropsy rate? *Lancet* **354**:2004.

Haque AK, Patterson RC, Grafe MR (1996). High autopsy rates at a university medical center: what has gone right? *Arch Pathol Lab Med* **120**:727–32.

Hooper JE, Geller SA (2007). Relevance of the autopsy as a medical tool. *Arch Pathol Lab Med* **131**:268–74.

Horowitz RE, Naritoku WY (2007). The autopsy as a performance measure and teaching tool. *Hum Pathol* **38**:688–95.

Huston BM, Malouf NN, Azar HA (1996). Percutaneous needle autopsy sampling. *Mod Pathol* **9**:1101–7.

Karunaratne S, Benbow EW (1997). A survey of general practitioners' views on autopsy reports. *J Clin Pathol* **50**:548–52.

Long Z, Lu P, Grooms T *et al.* (1999). Molecular evaluation of biopsy and autopsy specimens from patients receiving in vivo retroviral gene therapy. *Hum Gene Ther* **10**:733–40.

Lugli A, Anabitarte M, Beer JH (1999). Effect of simple interventions on necropsy rate when active informed consent is required. *Lancet* **354**:1391–2.

McPhee SJ, Bottles K, Lo B, Saika G, Crommie D (1986). To redeem them from death: reactions of family members to autopsy. *Am J Med* **80**:665–71.

Rutty GN (2007). Are autopsies necessary? The role of computed tomography as a possible alternative to invasive autopsies. *Rechtsmedizin* **17**:21–8.

Sonderegger-Iseli K, Burger S, Muntwyler J, Salomon F (2000). Diagnostic errors in three medical eras: a necropsy study. *Lancet* **355**:2027–31.

Squier W, Ironside J (2006). Falling necropsy rates and risks to public health. *Arch Dis Child* **91**:608–9.

Start RD, McCulloch TA, Benbow EW, Lauder I, Underwood JCE (1993). Clinical autopsy rates during the 1980s: the continued decline. *J Pathol* **171**:63–6.

Tester DJ, Ackerman MJ (2007). Postmortem long QT syndrome genetic testing for sudden unexplained death in the young. *J Am Coll Cardiol* **49**:240–6.

Chapter 3

THE ROLE OF THE AUTOPSY IN MEDICAL EDUCATION

Julian L Burton

You may take notes for 20 years, from morning to night at the bedside of the sick, upon the diseases of the viscera, and all will be to you only a confusion of symptoms, ... a train of incoherent phenomena. Open a few bodies and this obscurity will disappear.

Bichat (1771–1802)

Introduction

As discussed in Chapter 1, human dissection and the autopsy have always played a central role in medical education. With some notable exceptions, such as the application of imaging and more sophisticated toxicology, the technical aspects of the autopsy have changed little in 50 years. In contrast, undergraduate medical education has undergone dramatic changes during the past two decades. World-wide, there have been efforts to reduce information overload and to encourage students to be more self-directed in their learning.

The continuing decline in the autopsy rate and the modernisation of curricula mean that autopsies now play a less prominent role in the education of undergraduates and doctors. In many medical schools around the world students now graduate without ever seeing an autopsy. Some students find autopsies unpleasant, with concerns ranging from the minor – the unpleasant smell – to those suggest-

ing that the students were in considerable distress. However, to omit autopsy-based teaching is to lose a wealth of educational material.

This chapter considers the many and varied educational roles of the autopsy and discusses the advantages and disadvantages of using autopsies to teach undergraduates and postgraduates from outside the pathology department. In addition, the ways in which autopsy-based teaching can be successfully delivered are discussed.

Before the modern medical curriculum

Many students and clinicians believe that the only purpose of autopsies is to determine the cause of death (Benbow, 1990a). In a positivistic questionnaire-based study of medical student attitudes to the autopsy undertaken prior to the introduction of a 'modern' medical curriculum at the University of Manchester

(UK), Benbow demonstrated that students perceived the autopsy to be a valuable part of their training. In the early 1990s students reported that they found the autopsy useful because it increased their understanding of anatomy and of disease processes, and because attendance at such examinations would equip them with the knowledge needed to counsel relatives and seek consent for autopsies in the future (Talazaar *et al.*, 1987; Benbow, 1990a).

Not all students found the experience to be positive and rewarding. Some students objected to viewing autopsies, considering them to be distasteful, irrelevant to medical practice, an unnecessary mutilation. Additionally students raised religious objections or found it emotionally stressful to witness the autopsy of a patient they had cared for in life. Some students were concerned by the lack of respect shown for the deceased by both staff and students (Benbow, 1990a, 1991). Students' concerns ranged from the minor – the unpleasant smell – to those suggesting that the students were in considerable distress: 'attending a PM is the worst thing I have ever done', and 'overtaken with pain, grief and palpitations and burst into tears' (Benbow, 1990a).

At about the same time, on the other side of the Atlantic, Hill and Anderson (1991) identified a series of educational goals that could be achieved through the study of autopsies and which were regarded as important by a panel of 98 pathology educators attending an Association of Pathologists workshop in Colorado, USA. To a large extent the results mirrored those of earlier studies (DeRoy, 1976). These goals included using the autopsy to teach clinical pathophysiology and anatomy, clinicopathological correlation, the gross anatomy of disease, and the role of the autopsy in forensic medicine. Moreover, they found that the autopsy had a role in sharpening students' visual skills, and that it provided a medium by which students could learn about death certification, clinical audit, death statistics, the fallibility of medical diagnostics, the problem-based nature of medicine, the monitoring of new drugs and technology, and dealing with bereaved relatives (Hill and Anderson, 1991).

Medical education underwent dramatic reforms in the mid-1990s. In the UK, these were largely driven by the General Medical Council's publication *Tomorrow's Doctors* (1993), which called for a reduction in factual content and which limited the amount of staff–student contact time within the curricula. Similar changes were taking place around the world, and were associated with an increasing trend towards integrated self-directed and problem-based learning. A 1996/1997 survey in the USA revealed that there had been a decline in the amount of curricular time devoted to pathology teaching and that there was a move away from lecture-based teaching towards small-group discussion, with supplementary use of computer-assisted learning (Kumar *et al.*, 1998). Only 21 per cent of schools followed a 'traditional' didactic curriculum and 40 per cent of schools required students to participate in autopsies. Attendance at autopsies was optional in a further 52 per cent of US medical schools (Kumar *et al.*, 1998). Verma (1999), in contrast, found that medical students at the University College of Medical Sciences, Delhi, were knowledgeable about the procedures and values of autopsies.

In the UK, further curricular developments have followed the revision of *Tomorrow's Doctors* in 2002. Ongoing revisions and improvements can be expected for the foreseeable future. At the same time, autopsy rates – especially non-medicolegal autopsy rates – have declined around the world (Burton and Underwood, 2003, 2007). It has therefore been important to determine what roles, if any, the autopsy might continue to play within a modern medical curriculum.

Should students be exposed to autopsies?

The autopsy is still widely accepted as a powerful teaching tool. As discrete general and systems-based pathology courses have been removed from undergraduate medical curricula, and as clinically requested autopsies become infrequent, it has become more difficult to schedule time in curricula for students to encounter the autopsy. World-wide, there has been a shift towards student-centred problem-based self-directed learning. The autopsy is an ideal teaching tool in such circumstances – the autopsy process epitomises a problem-based approach. Ideally, all students will be exposed to autopsies during their undergraduate training. Autopsy findings can be used as the basis for problem-based learning projects. As a bare minimum, provision should be made for those students with a special interest to pursue a special study component that includes autopsy work (Nash, 2000). Currently, the 20 per cent of medical students in the USA who undertake pathology electives see an average of eight autopsies, but the remaining 80 per cent see an average of zero autopsies (Horowitz and Naritoku, 2007). Pathologists engaged in autopsy practice should charge themselves to expose students to autopsies to ensure that:

> *the autopsy becomes an essential part of the*
> *undergraduate medical curriculum so that*
> *medical students understand the role and value of*
> *an autopsy in the delivery of optimal health care,*
> *teaching, and for basic and applied research.*
>
> (Gotleib and Butany, 2005)

The autopsy as a sustainable teaching tool

Several studies (Welsh and Kaplan, 1998; Ferguson *et al.*, 2004) have indicated that residents – responsible for seeking consent for autopsies – must receive structured training which emphasised the importance of the autopsy if undergraduate autopsy teaching is to remain viable and sustainable. Sadly, Short *et al.* (2000) found that most residents attending the American Medical Association's Annual Meeting in June 1999 had not received formal training in the requesting of autopsies. Junior doctors in the UK are similarly unprepared for requesting autopsies (Carr *et al.*, 2004).

Consent and the educational autopsy

It has long been standard practice for consent to be sought before students examine patients as part of their training. Where intimate examinations are to be performed by the student while the patient is under general anaesthesia, the student or supervising clinician typically seeks written consent from the patient in advance. Traditionally, the autopsy has been used to teach students and junior doctors without the consent of either the deceased or the relatives of the deceased. Such a practice is now to be considered paternalistic and inappropriate. When consent from relatives is being sought for the performance of the autopsy, the opportunity should be taken to seek consent for students to be present to observe the examination. It must be remembered that in most, if indeed not all, jurisdictions medicolegal authorities do not themselves have the power to permit the autopsy to be used for teaching purposes. Here consent must be sought specifically from the relatives of the deceased to use the autopsy for teaching, with the permission of the medicolegal authority (Burton, 2001).

Occasionally, human tissues used to teach medical students themselves are brought for medicolegal autopsy (Bhardwaj *et al.*, 2007). Care must always be taken that human tissues used in teaching are retained only with appropriate consent and, at the end of their useful teaching lifetime, that they are disposed of appropriately.

Advantages and disadvantages of autopsy-based teaching

Curriculum design is, to some extent, an exercise in pragmatism because all teaching modalities have advantages and disadvantages. Those for the autopsy are listed in Table 3.1. For maximum benefit, exposure to autopsies must be relevant and, ideally, integrated with other activities in the curriculum, and included not just because the pathology department hopes that one student per year will become a pathologist! There should be specific educational aims and learning objectives for the inclusion of the autopsy in the curriculum: the amount of staff–student contact time is limited in many curricula and therefore time spent on one activity has the opportunity cost of time lost from another. Students should

Table 3.1 Advantages and disadvantages of autopsy-based teaching

Advantages	Disadvantages
Experiential learning	Time-consuming
Memorable learning experience	Health and safety risk
Problem-based learning in action	Physically unpleasant/frightening
May encourage students to become pathologists	May discourage students from becoming pathologists
May detect students with attitudinal problems	Expensive and underfunded
	Low caseload makes scheduling difficult
	Unsophisticated
	Presents a biased view of disease prevalence
	Demonstrations provide an artificially sanitised view of the autopsy

After Benbow (1990a,b); Morohashi (1998); Burton (2003); Fales-Williams et al. (2007); Horowitz and Naritoku (2007).

be prepared for their experience by giving them some notion of the sounds, sights and smells that will assail them in the post-mortem room (Burton, 2003).

Appropriately integrated, the autopsy is a powerful teaching tool. It is principally regarded as an opportunity for students to hone their anatomical and pathological knowledge and develop their skills in clinicopathological correlation (Box 3.1), but its uses are not limited to this. Traditionally it has formed a bridge between lecture- and laboratory-based didactic teaching and ward- and operating theatre-based experiential learning. Certainly it provides a link between the grey rigid tissues of the embalmed cadaver and the fresh living detail seen at surgery.

The newly dead can present an opportunity for the teaching of life-saving skills to medical students and junior doctors, either in the emergency room or at autopsy. Studies have suggested that practice is acceptable, particularly among those adults willing to volunteer their dead body for medical science, autopsy or organ donation, provided that consent is obtained (Oman *et al.*, 2002; Burton, 2003).

Autopsies and the hidden curriculum

The hidden curriculum runs alongside this and, while often forgotten, can have important impacts on the student that can be either positive or negative. 'Curriculum' is a complicated concept which includes not only what is to be taught (and what actually is taught) but also considerations of: to whom it is to be taught; how, when and where it is to be taught; and how the material is to be assessed (Burton and McDonald, 2001). The curriculum will have overtly stated aims (what the curriculum intends to deliver) and objectives (what the students can do having received the curriculum). By way of contrast, the hidden curriculum has been variously defined but can be simply regarded as the attitudes and values unwittingly transmitted to students both by what is (and is not) taught and how such teaching features in the curriculum (Burton, 2003). The students and staff may not be consciously aware that the hidden curriculum is being delivered.

The hidden curriculum sees attendance at an autopsy as a rite of passage, in which students experience something that sets them apart from the general population. The student gains a sense of belonging to the medical profession but at the cost of suffering an ordeal. Students are faced with their own mortality, and are encouraged to develop a

Box 3.1 What the autopsy can be used to teach

The autopsy provides opportunities to teach students about:

- gross pathology
- anatomy
- clinicopathological correlation
- the processes of death
- what happens to bodies after death
- an holistic approach to medicine
- what the autopsy entails (allows students to seek consent in the future)
- health and safety practices
- medical law
- practical procedures
- medical fallibility and medical errors
- medical ethics
- audit and clinical governance

After Oman et al. (2002); Burton (2003); Carr et al. (2004); Gotleib and Butany (2005).

sense of clinical detachment. Witnessing autopsies may encourage or discourage students in their desire to become pathologists, and may increase (or decrease) the credibility of their ward-based tutors. Presented appropriately, the autopsy encourages students to treat patients, be they alive or dead, with respect but there is a risk that students will be encouraged to view the body as an object. Some students will find the experience of autopsy-based teaching so unpleasant that they are discouraged from requesting autopsies when they have their own clinical practice (Burton, 2003).

Autopsy teaching modalities

The autopsy can be harnessed for teaching in several ways. Students may be invited to the mortuary individually or in pairs to witness the examination being performed *in toto* from external examination to reconstruction. Alternatively, many students experience the autopsy in the form of an autopsy demonstration, attending the mortuary in groups once the examination has been completed to discuss the clinical history of the patient and to view the gross (macroscopic) findings in organs and organ slices that have been laid out in trays. These can be difficult to schedule in mortuaries with a low case load. The pathologist may only become aware that an autopsy that can be used for teaching is available at the start of the day that it is to be performed. It can be difficult to have this information relayed to students. The pathologist will also need to be kept abreast of the students' timetables so that the demonstration is scheduled for a time that is amenable to both pathologist and students. In the most limited form of exposure, students encounter digital images or museum specimens retained (with appropriate consent) from autopsies either in tutorials or as part of collections held in museums or on-line. The choice of teaching modality has an impact on efficacy and efficiency (Fig. 3.1). Few students can attend an individual autopsy but each is likely to derive maximal benefit from this exposure. Images and museum specimens can be used to teach large numbers of students at once (they are time-efficient) but at the cost of a much lower impact.

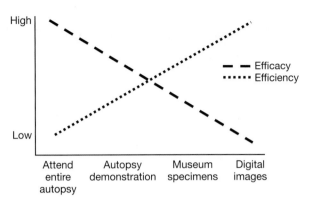

Figure 3.1 Efficacy and effectiveness of autopsy teaching modalities.

Relatively little has been published on the use of technology in autopsy teaching, although a small literature does exist on its use in teaching animal and human anatomy (which is analogous to autopsy teaching in the sense that a body is used for a practical demonstration). This suggests that computer-assisted learning techniques (Quentin-Baxter and Dewhurst, 1992, pp 27–33; Gunn and Maxwell, 1996, pp 205–15; Garvin and Carrington, 1997) and interactive laser video discs (Guy and Frisby, 1992; Quentin-Baxter and Dewhurst, 1995; Zirkel and Zirkel, 1997) may be successfully used to supplement or replace actual dissection, and support directed self-learning. Such resources can be time-consuming and expensive to produce.

As autopsy numbers decline, video presentations can be used to allow students to witness the components of an autopsy examination. They allow large numbers of students to receive a uniform experience, at a time that is suitable to the student; but they are expensive and time-consuming to produce and they lack the physical impact provided by being able to touch and smell the tissues (Burton and Rutty, 2000; Burton, 2003). Such videos can be used to prepare students for their experience in the post-mortem room. Videos can also be used to demonstrate specialised dissection techniques (such as those described in Chapter 11) to trainee pathologists (Burton *et al.*, 2004). Several studies (Goudie *et al.*, 1988; Brebner *et al.*, 1997a,b; Hunt *et al.*, 1997) have shown that autopsy demonstrations may be delivered via a video link to a classroom, obviating the need for students to come to a cramped mortuary viewing gallery. Indeed, there is no need for the autopsy and the students to be in the same building or even in the same country! Brebner *et al.* (1997a,b) demonstrated autopsies performed live in Aberdeen (UK) to students in Al Ain city in the United Arab Emirates via a telepathology link, though such methods are expensive.

Preparing students to see autopsies

Students who wish to attend a post-mortem examination should be reminded of the need to bring some form of identification with them (typically their student union membership card or hospital name badge) to confirm that they have a valid reason to be present in the mortuary. Photographic identification is preferable.

Some thought should be given to providing students with preparatory materials before they attend the mortuary to see an autopsy. The pathologist must be satisfied that the student is appropriately vaccinated to work in the mortuary. This is rarely a problem for students who are working on the wards, but may be of concern with students in the preclinical component of their studies. It must also be remembered that autopsies where the deceased is known to have a hazard group 3 pathogen (tuberculosis, HIV, etc.) are not suitable for student teaching (Chapter 6). Students should be asked to leave the mortuary if, on opening the body, it is discovered that the deceased has tuberculosis.

The pathologist who routinely works in the mortuary can easily forget how distressing it can be to see a 'fresh' human body dissected. Students should be advised that an autopsy comprises a review of the available clinical history, an external examination, evisceration of the internal organs, dissection and sampling of the internal organs, and reconstruction of the body. It can be helpful to remind them that the post-mortem suite is frequently noisy, that oscillating saws are used, that the body tissues will smell, that they will see blood, and that the incisions made

are large. Whether decomposed bodies are appropriate to be used for teaching is a matter best left to the discretion of the individual pathologist. Given the physically unpleasant nature of bodies in an advanced state of decomposition, such cases are probably best not used as a student's first encounter with the autopsy.

Students can be prepared for attending the mortuary by requiring them to view videos of an autopsy in advance. It should be made clear whether or not they will be expected to view the autopsy from the viewing gallery or to change into the appropriate personal protective equipment and attend on the autopsy room floor. The latter is practical when only one or two students are present. Larger numbers may be accommodated in the viewing gallery, particularly if audiovisual equipment is available to allow the dissection to be displayed on monitors.

On arrival, the student must be made aware of the health and safety regulations that apply in the mortuary, and the locations of the clean and dirty areas within the mortuary. The pathologist should ensure that students entering the 'dirty' areas of the mortuary are correctly attired in appropriate health and safety equipment. Ideally, the student will wear the same equipment as the pathologist performing the autopsy so that they may feel the pathological changes in the organs as well as see them.

Autopsy teaching and non-medical personnel

The autopsy has a valuable role in the teaching of non-medical personnel, including nurses, police officers, ambulance technicians, paramedics and scene-of-crime officers. All of these professional groups can be expected to have contact with the dead and some will be required to be present during the performance of autopsies. An understanding of the techniques employed during autopsy examination is therefore valuable. In addition, the autopsy can be used to teach nurses and paramedics the importance of leaving medical devices *in situ* when preparing the body for the mortuary. Police officers can be trained during autopsies on victim identification and can receive specialist training pertaining to handling bodies that have been contaminated chemically, biologically or by radiation. The latter should be extended to anatomical pathology technologists (and other autopsy pathologists), and this teaching can be undertaken using bodies that are not contaminated.

In this way, the various professional groups will have prior experience and will not face the dangers of having their first experience with an actually contaminated body.

Education through research

Ultimately, our knowledge of medicine is accrued through research, whether it be the study of books or the study of bodies. The use of the autopsy as an educational research tool, once common, has now declined. Autopsies remain a valuable source of research material. Pathologists can, with appropriate consent, play a valuable role in researching body storage systems, identification systems and body bags. The autopsy can provide biological material vital for one's own research (or the research of others) provided that ethical and consent issues are addressed appropriately.

Conclusion

The autopsy in all of its various guises is a valuable multi-functional teaching tool, but one which tends to be under-utilised. Pathologists engaged in autopsy practice face significant calls on their time, but the temptation to ignore the educational value of the autopsy should be strongly resisted. Although their use is not yet widespread the future may see modern technologies taking an increased role in the dissemination of autopsy-based teaching.

References

Benbow EW (1990a). Medical students' views on necropsies. *J Clin Pathol* **43**:969–76.

Benbow EW (1990b). Why show autopsies to medical students? *J Pathol* **162**:187–8.

Benbow EW (1991). The attitudes of second- and third-year medical students to the autopsy: a survey by postal questionnaire. *Arch Pathol Lab Med* **155**:1171–6.

Bhardwaj DN, Millo T, Lalwani S (2007). Skeleton used for anatomical study brought for medico-legal autopsy: a case report. *Med Sci Law* **47**:86–7.

Brebner EM, Brebner JA, Norman JN *et al.* (1997a). A pilot study in medical education using interactive television. *J Telemed Telecare* **3**(suppl 1):10–12.

Brebner EM, Brebner JA, Norman JN *et al.* (1997b). Intercontinental postmortem studies using interactive television. *J Telemed Telecare* **3**:48–52.

Burton JL (2001). Perhaps we should seek consent to show necropsies to students. *Br Med J* **323**:1426.

Burton JL (2003). The autopsy in modern undergraduate medical education: a qualitative study of uses and curriculum considerations. *Med Educ* **37**:1073–81.

Burton JL, McDonald S (2001). Curriculum or syllabus: which are we reforming? *Med Teacher* **23**:187–91.

Burton JL, Rutty GN (2000). *The Autopsy* (video series). University of Sheffield Television.

Burton JL, Underwood JCE (2003). Autopsy practice after the 'organ retention scandal': requests, performance and tissue retention. *J Clin Pathol* **56**:537–41.

Burton JL, Underwood JCE (2007). Clinical, educational and epidemiological value of autopsy. *Lancet* **369**:1471–80.

Burton JL, Diercks-O'Brien G, Rutty GN (2004). Videos have a role in postgraduate autopsy education. *J Clin Pathol* **57**: 877–81.

Carr U, Bowker L, Ball RY (2004). The slow death of the clinical post-mortem examination: implications for clinical audit, diagnostics and medical education. *Clin Med* **4**:417–23.

DeRoy AK (1976). The autopsy as a teaching–learning tool for medical undergraduates. *J Med Educ* **51**:1016–18.

Fales-Williams A, Danielson J, Myers R, Sorden S, Bender H (2007). The case correlation assignment: connecting antemortem and postmortem data in the senior year at Iowa State University. *J Vet Med Educ* **34**:183–93.

Ferguson RP, Burkhardt L, Hennawi G, Puthumana L (2004). Consecutive autopsies on an internal medicine service. *Southern Med J* **97**:335–7.

Garvin A, Carrington S (1997). Student-authored hypermedia in veterinary anatomy: teaching and learning outcomes of group project work. *Br J Educ Tech* **28**:191–8.

Gotleib AI, Butany J (2005). The academic autopsy: a patient safety issue. *Cardiovasc Pathol* **14**:47–8.

Goudie RB, Harris P, Patterson W (1988). How do we teach pathology? Post-mortems by video. *J Pathol* **154**:195–7.

Gunn C, Maxwell L (1996). CAL in human anatomy. *J Comput Assist Learn* **12**:205–15.

Guy JF, Frisby AJ (1992). Using interactive videodiscs to teach gross anatomy to undergraduates at the Ohio State University. *Acad Med* **67**:132–3.

Hill RD, Anderson RE (1991). The uses and value of the autopsy in medical education as seen by pathology educators. *Acad Med* **66**:97–100.

Horowitz RE, Naritoku WY (2007). The autopsy as a performance measure and teaching tool. *Hum Pathol* **38**:688–95.

Hunt NCA, James DS, Bull AD (1997). The still video camera: a suitable and convenient method of demonstrating post mortem findings. *Med Educ* **31**:386–9.

Kumar K, Daniel J, Doig K, Agamanolis D (1998). Teaching of pathology in United States medical schools, 1996/1997 survey. *Hum Pathol* **29**:750–5.

Morohashi Y (1998). Role of autopsy in medical practice. *Japan Hosp* **17**:1–5.

Nash JRG (2000). Pathology in the new medical curriculum: what has replaced the subject courses? *Pathol Oncol Res* **6**:149–54.

Oman KS, Armstrong II, JD, Stoner M (2002). Perspectives on practicing procedures on the newly dead. *Acad Emerg Med* **9**:786–90.

Quentin-Baxter M, Dewhurst D (1992). An interactive computer-based alternative to performing a rat dissection in the classroom. *J Biol Educ* **26**:27–33.

Quentin-Baxter M, Dewhurst D (1995). An interactive laser video disc to teach the functional anatomy of the rat. *J Biol Educ* **29**:34–9.

Short MP, Goldberg SA, VanGeest J (2000). Convenience survey regarding autopsy/organ donation education at the 1999 American Medical Association annual meeting. *Arch Intern Med* **160**:3167.

Talazaar HD, Schneiderman H, Yaremko L, Weinstein RS (1987). Medical student's attitudes toward the autopsy as an educational tool. *J Med Educ* **62**:66–8.

Verma SK (1999). Teaching students the value of autopsies. *Acad Med* **74**:855.

Welsh TS, Kaplan J (1998). The role of postmortem examination in medical education. *Mayo Clin Proc* **73**:802–5.

Zirkel JB, Zirkel PA (1997). Technological alternatives to actual dissection in anatomy instruction: a review of the research. *Educ Tech* **37**:52–6.

Chapter 4

AUTOPSIES AND THE LAW

Caroline Browne and Christopher P Dorries

Introduction

In England and Wales there are two key sets of legislation that govern autopsies (also referred to as post-mortems): the Human Tissue Act 2004 (hereafter, the 'HT Act') and the Coroners Act 1988. This chapter gives information on each of these and what they mean, both for the professionals undertaking post-mortem examinations and for the families of the deceased. The comparable legislation in Scotland, the Human Tissue Act (Scotland) 2006, has some differences, which are referred to later in this chapter. In Northern Ireland the comparable legislation is the Coroners (Northern Ireland) Act 1959 and the Coroners (Practice and Procedures) Rules (Northern Ireland) 1963 as well as the HT Act.

The request for a pathologist to undertake a post-mortem will generally come from one of two sources.

- *Request from a coroner.* This is required under the coroner's powers contained within the Coroners Act 1988. While issues of consent for the autopsy or initial tissue retention do not arise as coroners' autopsies are exempt from the consent requirements of the HT Act, there are requirements under the Coroners (Amendment) Rules 2005 in respect of tissue retention and under the HT Act as regards the storage and disposal of retained tissue.
- *Request from a clinician or clinical team.* Hospital (or consented) autopsies, now

comparatively rare, arise where clinicians have approached the next of kin or other appropriate person for permission to investigate issues where the cause of death is known and there is no other reason for coronial involvement. In these cases, issues of consent and other matters arise under the HT Act.

Because the HT Act is interwoven through the process of hospital autopsy and, from the pathologist's point of view, also through the coroner's autopsy, some explanation of that Act is set out to give the reader an initial understanding of its key requirements.

The Human Tissue Act 2004

In England, Wales and Northern Ireland, post-mortem examinations are subject to the requirements of the HT Act, which repealed and replaced the Human Tissue Act 1961, the Anatomy Act 1984 and the Human Organ Transplants Act 1989 as they related to England and Wales. Scotland has its own Act, the Human Tissue (Scotland) Act 2006, which is discussed separately here towards the end of this chapter.

The HT Act, which came into effect in full on 1 September 2006, provides the legal framework for the removal, storage and use of human organs and tissue for a number of purposes defined in the Act, referred to as *scheduled purposes* (one of which is determining the cause of death). It established the Human Tissue Authority (HTA; www.hta.gov.uk) as the regulatory body responsible for ensuring compliance with the HT Act and sets out the licensing framework which requires that a number of activities, including post-mortem examinations, can only be carried out under the authority of a licence granted by the HTA.

The change in the legislation resulted in part from two public inquiries that took place in England between 2000 and 2003, known as the Kennedy and Redfern inquiries, and the subsequent Isaacs Report, all of which established that the removal of organs and tissue from adults and children during post-mortem examination, and their subsequent storage and use without proper consent, had been common practice. An additional impetus was the 2001 publication of the report *The Removal, Retention and Use of Human Organs and Tissue from Post-mortem Examination*, which recommended a complete overhaul of the law on the removal and use of organs and tissue taken from people during surgery or after death. The resulting consultation document, *Human Bodies, Human Choices*, set out proposals on how the law might be changed; these proposals formed the basis of the new legislative framework.

The main body of the HT Act is divided into three parts.

- Part 1: *Removal, Storage and Use of Human Organs and Other Tissue for Scheduled Purposes*. This deals with consent, when it is required, and who may give it; it also sets out the offences under the Act and associated penalties. It is worth noting that, under section 5, the maximum penalty for an offence against the consent requirements is imprisonment for up to 3 years and/or a fine.
- Part 2: *Regulation of Activities Involving Human Tissue*. This establishes the Human Tissue Authority and its remit and, amongst other things, defines the regulatory and licensing system, including the penalties for breaching the licensing requirements.
- Part 3: *Miscellaneous and General*. This is concerned with various important supplementary issues and general provisions, including the HTA's powers of inspection.

This chapter of the book references relevant content in Parts 1 and 2 of the HT Act, and aims to provide simple guidance on the key statutory requirements relating to consent and licensing.

The HT Act's legislative framework for the storage and use of material from human bodies and the removal of material from deceased bodies requires that there be appropriate consent for these activities, and that establishments where removal, storage and certain other actvities take place be regulated through a system of licensing and inspection. (What is meant by 'appropriate' consent is explained later in this chapter.)

It is a complex piece of legislation and many of its requirements relate to several different sectors where the use of human organs and tissue is common (including research, anatomical examination and transplantation). For the purposes of this chapter, unless stated otherwise, explanation is given with reference to post-mortem examination only. Readers with interest in the use of organs and tissue in other areas should refer directly to the legislation and associated Regulations, and to the HTA's codes of practice for guidance.[1]

Section 1 of Part 1 of the HT Act lists the activities that are lawful if done with appropriate consent. These include the storage and use of bodies of deceased people for what is known as scheduled purposes and the removal, storage and use of tissue that has come from bodies of deceased people for use for scheduled purposes. Note that consent is not retrospective and an exemption under section 9 of Part 1 of the HT Act means that 'existing holdings' (e.g. blocks and slides held immediately before the day the HT Act came into force) are not subject to the consent requirements.

Scheduled purposes, which are defined in Schedule 1 of the HT Act and which are explicitly linked to licensable activities, are divided into two groups:

---

[1] Throughout this chapter, references are made to the HTA codes of practice on post-mortem examination and consent. HTA codes of practice give practical guidance to professionals carrying out activities that fall within the HTA's remit and adherence to them is assessed as part of the HTA's licensing and inspection process.

Box 4.1 Scheduled purposes in the Human Tissue Act 2004

Purposes requiring consent: general

1. Anatomical examination
2. Determining the cause of death
3. Establishing after a person's death the efficacy of any drug or other treatment administered to him/her
4. Obtaining scientific or medical information about a living or deceased person that may be relevant to any other person (including a future person)
5. Public display
6. Research in connection with disorders, or the functioning, of the human body
7. Transplantation

Purposes requiring consent: deceased persons

8. Clinical audit
9. Education or training relating to human health
10. Performance assessment
11. Public health monitoring
12. Quality assurance

purposes for which consent is always required and purposes for which consent is required only when the tissue is from the deceased. For ease of reference and for interest, they are listed in Box 4.1 as they appear in the Act.

Section 16 of Part 2 of the HT Act specifies the activities that can take place only under the authority of a licence. There are three that are relevant to post-mortem examination:

- 16(2)(b) – *the making of a post-mortem examination;*
- 16(2)(c) – *the removal from the body of a deceased person (otherwise than in the course of the carrying out of an anatomical examination or the making of a post-mortem examination) of relevant material of which the body consists or which it contains for use for a scheduled purpose other than transplantation;*
- 16(2)(e) i and ii – *the storage of the body of a deceased person or relevant material which has come from a human body for use for a scheduled purpose.*

An establishment licensed by the HTA for storage or removal may store or remove tissue for any of the scheduled purposes listed above (with the exception of anatomical examination) provided that appropriate consent is in place. (Further details about the licensing framework are given towards the end of this chapter.)

So, the HTA's role extends to ensuring that post-mortems and the removal and retention of any tissue are undertaken on suitable premises licensed for that purpose and with appropriate consent.

We have seen that under Part 1 of the HT Act, the removal, storage and use of organs and tissue from the deceased for scheduled purposes are all activities that require appropriate consent. Although *determining the cause of death* is one of the scheduled purposes, the HT Act goes further by defining *the making of a post-mortem examination* as an activity in its own right. In practical terms, this means that, where required, separate consent should be obtained for the post-mortem itself and for the subsequent storage and use of any tissue retained during the post-mortem.

A post-mortem takes place because it has been requested by a clinician and agreed to by the deceased person's relatives, or because the coroner considers it necessary, whether as part of a homicide investigation by the police or otherwise. Under the HT Act, the post-mortem must take place on licensed premises, whatever the reason for the examination. However, there are two exceptions to the consent requirements.

- The first is where the post-mortem and any removal and subsequent storage of organs and tissue are authorised by the coroner.
- The second is where there is retention of tissue beyond the coroner's remit as part of a homicide investigation by the police.

These are explained in detail later in this chapter.

Before beginning any post-mortem, the pathologist must be satisfied that the post-mortem and any removal, storage or use of tissue have been properly authorised, either by those close to the deceased (who have given their consent) or by the coroner. Although not a statutory requirement, the HTA recommends that wherever possible there should be written consent or instruction from the coroner.

The hospital post-mortem

A hospital post-mortem – that is, one that has been requested by a clinician for the purposes of learning more about the nature or progress of a disease – should be considered or requested only where the cause of death is already known in sufficient terms for the clinician to have completed a medical certificate as to the cause of death. If this cannot be done, the case should be referred to the coroner without discussing a hospital autopsy with the relatives.

Appropriate consent must be obtained from the relatives or those close to the deceased person before the post-mortem can be undertaken, unless the person who has died already consented while they were alive. It is usually the deceased person's clinician and members of the clinical team who will approach the family about the possibility of a post-mortem, knowing the patient's medical history and what learning might be gained from an autopsy. The HTA code of practice on consent gives detailed guidance on how to ensure that those giving consent have everything they need to enable them to make a fully informed decision. It advises that full details of the consent (including when it was obtained and the purposes for which it was given) should be noted in the patient's medical record, although ideally the consent should be given in writing. Consent must be obtained for all types of post-mortem examination, including those that are non-invasive.

In its code of practice on post-mortems, the HTA stresses the need for those taking consent to be competent to do so. It advises that

those seeking consent for hospital post-mortem examinations should be well informed, with a thorough knowledge of the procedure. They should be trained in how to seek consent and it is preferable for them to have observed a post-mortem examination and have had training in bereavement management.

In particular, they will need to understand the meaning of 'appropriate' consent.

In the HT Act, consent is appropriate if it has been given by a person identified in the Act as being able to give consent and there is a hierarchy that must be observed.

- First, consent may be given by the dying person.
- If consent from the person was not given, it may be given by his or her nominated representative.
- If there is no nominated representative, a person in a 'qualifying relationship' to the deceased immediately before death may give consent.

The HTA advises that, where an adult consented to a post-mortem before dying but those close to the person subsequently object

they should be encouraged to accept the deceased person's wishes, and it should be made clear that they do not have the legal right to veto or overrule those wishes.

In practice, healthcare professionals should make decisions on a case-by-case basis, mindful of the needs of the bereaved and the potential impact of proceeding with the post-mortem in light of strong opposition from the family.

Where consent for a hospital post-mortem has not been given by the person in life, the deceased person's nominated representative is the next in the hierarchy. When seeking consent from a nominated representative (or indeed from a person at the next level of the hierarchy, someone in a qualifying relationship), full and clear information should be provided about the post-mortem ensuring that they are able to make a properly considered decision.

Section 4 of Part 1 of the HT Act sets out how an individual can appoint one (or more) nominated representatives who may give consent. A nominated representative can consent to the autopsy itself and also to the removal, storage or use of tissue for any of the scheduled purposes (other than anatomical examination or public display). The HTA's code on consent advises that

if the deceased person appointed more than one nominated representative, only one of them needs to give consent, unless the terms of the appointment specify that they must act jointly.

Consent from a nominated representative cannot be overridden. However, the HT Act allows the nomination itself to be disregarded in some instances, for example if the nominated representative cannot be located.

Where there is no consent from the dying person and he or she has not appointed a nominated representative, consent may be given by someone in a 'qualifying relationship' to the deceased immediately before death. The HT Act lists those in a qualifying relationship to the deceased person in section 27 of Part 2. They are, in order of ranking:

- spouse or partner, including civil or same-sex partner;
- parent or child (in this context a 'child' can be over the age of 18);
- brother or sister;
- grandparent or grandchild;
- niece or nephew;
- stepfather or stepmother;
- half-brother or half-sister;
- friend of long standing.

The HTA code of practice on consent states that:

consent is needed from only one person in the hierarchy of qualifying relationships and should be obtained from the person ranked highest. If a person high up the list refuses to give consent, it is not possible to act on consent given by someone further down the list; for example, if a spouse refuses but everyone else would give consent, the wishes of the spouse must be respected.

It is important to note that if there is no one available in a qualifying relationship to give consent, the post-mortem examination cannot proceed.

Relationships listed together (e.g. 'brother or sister') have equal ranking, and consent may therefore be obtained from just one of them. For example, if the deceased person had no spouse but several children, the consent of only one of the children would be required. Difficulties may arise where there is conflict between individuals with equal ranking. The legal position is that the consent of only one of those ranked equally in the hierarchy is sufficient for the post-mortem to be undertaken. However, this situation needs to be handled with sensitivity and discussed with all parties and, as there is no legal requirement to undertake hospital post-mortems, the needs of the bereaved should be considered.

Under section 27(8) of Part 2 of the HT Act, a person in a qualifying relationship need not be taken into account if they do not wish or are unable to deal with the issue of consent, or *it is not reasonably practicable to communicate* with them in good time. In these cases, the next person in the hierarchy would become the appropriate person to give consent.

Section 2 of Part 1 of the HT Act relates to appropriate consent from children. The HT Act defines a child as someone aged under 18 years. (Under the HT (Scotland) Act, a child is defined as being under 16 years old.) Although a child cannot appoint a nominated representative, in all other ways the position of a child who, before dying, was competent to consent to the post-mortem is no different from that of an adult and the child could consent to the post-mortem itself and to the removal, storage or use of tissue for scheduled purposes. However, although the HT Act sets out the circumstances in which consent may be given by a child, it is unlikely that a child would be approached and appropriate consent would come from the person who had parental responsibility for the deceased child, usually a parent. In the absence of a person with parental responsibility, a person in a 'qualifying relationship' to the child may consent.

Note that anyone consenting to a hospital post-mortem has the right to change their mind, and the HTA recommends allowing 24 hours to pass before proceeding with the autopsy.

The HT Act does not deal with matters relating to the results of post-mortems and how these should be communicated to relatives, but the HTA gives the following guidance:

There may be occasions where the deceased person expressed a specific wish before death that information should not be shared with relatives and this should be respected as far as possible. Care should be taken regarding the possible disclosure of information, such as genetic information or HIV status, which the deceased person may not have wished to be disclosed, or which may have significant implications for other family members. Healthcare professionals should judge whether it is appropriate or not to disclose information about the deceased's medical history, as well as any other sensitive information that the hospital or coroner may hold about the deceased, that the family may not necessarily be aware of. In other circumstances, it may be necessary to share sensitive information with the family if the results of the post-mortem examination have the potential to affect them or other relatives. Legal advice should be sought on any legislative restrictions on disclosure.

The coronial autopsy

A coroner can require an autopsy to be undertaken to assist in his or her statutory function of establishing the cause and circumstances of any death where there is reasonable cause to suspect that the death is unnatural or of unknown cause.

It is sometimes said that the remit of a coroner's autopsy is limited to establishing whether a death is natural or unnatural. That is not strictly correct, for in general a specific cause of death will be necessary for the death to be registered. In those few cases where the cause remains unascertained, despite autopsy, an inquest must be held. Where the cause of death is unnatural, the autopsy is a valuable part of the coroner's inquiry to establish 'how' the death came about and evidence of injury or results of 'special examinations' such as toxicology often help establish far more than the bare medical cause of death.

Nonetheless, it is true that the coroner's autopsy is far removed from the academic hospital autopsy aimed at establishing precise details of medical science. The coroner's autopsy is sometimes criticised for this, being seen as a shortcoming, but it must be remembered that this is an examination directed by the state, often against the preferences of the family. It is therefore right that it is strictly limited by law, both as to need and extent.

Reform

The Coroners and Justice Act 2009 was given Royal Assent in November 2009 but most provisions will not come into effect until April 2012 at the earliest. The new Act, whilst it will eventually replace the 1988 legislation in its entirety, does not make wholesale practical changes to current practice in relation to autopsies. It remains to be seen what effect Rules and Regulations written to support the new Act will have; first consultations on these are likely in late 2010.

However, the plans to introduce a 'Medical Examiner' set out in the new Act may assist in narrowing the focus of autopsies to cases that are properly deserving. Further comment thereon is outside the remit of this chapter

The coroner's power to take jurisdiction and require an autopsy

The coroner does *not* have unlimited powers to inquire into a death or demand an autopsy. The basic right to take jurisdiction over a death is set out in section 8 of the Coroners Act 1988, which requires the coroner to hold an inquest if there is reasonable cause to suspect that the death:

- was violent or unnatural; or
- was sudden and of unknown cause; or
- occurred in prison.

Section 8(1)(c) also makes requirements where the death occurred 'in such circumstances as to require an inquest under any other Act' but there are no such other legislative needs at present.

Note that the custody provision applies simply by virtue of where the death occurs and there is no requirement for an unnatural or unknown cause, nor that the deceased is even a prisoner. However, the 1989 case of *R v. Inner North London Coroner* ex p *Linnane* [1989] 1 WLR 395 makes clear that the phrase 'in prison' should be widely interpreted and would include someone taken ill at a prison who later died in hospital, even if not guarded at the time.

The power to take jurisdiction carries two ancillary rights. Where a coroner needs to take possession of the body for a post-mortem examination the case of *R v. Bristol Coroner* ex p *Kerr* [1974] 2 All ER 719 allows him or her to exercise physical control over the body until the inquest is concluded – although it would normally be released much earlier. Further, section 22 of the Coroners Act gives the coroner power to order the removal of a body from where it lies to a mortuary, whether within the district or in an adjoining district of another coroner, for the purpose of a post-mortem examination, subject to the consent of the person providing the mortuary facility there. The restriction of movement to 'an adjoining district' is rather cumbersome in view of the modern trend towards centralisation of specialist mortuary facilities and the lack of paediatric pathologists.

Note that section 8 requires the coroner to conduct an inquest in *every* case where the cause of death is unknown or unnatural etc. Read in isolation, this would obviously bring tens of thousands more inquests than are properly required. However, the Act then goes on to make provision for autopsies in two distinctly differing circumstances.

- Section 19 gives the coroner power to require such an examination 'if of the opinion that it

Box 4.2 Section 19 of the Coroners Act 1988

Post-mortem examination without inquest

1. Where a coroner is informed that the body of a person is lying within his district and there is reasonable cause to suspect that the person has died a sudden death of which the cause is unknown, the coroner may, if he is of the opinion that a post-mortem examination may prove an inquest to be unnecessary: (a) direct any legally qualified medical practitioner whom, if an inquest were held, he would be entitled to summon as a medical witness under section 21 below; or (b) request any other legally qualified medical practitioner to make a post-mortem examination of the body and to report the result of the examination to the coroner in writing.
2. For the purposes of a post-mortem examination under this section, the coroner and any person directed or requested by him to make the examination shall have the like powers, authorities and immunities as if the examination were a post-mortem examination directed by the coroner at an inquest into the death of the deceased.
3. Where a post-mortem examination is made under this section and the coroner is satisfied as a result of it that an inquest is unnecessary, he shall send to the registrar of deaths a certificate under his hand stating the cause of death as disclosed by the report of the person making the examination.
4. Nothing in this section shall be construed as authorising the coroner to dispense with an inquest in any case where there is reasonable cause to suspect that the deceased: (a) has died a violent or an unnatural death; or (b) has died in prison or in such a place or in such circumstances as to require an inquest under any other Act.

may prove an inquest unnecessary' by establishing a (natural) cause of death (Box 4.2).
- Section 20 allows an autopsy where it is already clear that an inquest will be needed because the cause of death is clearly unnatural (Box 4.3).

These are quite different powers. The authority under section 19 is comparatively limited – simply to

Box 4.3 Section 20 of the Coroners Act 2008

Request to specially qualified person to make post-mortem and special examinations

1. Without prejudice to the power of a coroner holding an inquest to direct a medical witness whom he may summon under section 21 below to make a post-mortem examination of the body of the deceased, the coroner may, at any time after he has decided to hold an inquest: (a) request any legally qualified medical practitioner to make a post-mortem examination of the body or a special examination of the body or both such examinations; or (b) request any person whom he considers to possess special qualifications for conducting a special examination of the body to make such an examination.
2. If any person who has made a post-mortem or special examination in pursuance of such a request is summoned by the coroner as a witness, he may be asked to give evidence as to his opinion upon any matter arising out of the examination, and as to how, in his opinion, the deceased came by his death.
3. Where a person states upon oath before the coroner that in his belief the death of the deceased was caused partly or entirely by the improper or negligent treatment of a medical practitioner or other person, that medical practitioner or other person: (a) shall not be allowed to perform or assist at any post-mortem or special examination made for the purposes of the inquest into the death; but (b) shall have the right, if he so desires, to be represented at any such post-mortem examination.
4. In this section 'special examination', in relation to a body, means a special examination by way of analysis, test or otherwise of such parts or contents of the body or such other substances or things as ought in the opinion of the coroner to be submitted to analyses, tests or other examination with a view to ascertaining how the deceased came by his death.

establish a cause of death which is natural. This contrasts with the powers under section 20 where the examination is to provide evidence for the inquest and a wider range of investigations can be made. Section 20 allows the coroner to request any person (i.e. not necessarily a doctor) whom he or she considers to possess appropriate qualifications to make a 'special examination'. This is defined as an analysis or test of such parts or contents of the body as the coroner thinks ought to be submitted to analysis, test or other examinations with a view to ascertaining how the deceased came to die. Any decision on a special examination might commonly be on advice from the pathologist conducting the post-mortem.

Confusingly, section 21 (not shown here) then allows the coroner to summon in evidence at an inquest:

- a doctor who attended at the death or during the last illness; or
- a doctor in practice in or near the place where the death occurred.

This medical witness may be asked to give an opinion on how the deceased came to die. Further, the coroner may direct such a medical witness to make a post-mortem examination of the body of the deceased. This appears to be an anachronism, said to be taken almost verbatim from the Coroners Act 1836. It is not clear, in modern society, how a doctor 'in practice nearby' is going to be able to assist. Nor does the power to direct a medical witness to perform a post-mortem add anything to section 20. Further, section 21 adds nothing in practical terms to section 11(2), which requires the coroner to examine on oath all who have knowledge of the facts of death – a clear power to summon any witness (medical or otherwise) who can give relevant evidence.

The Coroners Rules 1984

A number of rules in the subordinate legislation are relevant to the pathologist.

Rule 5

Any post-mortem is to be made as soon after the death as reasonably practicable. There is therefore a specific requirement for expediency.

Rule 6

This sets out the matters to be taken into account by the coroner when deciding who should be requested to perform the post-mortem.

- Rule 6(i)(a) states that the examination should be made by a pathologist with suitable qualifications and experience.
- Rule 6(i)(b) requires the coroner to consult with the Chief Officer of Police as to the identity of the pathologist if the death is suspicious. While the coroner is not obliged to follow the wishes of the police, in reality it is virtually inevitable that the pathologist would be from the Home Office list of accredited forensic pathologists.
- Most significantly, rule 6(i)(c) directs the coroner not to instruct a pathologist on the staff of a hospital if the death has occurred there and the conduct of any member of the hospital staff is likely to be called into question. While there is a saving clause concerning 'undue delay', the requirement for overt independence is important.

Rule 10

There is no statutory requirement as to the actual nature of the work undertaken in the examination. The nearest to legislative guidance is contained in rule 10(1), which requires the pathologist to report to the coroner in a form similar to that set out in Schedule 2 of the *Rules*. The schedule contains a detailed list of all the major organs of the body, which at the very least implies that these should be examined. The provisions of rule 10(2) in relation to the release of reports are considered further below.

Rule 11

In terms of premises, rule 11(1) forbids a post-mortem to be performed in a dwelling house or in licensed premises, surely an anachronism in the days of HTA licensing. By rules 11(2) and 11(4) the post-mortem must be in adequately equipped premises, that is to say 'supplied with running water, proper heating and lighting facilities and containers for the storage and preservation of material'. Rule

11(3) requires that, if a person has died in a hospital 'so equipped', any post-mortem examination shall be made in those premises – but even this is unless the coroner otherwise decides.

The autopsy report

While the format and content of the autopsy report are generally outside the remit of this chapter, some legal issues arise.

The HTA indicates that, before the post-mortem is carried out, relatives should be told when the results are likely to be available. This places some responsibility on the pathologist to (a) communicate a short cause of death promptly to the coroner's officer, and (b) provide the final report within a normal timescale.

By 10(2) of the Coroners Rules 1984, unless authorised by the coroner, the pathologist must *not* supply a copy of the report to any person other than the coroner. Rule 13 makes similar provision in respect of special examinations. Thus, in theory at least, a pathologist reporting on a coroner's post-mortem in a hospital may not give the clinicians involved in the case a copy of the report unless and until the coroner agrees.

In the past there has been a division of opinion between coroners as to whether post-mortem reports should be made freely available. Most (but not all) coroners now take a view towards appropriate disclosure. Thus it would now be common for a hospital pathologist to be allowed to provide the clinicians with a copy of the report in all deaths occurring within the hospital. By extension this could also apply to hospital risk managers, who might need prompt information on causes of death etc.

Further, Home Office Circular 62/1994, issued following the Clothier Report (into the deaths of children at Grantham Hospital), recommended that:

in every case coroners should send copies of post-mortem reports to any consultant who has been involved in the patient's care prior to death, whether or not demanded under rule 57

and the Home Secretary asked that coroners review their procedures to ensure that access to reports was facilitated and dealt with as speedily as possible. The Model Coroners Charter produced by the Home Office in 1999 in an effort to promote consistency also suggests that a copy of the report should be made available to the family.

All this leaves rule 57(1) of the Coroners Rules somewhat in isolation. This rule provides that the coroner must, on payment of the appropriate fee, supply to any person who in his or her opinion is a properly interested person (i.e. a participant at the inquest) a copy of any report of the post-mortem or special examination. It is not made clear whether this entitlement arises at the time the report is received by the coroner (i.e. before any inquest) or only after proceedings are completed. The normal exceptions to disclosure would be cases of suspicious death or where release of information may hinder an on-going police enquiry.

In releasing a post-mortem report prior to an inquest, it may be appropriate for the coroner to make it clear that the report is on a preliminary basis. The pathologist may wish to alter the conclusions having heard the results of other enquiries or medical investigations and the evidence given at the inquest hearing.

Tissue retention in the coronial autopsy

While it is generally recognised that some histology is a normal part of an autopsy conducted under section 19 of the Coroners Act 1988, the power to retain significant amounts of tissue, or whole organs, for 'special examination' only arises under section 20 of that Act.

Whatever the power used, tissue retention in a coroner's autopsy does not fall under the HT Act but is instead governed by changes to the Coroners Rules 1984 set out in the Coroners (Amendment) Rules 2005 – a short but complex piece of subordinate legislation. The requirements are listed in simple terms in Box 4.4.

A number of issues arise, of varying complexity. First, although the coroner (at step 2 in Box 4.4) will set a maximum period for retention, the coroner's power to allow retention actually ceases when his or

Box 4.4 Tissue retention

Requirements of the Coroners (Amendment) Rules 2005

1. The pathologist must tell the coroner the exact details of the material to be retained and for how long it is required.
2. The coroner then authorises the specific retention and sets a maximum period (as to which see below).
3. The coroner must tell the family of the retention and, where possible, gain their instruction as to disposal. The choices given in the Rules are:
   - return of the material to the family
   - allowing retention for research or other purposes
   - respectful disposal by the pathologist.
   Although it is not a requirement of the Rules, coroners may give the additional option of delaying the funeral pending the later return of the material to the body.
4. The family's decision should be communicated to the pathologist, although there is actually no requirement in the Amendment Rules for such a notification, an issue which has caused some difficulties.
5. The pathologist must keep a record of the details of the retention or disposal of material.
6. The autopsy report must declare the retention and disposal.

her interest in the case finishes. With an autopsy (inquest) under section 20 of the Coroners Act this is straightforward enough; the coroner's powers cease when the inquest is concluded, although the pathologist must obviously be notified that such has happened as they may well not be aware of the inquest unless called to give evidence.

The situation is more difficult where the autopsy was under section 19 (to show an inquest is unnecessary by proving the death is of a known, natural cause). There is no obvious point at which the coroner's interest ceases. Indeed, the coroner is always able to return to such a case and declare that an inquest will be held if it becomes apparent that the death may be unnatural. In general, the point at which the coroner receives the pathologist's final report and completes a notification to the Registrar General of whether or not there is a revised cause of death is taken as the relevant time for disposal. Clearly this also requires notification to the pathologist.

Finally, it is increasingly common that the 'allowing retention for research or other purposes' option is subdivided to allow the relatives to opt for the material being kept as part of the deceased's medical record, possibly for a set period, for use for specific scheduled purposes defined in the HT Act. This allows the advantage of retention for audit or later review of cause without going to a point where relatives may feel uncomfortable. Disposal is dealt with in more detail below.

Coronial autopsies and the Human Tissue Act

In the case of coronial autopsies, the post-mortem examination itself and the removal and use of organs and tissue to determine the cause of death do not require consent from the relatives, *as anything done for purposes of functions of a coroner or under the authority of a coroner* is exempt from the consent requirements of the HT Act (section 11 of Part 1).

Although the consent of relatives is not required, the HTA advises that the reasons for the post-mortem and the process that will be followed should be explained to the family at whatever level of detail they seek. As a minimum, they should be told when and where the examination is to be performed, and informed of their right to be represented at the post-mortem by a registered medical practitioner.

When the coroner's authority has ended (see Box 4.4), if the material is not disposed of, the further storage of post-mortem samples falls within the remit of the HT Act and it is unlawful to continue to retain material for a scheduled purpose without appropriate consent or on unlicensed premises.

Tissue retention in criminal cases

Different questions arise where tissues need to be retained in connection with the investigation of homicide, a situation that may cause families some distress.

In such cases, the retention of relevant tissues may be of extreme importance. First, it will be necessary in order to ascertain the cause and circumstances of the death to satisfy a court 'beyond reasonable doubt'. Second, in the interests of fairness to any prospective defendant, it is essential that experts instructed by the defence lawyers can conduct their own scientific examination of the tissues if they wish.

Notwithstanding that there is a homicide investigation, the body is in the possession and control of the coroner and any autopsy can only be done on his or her order, generally under the power in section 20 of the Coroners Act 1988 (see above). The police do not have a power to require an autopsy themselves.

Much of any material retained at such an autopsy will relate to the cause of death and will, initially, fall within the changes to the Coroners Rules 1984 set out in the Coroners (Amendment) Rules 2005 described above. But there will also be material retained purely for the purposes of the police investigation (typically fingernail scrapings or body cavity swabs) that might relate to identifying the offender rather than the direct cause of death. While it may be hoped that such items will contain material from the offender, they will also undoubtedly contain material from the deceased. When the coroner's interest finishes (see above), these items may well be held by the police for their own purposes.

In addition, material properly taken in relation to the cause of death may also be required for the criminal process after the coroner's interest has finished. The Code of Practice issued under the Criminal Procedure and Investigation Act 1996 provides for the following minimum retention periods for material considered relevant to a prosecution:

- 3 years in respect of a conviction after a not guilty plea at a trial on indictment;
- if an appeal is lodged, until after the appeal is determined.

Many would now argue that longer periods are appropriate.

Section 39 of Part 2 of the HT Act contains exceptions for criminal justice purposes. Consent is not required to retain material for the purposes of a criminal investigation, nor does material taken for this purpose need to be held on licensed premises. Where material is held under the authority of a coroner and the police simultaneously, the section 39 exemptions of the HT Act apply.

Material taken and/or retained under police authority only is not subject to the provisions of the HT Act with regard to disposal. However, Home Office guidance provides that the police, so far as is practicable, will dispose of the material in compliance with the requirements of the HT Act.

If following the cessation of a police investigation continued retention of tissue is authorised by the coroner, it must then be held on licensed premises and in accordance with the Coroners (Amendment) Rules 2005.

Those requiring a more detailed analysis of material retention in criminal cases are directed to 'Police and coroners approach to pathology (issue 1)', which is available on the Home Office website at www. homeoffice.gov.uk.

Disposal

Section 14 of Part 2 of the HT Act lists among the activities within the remit of the HTA the disposal of the body of a deceased person which has been stored or used for a scheduled purpose and the disposal of material which has been removed from the body of a deceased person for various purposes, including post-mortem examination. The HTA provides guidance on disposal in a code of practice on this topic.

The point for the pathologist to note is that, when the coroner has communicated the family's wishes to the pathologist holding the material, the pathologist should act on this information without unreasonable delay. Establishments should ensure that there are systems in place to dispose of the tissue in accordance with the wishes of the next of kin and in line with the HTA's code of practice, which states that:

if the wishes are to reunite organs and tissue with the body before burial or cremation, there should be a system of checking that any retained tissue is accounted for before the body is released to the family. If there is tissue not accounted for, there should be a clear procedure for detailing the course of action to be followed. Efforts should be made to keep the relatives informed throughout the process.

Licensing

As mentioned earlier in this chapter, the HT Act sets out the licensing framework for establishments where post-mortem examinations take place. Pathologists and others working in this field need to be aware of the licensing requirements and the statutory duties they place on individuals working under the licence.

Section 16 of Part 2 of the HT Act makes post-mortem examination an activity that can take place only under the authority of a licence granted by the HTA. There are no exceptions to this requirement so, as mentioned earlier, whatever the circumstances of or reasons for the post-mortem, a licence will be required. In addition, a licence is required for the storage of organs and tissue (including in the form of blocks and slides) taken at post-mortem for use for scheduled purposes.

Under Regulations made by the Secretary of State, the storage of post-mortem tissue for use for research which is ethically approved by a Research Ethics Authority[2] (or for which ethical approval is pending) is exempt from licensing. Also exempt is the storage of post-mortem tissue for the sole purpose of analysis for a scheduled purpose (other than research), where the tissue has come from and will be returned to licensed premises – for example, post-mortem specimens sent to a specialist testing facility. These exemptions are set out in the HT Act (Ethical Approval, Exceptions from Licensing and Supply of Information about Transplants) Regulations 2006. Finally, tissue stored by the police for criminal justice purposes is not required to be stored on HTA-licensed premises (see section 39 of Part 2 of the HT Act).

The HT Act identifies persons working under the licence, including the Designated Individual, who has a statutory duty under section 18 of Part 2 of the HT Act to secure:

- *that the persons to whom the licence applies are suitable persons to participate in the carrying on of licensed activity;*
- *that suitable practices are used in the course of carrying on that activity;*
- *that the conditions of the licence are complied with.*

The role of the Designated Individual is thus an important one, which must be undertaken by someone with a sound knowledge and understanding of the licensed activities and associated operational procedures.

Section 16(1) prohibits licensable activities from being carried on without a licence and, under section 25, the maximum penalty for such an offence is imprisonment for up to 3 years and/or a fine.

Schedule 3 of the HT Act lays down the characteristics of a licence as well as the HTA's power to grant, revoke, vary and suspend licences. This section may be of interest to readers who would like information about the detailed aspects of the licensing process.

The Human Tissue (Scotland) Act 2006

Consent is the key principle governing the use of human tissue for certain purposes in Scotland, although different terminology is used in the Scottish legislation. The HT (Scotland) Act refers to 'authorisation' rather than 'consent' and the activities of the coroner are undertaken by the procurator fiscal.

In the HT (Scotland) Act, 'post-mortem examination' refers to:

examination of the body of a deceased person involving its dissection and the removal of organs, tissue samples, blood (or any material derived from blood) or other body fluid which is carried out for any or all of the following purposes:

- *providing information about or confirming the cause of death;*
- *investigating the effect and efficacy of any medical or surgical intervention carried out on the person;*

---

[2] Defined in regulation 2 of the HT Act 2004 (Ethical Approval, Exceptions from Licensing and Supply of Information about Transplants) Regulations, 2006.

- *obtaining information which may be relevant to the health of any other person (including a future person);*
- *audit, education, training or research.*

As in the HT Act, post-mortems carried out *for the purposes of the functions or under the authority of the procurator fiscal* are exempt from the 'authorisation' requirements.

The HT (Scotland) Act is another complex piece of legislation, and space precludes detailed analysis of its contents. However, a key difference between it and the HT Act is that it allows the continued storage of tissue samples, blood (or any material derived from blood) and other bodily fluid removed during the post-mortem under the authorisation of the procurator fiscal – to be retained as part of the medical record when the procurator fiscal's purposes have ceased, without the need to obtain further authorisation. Tissue held as part of the medical record can then be used for the following purposes:

- providing information about or confirming the cause of death;
- investigating the effect and efficacy of any medical or surgical intervention carried out on the person;
- obtaining information that may be relevant to the health of any other person (including a future person);
- audit.

Further reading

Online

www.homeoffice.gov.uk/documents/approach-to-pathology1.pdf

www.opsi.gov.uk/si/si2006/20061260.htm

www.hta.gov.uk

HTA codes of practice

Consent, code 1.

Post-mortem examination, code 3.

Disposal, code 5.

General

Learning from Bristol: Report of the public inquiry into children's heart surgery at the Bristol Royal Infirmary 1984–1995, Bristol Royal Infirmary, July 2001.

Report of the Royal Liverpool Children's Inquiry, January 2001.

Investigation of Events that Followed the Death of Cyril Mark Isaacs, Department of Health, Issacs Report Response, July 2003.

Removal, Retention and Use of Human Organs and Tissue from Post-mortem Examination – advice from the Chief Medical Officer, Department of Health, Department for Education and Employment and Home Office, TSO, 2001.

Human Bodies, Human Choices: The law on human organs and tissue in England and Wales – a consultation report, Department of Health, 2002.

Chapter 5

RELIGIOUS ATTITUDES TO DEATH AND POST-MORTEM EXAMINATIONS

Jane E Rutty

Religion is like going out to dinner with friends. Everyone may order something different, but everyone can still sit at the same table.

HH The Dalai Lama

Introduction

Religion is often expressed as stories, symbols, beliefs and practices, through the conviction that there is an ultimate power or reality that is often mystical in nature, giving meaning to the life experience of the individual. Prayers, rituals, meditation and music are ways of expressing such beliefs both personally and publicly. Such beliefs also have an effect on individual moral behaviour, in turn setting religious laws and traditions. This includes how individuals cope with serious illness and prepare for death.

Death, on the other hand, is described from a scientific viewpoint as the permanent termination of the biological functions that define a living organism; in other words, physical death. Yet the true nature of death has for thousands of years been the central concern of all religions from around the world as they concentrate not only on the physical death and the effects thereof, but on the non-physical mind and/or soul too.

This chapter therefore aims to provide pathologists engaged in autopsy practice with an overview of religions from around the world and their held beliefs and attitudes to not only death but also the care after death, including post-mortem examinations from both the physical and non-physical viewpoints. The intention is for this chapter to be easy to access so that it can be used for reference purposes concerning the sensitive holistic medical care of the deceased and his or her family.

Background to religious attitudes

Everyone from around the globe it seems holds a system of beliefs about the cause, nature and purpose of the universe. In addition, the majority of us also hold these values with reference to a God or gods. The modern example of this can be seen when reviewing the leading religion for each country around the world (Fig. 5.1; Matthews, 2009). However, the world has also seen movement of people between countries. Such people bring with them their own distinct culture and sometimes their own language or religion.

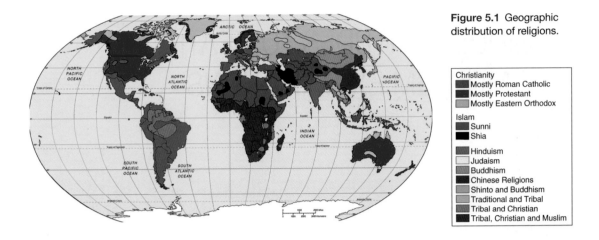

Figure 5.1 Geographic distribution of religions.

A prime example is the UK, which has welcomed newcomers for centuries, thus boasting a multi-cultural society. The nineteenth century, for instance, witnessed the arrival of Jewish people escaping persecution from Russia and Poland and Irish people escaping poverty in rural Ireland. The twentieth century observed the influx of Caribbean workers invited to help rebuild Britain after the Second World War; Asians from India, Pakistan and Bangladesh who escaped poverty; East African Asians who fled persecution; and Eastern European refugees who came following war and political unrest in Romania and the former Yugoslavia (Migration Statistics Unit, 2007).

The twenty-first century is now seeing an estimated 577 000 people arriving to live in the UK per year (according to 2007 National Statistics); in other words, around 1580 per day. An example of this is an estimated 96 000 Polish citizens who migrated into the UK in 2007, the highest inflow of any individual citizenship. In contrast an estimated 340 000 people are emigrating per year from the UK: 932 per day. Reasons for entering or leaving the UK range from work, study, marriage, asylum seeking or long holidays, to coming or going home to live. In summary, this means that 237 000 more people enter than leave the UK annually, the equivalent of adding 650 people a day to the population (Migration Statistics Unit, 2007).

In part this has led to a multi-religious identity within the UK, even though Christianity is the leading religion at 71.6 per cent (Fig. 5.2). After Christianity, Islam was the most common faith with 2.7 per cent describing their religion as Muslim

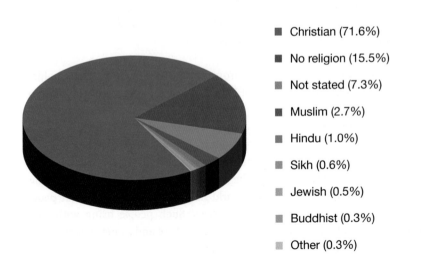

- Christian (71.6%)
- No religion (15.5%)
- Not stated (7.3%)
- Muslim (2.7%)
- Hindu (1.0%)
- Sikh (0.6%)
- Jewish (0.5%)
- Buddhist (0.3%)
- Other (0.3%)

Figure 5.2 The UK population by religion.

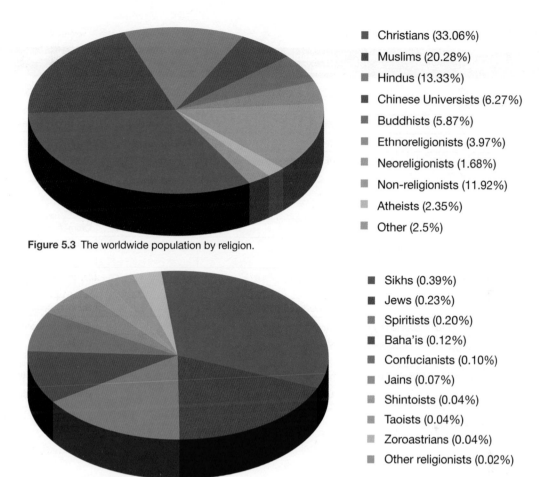

Figure 5.3 The worldwide population by religion.

■ Christians (33.06%)

■ Muslims (20.28%)

■ Hindus (13.33%)

■ Chinese Universists (6.27%)

■ Buddhists (5.87%)

■ Ethnoreligionists (3.97%)

■ Neoreligionists (1.68%)

■ Non-religionists (11.92%)

■ Atheists (2.35%)

■ Other (2.5%)

■ Sikhs (0.39%)

■ Jews (0.23%)

■ Spiritists (0.20%)

■ Baha'is (0.12%)

■ Confucianists (0.10%)

■ Jains (0.07%)

■ Shintoists (0.04%)

■ Taoists (0.04%)

■ Zoroastrians (0.04%)

■ Other religionists (0.02%)

Figure 5.4 The worldwide population of other religions (total 2.5 per cent).

(1.6 million). The next largest religious groups were Hindus (559 000), followed by Sikhs (336 000), Jews (267 000), Buddhists (152 000) and people from other religions (179 000). These groups together accounted for 2.7 per cent of the UK population. About 15.5 per cent of the population stated that they had no religion. This category included agnostics, atheists, heathens and those who wrote 'Jedi Knight' (Office for National Statistics, 2001).

Religion is significant for the majority of individuals internationally. It is vital, therefore, never to assume that the previous picture put forward regarding religious statistics is the everyday make-up of UK society. The increase in international travel gives us a slightly different picture (Figs 5.3 and 5.4; Encyclopaedia Britannica, 2006). The vital importance of being aware of key beliefs to such religions allows the

care of the deceased and relatives to remain respectful and spiritually sensitive. This is especially so as death has a tendency to lead religious customs and it is exceptionally unusual for funerals not to be associated with religious rites. However, the world's religions are so varied that it is not that astounding in such a mixed multi-cultural civilisation that it is enormously simple to bring about offence unintentionally.

The intention of this chapter is not to present a theological examination, but to give an explanatory description that can be simply accessed and employed for reference purposes on the subject of spiritual care after death by pathologists and others working in the mortuary. For ease, the chapter has been separated into the three broad groupings of contemporary faiths – the Abrahamic, Dharmic and

Table 5.1 Summary of religious attitudes to death

Religion	Agreeable to last offices?	Agreeable to organ donation?	Agreeable to autopsy?	Body disposal
Atheism	Yes	Yes	Yes	Burial or cremation
Bahá'í	Yes	Yes	Yes	Burial
Buddhism	Yes	Yes	Yes	Cremation preferred
Christianity	Yes	Yes	Yes	Burial or cremation
Confucianism	May prefer to be washed by family	Yes, but traditionalists may be superstitious		Burial preferred
Hinduism	No	Yes	Disliked	Cremation
Islam	No	Yes	Yes	Burial
Jainism	Yes	Yes	Yes	Cremation
Judaism	Should be handled as little as possible	Yes	No	Burial
New Age Spirituality	Dependent on underlying religion followed			
Rastafarian	Yes	Considered distasteful		Burial preferred
Shintoism	Prefer to be washed by family	Yes, but traditionalists may be superstitious		Cremation preferred
Sikhism	May prefer to be washed by family	Yes	Yes	Cremation
Taoism	Prefer to be washed by family	Yes, but traditionalists may be superstitious		Burial or cremation
Zoroastrian	Yes	Unwilling	No	Burial or cremation

Adapted from Rutty (2001, 2004).

Far Eastern – and other traditions. The brief key beliefs concerning death and care after death that will incorporate information on funerals, organ donation and autopsies are given. A very brief summary of this can be found in Table 5.1.

The Abrahamic faiths

The Abrahamic faiths are monotheistic in that their doctrine or belief is that there is only one God. Four well-known monotheist traditions are Judaism, Christianity, Islam and the Bahá'í faith, all of which arose in the Middle East and are inextricably related to one another, being traceable back to Abraham (around 2000 BC). Christianity originated within the Jewish tradition and Bahá'í within the Islamic. The Abrahamic faith is considered to be a young faith compared with Egyptian society, which had already built the pyramids by 3000 BC (Kramer, 2003).

Judaism

Judaism is regarded as the oldest religion within the Abrahamic faiths and is entwined with culture. However, it has gone through a number of phases, developments and changes that have led to today's Rabbinic phase of three diversities, these being the Orthodox Tradition, Conservative Judaism and Reform Judaism. The Orthodox Tradition is usually much more customary and observant of religious and dietary laws than other sects that fit their religious rites into contemporary society.

Overall, Judaism believes that there is one God, Creator and Lord of the universe, otherwise known as the Covenant which guides their way of life. The first five books of the Old Testament (the Torah) contain laws and rules for everyday life, principal among which are to worship one God and obey the Ten Commandments and the practice of charity and tolerance towards other people.

Life is considered to be sacred and death is viewed as being controlled by the Omnipotent One (i.e. God, who has absolute and unlimited power). Judaism holds a firm belief in the afterlife, where those who have lived a worthy life will be rewarded. Death according to Judaism is not a tragedy, even when a young child dies or when someone dies through adverse or disastrous circumstances. Instead, death is considered to be natural, like our lives, in that it has meaning and is part of God's plan. Two of the most important commandments are to honour the dead and to comfort the mourner. Hence, deep religious meaning is invested in death and dying rituals based around the concepts of ritual, community and memory (Solomon, 2000; Nazarko, 2006).

Care after death

Throughout the entire period between death and the funeral, the body is never left unattended. Very importantly, the body is guarded or watched as it is believed to be vulnerable and unable to watch over itself until it has 'come home' to its final resting place within the grave.

The body must be handled as little as possible, as considerable importance is attached to the ritual cleansing and clothing of the body. This is undertaken by Jews who are specially qualified and of the same sex as the deceased. Hence limited laying out should be performed by healthcare staff. However, if members of the family are not present, most non-Orthodox Jews would accept the usual washing and last rites performed by hospital staff. Otherwise, once death has been established, the eyes and mouth of the deceased must be closed by a child, a relative or a close friend – in that order of preference. Healthcare staff should ensure the jaw is supported and limbs are straightened with the arms placed by the sides. The body is then labelled and covered with a white sheet. If the family wish to view the body, mortuary staff should ensure that the room is free from any religious symbols (Nazarko, 2006).

The immediate family will contact the local Jewish undertaker and synagogue and put the ritual proceedings in motion. Judaism believes it to be a humiliation to the dead to leave them unburied. Therefore, arrangements to bury the deceased, ideally within 24 hours, are of upmost importance, being delayed only for the Sabbath and other major festivals. Cremation is most unusual, as historically it is frowned upon as an unnatural means of treating the human body, but non-Orthodox Jews allow cremation (Cytron, 1993).

The preservation of life is an important guiding principle in Judaism and so there is no objection to the principle of organ donation. However, Orthodox Jews may be less willing. With regard to autopsies, Jewish law requires that after someone has died the body be buried in its entirety. Judaism believes that man was created in God's image and so any mutilation of the body is loathed strongly. Therefore, autopsy examinations are not permitted in Jewish law unless required by civil law (Green and Green, 2006).

Christianity

The term 'Christianity' comes originally from the Hebrew word *Messiah*, meaning 'The Anointed One'. The Greek translation *Christos* was the foundation of the English translation 'Christ'. Based on the writings of the New Testament, Christians believe that Jesus Christ (first century AD), who was born a Jew in the Roman province of Palestine (now known as Israel, Palestine and Jordan), was the divine son of God who became man on Earth. The central belief of Christianity is that God is the one God who reveals himself as the Trinity of the Father, the Son and the Holy Spirit. Christians believe that Jesus was conceived by the Holy Spirit and born of the Virgin Mary. Following his baptism by the prophet John the Baptist he became a preacher and healer, teaching people how to live godly lives, suffering himself the pains and temptations of a mortal man but without sin. According to the Gospels of the New Testament, he went to observe Passover in Jerusalem and on arrival was met with people celebrating his doctrines about death, judgement, heaven and hell. This led to his arrest for blasphemy, for which he was tried and crucified. Following his death, his disciples were convinced that God raised him from the dead on the third day after his burial and ascended him into Heaven where he is now seated at the right side of the Father (God). They converted others to believe, which eventually founded Christianity (Toropov, 2004).

Today, Christianity is practised all over the world. It believes that the death and resurrection of Jesus is not only an important event but also a demonstration that Jesus has the power over life and death and the ability to give people eternal life. However, despite major commonalities many doctrine disagreements have taken place over the last two millenia. This has resulted in differing traditions that, in turn, have placed varied significance on the rituals of caring for the dead. The three main forms of Christianity – Roman Catholicism, the Anglican Communion and the Free Churches – will now be presented in turn, along with information on the Afro-Caribbean Community, Church of Jesus Christ of Latter Day Saints and Jehovah's Witnesses.

Roman Catholicism

The Roman Catholic Church is the single largest Christian church, claiming more than a billion members. Catholics believe that the Pope, the Church's highest authority, is the true successor to Saint Peter the apostle appointed by Jesus Christ to be its head (O'Collins, 2008). Of great meaning to Catholics is the sacrament of Baptism. Children especially will be baptised before or even at death if needed. Otherwise, Catholic sacraments most associated with the end of life are Reconciliation (Confession or Penance), Holy Communion (Eucharist) and the Anointing of the Sick (Last Rites) (Kemp, 2002). A Catholic priest should always be called to enable these sacraments to be given either at the point of death or up to 3 hours after.

Care after death

Routine last offices are appropriate. Within Irish communities, it is traditional to exhibit the body after death before the funeral. Therefore, particular care should be taken if the next of kin consent to organ donation or post-mortem examination. Catholics overall are traditionally buried rather than cremated, but there are no religious objections to cremation.

The Anglican Communion

The Anglican Communion is the third largest Christian communion in the world and incorporates a wide spectrum of beliefs and practices. In summary, there is no single Anglican church with universal authority. While they believe many Catholic doctrines, they reject the power of the Pope. Instead, all churches within the communion are independent, but in communion with the Church of England. The Archbishop of Canterbury is the religious head of the Church of England. He has no formal authority outside this jurisdiction, but is symbolically recognised worldwide as the head of the communion. There are many churches within the communion such as the Church of Ireland and the American Episcopal Church, each of which has its own doctrine and liturgy underpinned by the Church of England. Anglicans believe that everyone baptised will share in Christ's resurrection and eternal life after death. As with Catholicism, should a child die without being baptised the family may feel their child will be prevented from entering the family of God. Baptism can be performed soon after death by an Anglican priest (Toropov, 2004).

Care after death

Routine last offices are fitting with no objection to organ donation or post-mortem examination. Both burial and cremation are acceptable.

The Free Churches

Free Churches are Christian churches that evolved in the USA where they were founded outside the state system with no ties to Rome. They do not conform to Catholic or Anglican traditions. In essence, Free Churches are free from state interference in internal affairs. The majority of members portray themselves as Protestants or Chapel. Examples of Free Churches include Methodists, Baptists, Salvation Army, Quakers, Seventh Day Adventists and the United Reform Church (Cracknell and White, 2005; Dandelion, 2008). Less importance is put on the administration of sacraments than for Catholics or Anglicans, with the example of some groups not seeing the baptism of a sick or dead child as critical. Instead, it is more likely that a minister will be invited to pray with the patient and family.

Care after death

Routine last offices are appropriate with no religious disapproval to organ donation or autopsies. Burial or cremation is considered acceptable

Afro-Caribbean Community

The main religion of the West Indies is a form of Christianity, the main Christian churches being Anglican, Methodist and Pentecostal, but there is an extensive difference in how it is practised from island to island. The one commonality is that they are observed as being much more expressive in how they worship compared with other Christian faiths. It is important to note that Baptism for the Afro-Caribbean Community is very important as it involves the naming of the child. They believe that all children should be named before death. When a person is dying or deceased then it is not unusual for a large number of family members to visit as they like to be near the individual at the time of death (Green and Green, 2006).

Care after death

Last offices are considered appropriate, but the ideal would be for them to be performed by an individual from a similar ethnic background. Traditionalists are less likely to agree to organ donation than the younger generation. In addition the older generation are unlikely to consent to an autopsy except in coroner's cases, as they believe that the body should be intact for the afterlife and so any disfigurement will be very distressing – especially as the body may be viewed before and during the funeral service. For this very reason, embalming is preferred if the funeral is to be delayed for some reason. Burial is favoured over cremation. For the extended family and friends of the deceased, the funeral is an important and decorative occasion (Green and Green, 2006).

Church of Jesus Christ of Latter Day Saints

The Church of Jesus Christ of Latter Day Saints, commonly called the Mormon Church, was founded in 1830 AD by the prophet Joseph Smith, a farm labourer. It is held that Joseph Smith found hieroglyphic scripts on golden plates in a nearby hill disclosed to him by an angel. Following its translation, the Book of Mormon is believed to be the literal record written by prophets and followers of Jesus Christ of God's dealings with civilisations from around 2600 BC through to 420 AD in the Americas.

It is understood to be a holy scripture, another witness of Jesus Christ, comparable to the Bible. With over 11 million members worldwide today and a predicted 265 million by 2080, Mormons embrace the idea that they have reinstated the Church as created by Christ where other Christian churches have gone off course.

Mormons believe that there are three stages to life: pre-existence as a spirit child (prenatal), probation on Earth, and finally eternal life with the Heavenly Father. Death is thought to be a blessing and a purposeful role to eternal existence. At some time after death, the spirit and the body will reunite and be resurrected to the spirit world, which is separated into two: Paradise, where the good spirits wait for resurrection, and Spirit Prison, where the unrighteous spirits live in darkness. The good spirits are able to visit the Spirit Prison and preach the gospel. If one of the unrighteous spirits accepts the gospel and repents they are able to progress to Paradise (Green and Green, 2006).

Care after death

There are no formal procedures in caring for the dying or dead, so routine last offices are appropriate – with the exception that if the sacred garment is removed then it must be replaced on the body. Reassurance and practical help regarding funeral arrangements will be offered by the Bishop. Before making a final decision about organ donation and autopsies, Mormons will be expected to ask the Lord for inspiration while assessing the benefits and counter arguments. It is worthy to note here that the body may be viewed before the funeral at the church meeting house. Concerning disposal of the body, burial is preferable with cremation being discouraged rather than being ruled out (Green and Green, 2006).

Jehovah's Witnesses

The Christian sect Jehovah's Witnesses was founded in 1872 AD by the American clergyman Charles Taze Russell in Pennsylvania, USA. Deeply committed Jehovah's Witnesses endeavour to live their lives as directed by the Old and New Testaments. Such messages are spread mostly by members who preach from door to door and distribute literature. They believe that Jehovah is the Supreme Being and that Jesus is the Son of God who was a created being who was formerly in a pre-human state as the Archangel Michael. In 1914 AD, the Heavenly Kingdom resulted in the invisible enthronement of Christ as King. Very importantly, they recognise faithfulness and duty only to the kingdom of Jesus Christ, regarding the world currently as being under the control of Satan. They reject to salute any flag, vote, run for public office or join the Armed Forces. Jehovah's Witnesses believe that in the near future the battle of Armageddon will commence, where Jesus under Jehovah's divine rage will perform retribution upon supporters of all other religions (i.e. false religions), resulting in the world being cleansed and God's Kingdom being created on Earth (Green and Green, 2006).

Care after death

No official last rites are practised when death occurs, so routine last offices are proper. A matter for individual conscience is the issue of organ donation or autopsy, as it is not promoted either way. Of special note is that, should Witnesses agree to organ donation, then before transplantation all organs and tissues must be completely drained of blood as blood represents life itself and must be respectfully handled. Witnesses will not consent for blood to be stored or reused in any way. The funeral is prepared with respect to the individual rather than a formal written service with both burial and cremation being acknowledged (Green and Green, 2006).

Islam

The conception of Islam is officially deemed to have occurred in 610 AD when the Angel Gabriel began to reveal the Word of God to the prophet Muhammad. Islam in Arabic means 'to submit', specifically to God, and a Muslim is 'one who submits'. There are three main branches of Islam – Sunni, Shi'ite and Sufi – but none is considered to have overall authority for all Muslims. Muslims hold that God has sent prophets such as Abraham, Moses and Jesus, but followers of these and other prophets have corrupted their teachings through mistakes and distortion and so God sent Muhammad to remind man again of the truth. It is believed that God's message was written down as soon as it was revealed and passed on as intended by God through the Qur'an. The essence of Islam is that there is one God (Allah), the creator and ruler of the Universe who is all powerful and has no equal. In practice, adherents demonstrate their beliefs by living their life according to Islamic law (Shari'ah) usually within an Islamic community through the traditional duties of the five pillars of Islam: bearing witness to the unity and uniqueness of God and to the prophet Muhammad; prayer at prescribed times each day; fasting during the month of Ramadan; pilgrimage to Mecca; and paying a certain amount of one's own wealth as alms for the poor (Robinson, 2007).

Death is considered to be an element of God's overall plan. In general, Muslims believe that after death everyone is judged and will go either to Paradise or to the Fire according to their good and bad deeds during life. Death should not be feared as it is assumed that an observant Muslim will achieve salvation, and hence extreme grief is suppressed for this very reason (Sarhill et al., 2003).

Care after death

Following death, enormous respect should be shown. Non-Muslims should not touch the body. Normally, the body is ceremonially washed at least three times with soap and specially wrapped with three pieces of white cotton cloth (Kafan) along with scent or perfume, so last offices by healthcare staff should not be performed unless the family are unavailable. Even then healthcare staff should always wear disposable gloves and last offices must be minimised by closing the eyes, bandaging the lower jaw to the head so that the mouth does not gape, straightening the body at the elbows, shoulders, knees and hips (thus enabling washing and enshrouding of the body later), and turning the head towards the right shoulder (so the body can be buried with the face towards Mecca). Do not wash the body, nor cut hair or nails. Cover the deceased with a sheet ensuring that the whole of the body is covered (Sarhill et al., 2003; Green and Green, 2006).

As the body is believed to belong to God, strict Muslims are opposed to organ donation, and so the matter should not be discussed unless the family initiates the possibility first or if the deceased has consented in writing beforehand. If organ donation is approved, the organs must be transplanted instantly and not kept in organ banks. Apart from when ordered by the coroner, autopsies are prohibited within the Islamic faith. However, if an autopsy is required the ceremonial preparations in caring for the body will begin after the autopsy. The funeral should take place within 24 hours and delays cause anguish to families. As Muslims believe there will be a bodily resurrection, bodies are buried rather than cremated.

The Bahá'í Community

Arising out of Islam in 1863 AD and being one of the youngest of the world's major religions, the Bahá'í Community was founded by the Persian Mirza Husayn Ali in present-day Iran. Believed to be a prophet sent by God, he is recognised today as Baha'u'llah, which means 'the Glory of God'. The Bahá'í faith tries to encompass all religions into one faith in that there is simply one God who is the creator of life, advocating world peace. The purpose of life is to know and love God through the acquisition of virtues and spiritual qualities so as to carry forward an ever-advancing civilisation and in preparation for the next world. The faith has no clergy or individuals in positions of personal leadership, and is administered by elected bodies at local, national and international levels. It now has around 5 million followers throughout the world. The Bahá'í believe that one's soul comes into existence at conception and is immortal. Because everyone has an eternal soul it is not subject to decomposition at death. Instead the soul is able to journey around the spirit world, an eternal extension of our own universe. There are no official last rites practised when death occurs (Momen, 2008).

Care after death

Last offices by healthcare staff are accepted. Bahá'ís from Iran and some other countries within the Middle East are required to observe certain procedures. This may include the body being washed carefully by the family, being wrapped in a shroud of white silk or cotton and a Bahá'í burial ring being placed on the finger. With the Bahá'í faith having no disagreements between modern medicine and religion, there is no objection to organ donation or autopsies. Simple funerals are arranged by relatives of the deceased in consultation with the local Bahá'í community, each being unique in nature. Burial is preferred, as cremation is not permissible, observing the following burial laws: no embalming unless required by law, no means of speeding up the natural process of decomposition, such as calcinations, and interment within 1 hour's journey from the city or town where death occurred. This includes all remains donated to medical science. The body should be placed so that the feet face the tomb of Baha'Allah near Acre (Smith, 2008).

Rastafarianism

Rastafarianism is considered to be a political–religious movement that began during the 1930s in the West Indies among the descendents of African slave families. It began with the 'Back to Africa' campaign of Marcus Garvey advocating the repatriation of black people to Africa, their true home and heaven on Earth. It was in 1966, though, that Haile Selassie visited Jamaica and convinced the Rastafarians not to immigrate to Ethiopia until they had liberated the people of Jamaica. Rastafarians believe that they are reincarnated from the Lost Tribes of Israel and that their redemption will be through an exodus led by God back to Africa (the homeland) which will be a heaven on Earth where black superiority will be claimed over the whites. Frequently linked with dreadlocks, marijuana and reggae music, Rastafarianism currently has a following of over 700 000 worldwide. Dreadlocks or 'locks' are a symbol of their faith and a sign of black pride. The smoking of marijuana, the 'holy herb', is a holy sacrament to many, believed to be the key to new understanding of the self, the universe, and God being the vehicle to cosmic consciousness. It was the popular reggae singer Bob Marley in the 1970s and 1980s who assisted the message of Rastafarianism to become widespread. Rastafarianism has no centralised organisation or formal church. Instead it is practised as a personal religion where members share in a deep love of God and the belief that the Temple is within each person. Rastafarians believe in the resurrection of the soul after death and so families may pray by the bedside of the dying. There are no formal last rites (Green and Green, 2006).

Care after death

Routine last offices are appropriate, but it is to be noted that Orthodox members may not permit their hair to be cut. Both organ donation and autopsy are considered distasteful with few agreeing to either, except when ordered by the coroner. The funeral is plain and simple and attended only by intimate family and friends, with burial being preferred, but cremation is not forbidden (Green and Green, 2006).

The Dharmic faiths

The Dharmic religions, sometimes referred to as traditions, are a group of religions whose theology and philosophy centre on the concept of Dharma, meaning 'fixed decree, law, duty' in the spiritual sense of 'natural law and reality'. All Dharmic religions originate from India, but can now been seen all over the world, but especially so around the Indian subcontinent, East Asia and South East Asian. One of the main religions within this group is Hinduism, out of which grew Buddhism, Jainism and Sikhism. These four faiths will now be discussed in turn.

Hinduism

Hinduism was originally a term used to describe people who lived east of the River Indus. Today, Hinduism is the oldest religion practised in the world with its roots traced back to at least 2500 BC. Like many other faiths and traditions, it is not just a religion but a way of life that is steeped in culture. There are believed to be around 1 billion adherents to Hinduism, of whom 890 million live in India. Followers of Hinduism believe in one ultimate Supreme being who has unlimited forms and who can be identified with and venerated in various ways. The overall aim of Hinduism is freedom of the soul from endless reincarnation in differing forms and the sufferance inherent in existence (Kemp, 2002). These differing

reincarnated forms are dependent on how faithful one has been concerning religious duties. It is thus possible that those who have been inattentive or remissive of their duties may be reborn into a lower caste.

The majority of Hindus prefer to die at home as there is great religious significance in this for them. Death in a hospital can be deeply distressing to the family. Some Hindus will prefer to return to India to the sacred city of Varanasi on the north bank of the River Ganges to die. A person near death should be placed with his or her head facing east and a lamp placed near the head. As death nears, large numbers of family members will be present. Along with chanting and prayers, a few drops of Ganges water, the leaves of the sacred tilsi plant and a piece of gold are placed in the mouth of the dying person before death – that is, before the soul leaves the body (Breuilly and Palmer, 1999; Bauer-Wu et al., 2007).

Care after death

Last offices by healthcare staff are inappropriate as the body should not be washed by non-Hindus. Instead it is the family who bathe, dress and wrap the body in a piece of new cloth. However, if it is necessary for healthcare staff to be involved then it is essential that disposable gloves be worn, the eyes closed, the limbs straightened and the body wrapped in a plain sheet with no religious emblems or artefacts. All jewellery, sacred threads and any other religious objects should not be removed. Although they are rather unpopular, there is no resistance to organ donation or autopsies; should either occur then the ritual preparation of the body will begin afterwards. Hindus favour that, as in India, funerals take place within 24 hours of death. The body is cremated as only the soul is needed for reincarnation. The eldest son as part of the funeral rites would light the funeral pyre in India or stand by the coffin as it passes through the furnace. The ashes are thrown into a river, preferably the River Ganges, on the third day and then later the ceremony shraddha marks the end of the deceased soul's journey and family mourning (Green and Green, 2006; Klostermaier, 2007).

Buddhism

As a reform of Hinduism, Buddhism was founded by Siddhartha Gautama, a Hindu Prince in the sixth century. He was given the name of Buddha, meaning 'Enlightened One' or 'The Awakened'. Today Buddhism is the second largest Dharmic tradition with over 700 million adherents across East Asia and South East Asia. Buddhism is the most popular eastern philosophy in western countries with three formal schools: Theravada, Mahayana and Tibetan. While Buddhists believe in many of the fundamental values of Hinduism, including reincarnation, they do not acknowledge the caste system. Buddhists believe that there is no god or divine judgement, instead recognising that it is the law of 'Dharma' (cause and effect) that affects each and everyone's future and fate. Buddha is revered, therefore, as a model of everyday life underpinned by the Four Noble Truths: all sentient beings suffer, the cause of suffering is desire, the way to end suffering is to cease to desire, and the way to cease to desire is to follow the Eightfold Path – 1, right belief; 2, right intent; 3, right speech; 4, right conduct; 5, right endeavour; 6, right effort; 7, right mindfulness; and 8, right meditation (Kemp, 2002). Following this Eightfold Path will lead to emancipation from rebirth. Death according to Buddhism is considered to be a time to progress into something better, so it is important for the dying patient and his or her family to be in a quiet place so that wholesome thoughts and past good deeds can be reflected upon (Rinpoche, 2008).

Care after death

Last offices by healthcare staff are considered appropriate as there are no official Buddhist rites following death, although a Buddhist minister or monk of the same school as the deceased should be notified of the death directly. There is no objection to organ donation or autopsies, given that serving others is elemental in Buddhism, demonstrating compassion. However, if the death was sudden or concerned a small child, Buddhists will be troubled about the deceased's rebirth as the person's mind will not have been prepared prior to death. The funeral service can be of any order as long as Christian doctrine or the Deity are not incorporated. Pregnant women will not attend the service though, as Buddhists believe this could cause bad luck to the baby. It is customary for cremation to take place 3–7 days after death since there is no belief in the resurrection of the body, although burial is acceptable (Truitner and Truitner, 1993).

Sikhism

Sikhism is a religious tradition based on the teachings of 10 Gurus who lived in northern India during the seventeenth and eighteenth centuries who abandoned the traditions of fifteenth century Muslim and Hindu faiths. Founded by Guru Nanak in what is now Pakistan, it has today around 20 million adherents, of whom 80 per cent live in Pakistan and India. Britain has the next leading adherent population. The word 'Sikh' in the Punjabi language means 'disciple'. Sikhs believe that they are the disciples of God following the writings of the Ten Sikh Gurus. The main philosophy and beliefs centre on there being only one God, the same for all people of all religions, who created everything. Life then is considered to be something that should be practised virtuously and truthfully while maintaining a balance between spiritual and temporal obligations. Attachment to material things can lead to reincarnation and rebirth. Only when the soul is pure enough can it achieve salvation and mergence with God. In addition, Sikhs believe intently in protecting religious freedom. This is demonstrated through the establishment of the Khalsa order, which upholds the highest Sikh virtues of commitment, dedication and social conscience. The order encompasses both men and women who have undergone the Sikh baptism ceremony and follow the Sikh Code of Conduct and Conventions by wearing the five signs of their faith, otherwise known as the Five Ks: Kesh, uncut hair; Kanga, a comb to keep the hair in place; Kara, a steel bangle; Kirpan, a small sword or dagger; Kachera, short trousers or breaches. After death, it is understood that behaviour during life is determined by God, resulting in either being in eternal union with God or being reborn. Either way Sikhs hold that it is wrong to mourn excessively for the deceased as they will exist in a different body (Breuilly and Palmer, 1999, Kalsi, 2007).

Care after death

More often than not families prefer traditionally to lay out the body. After death, the body is washed. If the deceased was a member of the Khalsa then he or she will be dressed in the Five Ks. The deceased's face may be viewed on many occasions prior to the funeral so a peaceful appearance is desirable. After touching the body the family will probably like to take a bath or wash their faces, hands and feet before going home. If the family are not available then there is no objection to limited last offices being undertaken by healthcare staff. This includes leaving the Five Ks intact, the hair kept covered with no trimming of either hair or beards, the eyes closed, the jaw supported, limbs straightened and then covered with a white sheet with no religious emblems. Both organ donation and autopsies are considered acceptable, but any incisions should be carefully sutured, so that any bathing or dressing does not cause wound dehiscence during ritual proceedings. Should organ donation be granted or an autopsy required, then such ritual proceedings will begin afterwards. Preferably then, within 24 hours, the body is cremated (Green and Green, 2006; Nazarko, 2006).

Jainism

There are more than 8 million Jains world-wide, 98 per cent of whom live in India, with the biggest Jain communities outside India being within the UK, USA, the Far East and Australia. The true meaning of Jain is 'those who are able to overcome their innermost feelings of hate, greed and selfishness'. Also a Dharmic religion emerging from Hinduism around 800 BC, Jainism denies the idea of a supreme being and believes instead in a deep respect for all living things, describing a path of non-violence. Jains believe that countless numbers of souls are trapped in our world and are considered to be evil and tied in a cycle of reincarnation due to accrued moral behaviour demonstrated in previous lives, otherwise known as 'karma'. In other words, karma is the quality of our current and future lives as determined by our behaviour in this and previous lives. The aim of

a Jain is to eliminate this karma through good behaviour in order to achieve liberation of the soul, transcend the world and achieve eternal spiritual bliss, 'moksha'. Jainism believes that death is a mysterious event that can be experienced by both ordinary and higher types of souls, describing 17 different types of death. Two of these in particular are considered to be very important. Akama Marana refers to someone who has attachment to life and does not want to die, probably as a result of being unsure as to the concepts of reincarnation. Sakama Marana, in steep contrast, refers to someone who is not afraid of death and accepts it, knowing that it is a natural process. Of note, Jainism is quite different from other traditions in that to hasten one's own death normally through starvation is acceptable to those considered as having superior spiritually. Again unlike other religions, Jains will not cry for the deceased as this is believed to prevent the dead from rising (Rees, 2001; Long, 2009).

Care after death

Family members may wish to wash the body after death. The body will be dressed in new clothes. The exception is in India, where the body will be shrouded by a white cloth and new clothes instead are given to the poor. If the family are unavailable then last offices by healthcare staff are appropriate. On the day of the deceased's death a service will take place in the temple. Organ donation or autopsies are not objected to as Jains believe that it is a good thing to assist in helping better other people's lives and in developing new knowledge. The body in its coffin will be taken home before the funeral to enable relatives and friends to look at the deceased's face for the last time and to pray for their soul. Jains will dispose of the body through cremation, usually within 24 hours. For the funeral a flower will be placed on the coffin to resemble life, but removed just before the cremation as it is believed to be morally wrong to intentionally hurt a living thing (Nazarko, 2006).

Far Eastern traditions

Far Eastern Traditions, sometimes referred to as East Asian religions, focus on the concept of Tao or

Dao (The Way) and include Taoism, Shinto and Confucianism. Today there are many Chinese community adherents all over the world, but it is important to note that, due to interpretation, they may differ significantly from traditional culture.

Taoism

Believed to have originated in pre-history China, the fundamentals of Taoism were defined by Lao Zi in the sixth century BC. It has around 20 million followers. Taoists hold that all events are divine and that a life of quiet contemplation will achieve oneness with Dao. Central to their beliefs is the Chinese concept of 'Yang' and 'Yin', which are the male and female opposites of personality and which bring balance to the universe, giving order to life. Supporters of Taoism trust that an individual has no less than one soul, with more than one being male and one female (Yang and Yin). At death the souls separate, the female soul sinks into earth as a ghost (kwei) and the male soul rises and becomes a spirit (shen). After death, souls are judged and punished, where one of the souls will go to Hell before being able to go to its allotted place. Here souls can bribe keepers to receive better care. It is important, therefore, that the living family supply their deceased with liberal resources. In response, spirits will pledge victory in life if they are content or tragedy if not. Traditionally the Chinese who follow Taoism have an aversion to death (Fisher, 1997).

Care after death

Limited last offices should be undertaken by healthcare staff as the deceased will be washed ritually and cleansed with incense. Some may even be embalmed. To represent purification and protection from the influences after death, layers of white paper money or talismans are put over the deceased. A deceased child would be dressed in new clothes just before or after death. Traditionalists will be superstitious of organ donation and autopsies. This is because they believe that it is critical to appease the evil spirits and ghosts who are everywhere, and with the heart being central to all life it will be difficult for relatives to give consent. Otherwise there is no objection. Funeral rites are very ritualistic, providing comfort

and support to the family, an example being waiting for the most favourable date and place for the burial, although modern followers of Taoism prefer cremation. During the funeral special Bank of Hell notes, paper houses and other goods are burnt to enable the soul to pay for an early release from the various Hells, of which there are 10. Customarily, the bones are exhumed around 10 years later, when they are cleaned and re-buried at a site chosen by a feng shui expert (Woo, 1992; Gudmundsdottir *et al.*, 1996; Rees, 2001).

Shintoism

An indigenous Japanese religion with more than 3.2 million followers, Shinto means 'the way of the gods' or 'kami'. Kami are the sacred energies found in nature such as trees, rocks and water to name only a few. The Japanese do not regard kami just as divine Gods, as many kami are ancestors who remain close to the earthly world. Vitality, growth and prosperity will be asked of the kami through ceremonies that involve the rituals of purity, loyalty and sincerity. Dissimilar to other traditions, death – while accepted as being inevitable, irreversible and heartbreaking for everyone involved – is considered to be an evil. After death the spirits of the dead move into a land that is no longer pure, but a place of decay and corruption, where they are finally released from all physical limitations and again become part of the universal life force. Just as heaven and the underworld are close to the middle land (Earth), so the dead remain close to the living. Shinto rituals provide the dead with a means of escape from decay and corruption, enabling them to grow into exalted beings to become part of the world of kami (Fisher, 1997; Rees, 2001; Reader, 2007).

When communicating with families who follow Shintoism, physical contact should be avoided as the Japanese customarily do not gaze into another person's eyes. This is considered offensive in their culture. Of note, too, is that a Japanese person may in respect say 'no' three times before giving you their genuine reply, which should be taken into particular consideration with concerning the care after death. Do not presume that a nod or a smile means agreement, but ask the person if he/she comprehends what you have said.

Care after death

It is extremely important after death that respectful words be exercised. Never use the word 'body' (*Shitai* in Japanese) to relatives. Instead use Japanese comparables for the deceased, *Itai* and *Go-Itai*. *Go* is a prefix which further raises *Itai*. In addition, when talking about the deceased ensure that flattery is included as part of the conversation, particularly so if the person died in a tragic accident. The only exception would be if the deceased had performed vicious offences. The souls of those who died violently are believed to be restless and potentially hazardous to the living unless they are calmed by food and purification. Last offices are considered inappropriate within Shintoism and therefore should be avoided. Instead the family will bathe the body in a bath of warm water performing purification rites, before wrapping the body in a white kimono. As in Taoism, some traditionalists may be superstitious of organ donation and autopsies, but overall there is no opposition as such. Family and friends will then traditionally visit the deceased for around 2 days. Shinto funerals are held for Shinto priests, important Shinto devotees and the Emperor and his family only. All other followers follow the Buddhist funeral customs with cremation being preferred to burial (McQuay, 1995; Woo, 1992).

Confucianism

Confucianism, founded by Kong Fuzi (Confucius) in fifth century BC China, has a following of around 6 million that has spread from China to Korea, Japan and Vietnam. There is also great interest among Western countries. Confucianism is a major thought system in relation to the principles of good conduct, practical wisdom and proper social relationships. Stability, happiness and prosperity lie in conforming to the 'Will of Heaven', a spiritual principle that regulates the course of events. Confucianism has influenced the Chinese attitude towards life by emphasising personal control, adherence to social hierarchy and social and political order, which in

turn has provided the background for political theories and institutions. After the death of Confucius, various schools of Confucian thought have emerged through the centuries including Mencius, Hsun-tzu, Han Confucianism and Neo-Confucianism. Beliefs about death will vary depending on the school of Confucian thought followed (Yao, 2000; Coogan, 2005).

Care after death

Funeral and mourning customs will vary from family to family, so it is best to be guided by the family concerning last offices. Traditionally, at death relatives will cry out loud to inform the neighbours and the family will begin mourning by wearing clothes made of course material. There is no aversion to organ donation or autopsies by Taoists, although again conservatives may be rather superstitious. After this, the body is washed and put in a coffin, where both food and significant objects of the deceased will also be placed such as lucky charms. Families will be deeply offended if this is refused. Incense and money will be brought by mourners to assist with the funeral costs. A Buddhist, Taoist or even a Christian priest will perform the burial ritual. Friends and family follow the coffin to the cemetery with a willow branch symbolising the soul of the person who has died. This willow branch is carried back to the family altar where it is used to 'install' the spirit of the deceased. Liturgies are performed on the seventh, ninth and forty-ninth days following the burial and on the first and third year anniversaries of the death.

Other traditions

As well as the faiths within the Abrahamic, Dharmic and Far Eastern religions covered in this chapter there are a large number of so-called new religions, which are listed in Box 5.1. These, however, follow the same principles in relation to death as their principal faiths. In addition to these there is an enormous number and wide variation of faiths outside these traditions such as atheism, New Age Spirituality and Zoroastrian which will now be presented.

Box 5.1 Religions, sects and alternative spiritualities

CHRISTIANITY

Christadelphians
Christian Science
Church of Jesus Christ of Latter Day Saints
  (Mormonism)
Exclusive Brethren
Jehovah's Witnesses
New Apostolic Church
The New Church
Unity School of Christianity

African independent churches
Nazareth Baptist Church (Shembe)
Oneness Pentecostalism

The anti-cult movement
Branch Davidians
People's Temple

Celt Christian spirituality
The Family (Children of God)
Holy Order of MANS
Jesus Fellowship (Jesus Army)
Jesus Movement
Word of Faith Movement

Communal groups
Brotherhood of the Cross and Star
Family Federation for World Peace and Unification
  (Unification Church)
The Way International

Global network of Divergent Marian Devotion

Ngunzism
Celestial Church of Christ (Aladura)
Church of the Lord (Aladura)
Iglesia ni Cristo
Kimbanguism
Rastafarianism
Worldwide Church of God
Zion Christian Church

Prosperity spirituality
Creation Spirituality
Embassy of Heaven Church
International Churches of Christ

JUDAISM

Lubavitch Movement
Reconstructionist Judaism

Kabbalism
ALEPH: Alliance for Jewish Renewal
Gush Emunim
Havurot Movement
Humanistic Judaism
Meshihistim

ISLAM

Bahá'í Faith
Halveti-Jerrahi Order of Dervishes
Haqqani Naqshbandis
Shadhili-Akbari Sufi Order

Contemporary Sufism
Bawa Muhaiyaddeen Fellowship
Nation of Islam
Subud
Sufi Movement (International Sufi Movement)
Sufi Order of the West (Sufi Order International)
United Nuwaubian Nation of Moors

ZOROASTRIANISM

Parsee Theosophy
Mazdazan
Ilm-e Khshnoom

INDIAN REGIONS

Ananda Marga
Brahma Kumaris
Church of the Shaiva Siddhanta
Hao Hoa
Meher Baba Movement
Muttappan Teyyam
Radhasoami Tradition
Ramakrishna and the Ramakrishna Mission
Satya Sai Baba Society
Self-Realization Fellowship
Self-Revelation Church of Absolute Monism
Swaminarayan Movement
Transcendental Meditation

Tantric spirituality
Adidam
Autoville
Consciousness (Hare Krishna Movement)
Dhammakaya Foundation
Eckankar
Elan Vital
Friends of the Western Buddhist Order
ISKCON: International Society for Krishna
Krishnamurti and the Krishnamurti Foundation

continued ➤

Box 5.1 *continued*

Lifewave
Mata Amritanandamayi Mission
Mother Meera
New Kadampa Tradition
Osho Movement
Santi Asoke Movement
Shaja Yoga
Shambhala International
3HO Foundation (Healthy, Happy, Holy Organisation)

RELIGIONS OF EAST ASIA

Cheondogyo
Nichiren Shoshu
Omoto
Quan Zhen
Tenrikyo

Chinese new religions
Rissho Koseikai
Sekai Kyuseikyo
Shinnyoen
Yiguandao (Tian Dao)

Feng Shui
Agonshu
Ananaikyo
Aum Shinrikyo
Byakko Shinkokai
Daesunjinrihoe
Falun Gong (Falum Dafa)GLA (God Light Association)
Kofuku no Kagaku
Mahikari
Suma Ching Hai

Japanese new religions
Cao Dai
Gedatsukai
Perfect Liberty Kyodan
Reiki
Reiyukai
Seicho no Ie
Soka Gakkai

Martial arts
Bentenshu
Cult of Mao and the Red Guards
Kodo Kyodan
Tensho Kotai Jingukyo

INDIGENOUS AND PAGAN TRADITIONS

Cargo cults
Druidry
Santeria (La Regla de Ocha)

African neo-traditional religions
Candomble
Kardecism
Heathenism
Native American Church

Shamanism
Church of All Worlds
Covenant of the Goddess
Eco-Paganism: Protest movement
   Spiritualities Umbanda
Fellowship of Isis
Wicca

WESTERN ESOTERIC
Western esotericism

NEW AGE TRADITIONS
Anthroposophical Movement
Arcane School
Grail Spirituality
Emissaries of Divine Light
Freemasonry
Gurdjieff and Ouspensky Groups
'I AM' Religious Activity
Neo-Templar Orders
Ordo Templi Orientis (OTO)
Rosicrucianism
Society of the Inner Light
Spiritualism
Hermetic Order of Golden Dawn
Theosophical Society

Astrology
A Course in Miracles
Celestine Prophecy
Company of Heaven
Damanhur
Fiat Luz
Impersonal Enlightenment Foundation
Jasmuheen and the Breatharians
Movement of Spiritual Inner Awareness
Order of the Solar Temple
Servants of the Light
Share International Foundation
Temple of the Vampire
Universal Christian Gnostic Church

continued ➢

Box 5.1 *continued*

The Tarot Church Universal and Triumphant (Summit Lighthouse) Findhorn Foundation School of Economic Science	Transpersonal Psychologies URANTIA

Celebrity-centric Spirituality	*Ufology and UFO-related movements* Silva Mind Control
Apocalipticism and Millenarianism Synanon Church Unarius Academy of Science	*Implicit religion* Chen Tao (God's Salvation Church) Doofs and Raves in Australia Emin
Feminist and eco-feminist spirituality Aetherius Society Church of Scientology	Heaven's Gate Human Potential Movement Landmark Forum Neuro-Linguistic Programming
Postmodern Spirituality Psychedelic Spirituality	Thee Church ov MOO Raelian Religion

Adapted from Partridge (2004).

Atheism

There are numerous forms of atheism, including humanism, secularism, rationalism, humanistic Judaism, Christian non-realism, postmodernism and unitarian universalism. The term 'atheism' comes from the Greek word meaning a lack of belief in any form of deity. It is not a religion or philosophical system, but a belief that people can formulate their own appropriate moral codes. Atheists believe that people's attitudes to deities and gods are the same as believing in the tooth fairy in that such beliefs are merely based on superstition. Of interest, research does show that followers of atheism have the lowest divorce rate compared with other religious groups, demonstrating sound family ideals (Religious Tolerance, 2009).

Care after death

Last offices by healthcare staff are considered appropriate. It is an individual choice as to whether to agree to organ donation or autopsies. As an alternative to a religious funeral a humanistic funeral is preferred where the life of the deceased is recollected. There are no hymns or prayers included as atheists feel that religion has no importance. However, music, reflections on death, poetry and prose, a eulogy, candle lighting and formal words of goodbye form the basis of the funeral (Wilson, 2004). Again it will be the individual's choice whether to be buried or cremated.

New Age Spirituality

New Age Spirituality – sometimes called the New Age Movement – is a complex system of people who share similar philosophies which they incline to add to whatever other religion they respect. Therefore there are no holy scripts, principal organisations, membership, formal clergy or doctrine. Beliefs tend to embrace astrology as a means of projecting the future, crystals as a basis for healing, and Tarot cards for life decisions. They trust moreover that God is a state of higher consciousness and that a person may reach the total understanding of personal, human potential. There are a number of essential values, although individuals are supported to decide which agree with them best – for example, monism, pantheism, panentheism, reincarnation, karma, aura, personal transformation, and holistic health. Viewpoints about death are reliant on what underlying religion New Age Spiritualists abide by (Partridge, 2004).

Care after death

Specific care of the body, organ donation and consent for autopsies are dependent on which underlying religion New Age Spiritualists follow.

Zoroastrianism

Zoroastrianism was the dominant religion of Persia, originating in the sixth century BC until the rise of Islam. Based on the teachings of Zoraster, the religion's prophet and founder, today the largest communities can be found in India (92 000) and Iran (around 30 000), and it is estimated that there are about 7000 Zoroastrians in Britain, about 5000 of whom live in London. Offshoots of Zoroastrianism include Mithraism and Manichaeanism. Zoroastrians believe that there is only one Creator and supreme force. It has important texts rather than scriptures known as the 'Avesta' maintaining a dualistic doctrine, contrasting the force of light and good in the world with that of darkness and evil. With regard to death, they hold that their soul is allowed 3 days to meditate on their life. Following this their soul will be judged in that, if good thoughts, words and deeds outweigh the bad, the soul is taken into heaven. The alternative is the soul being led to hell. There are no last rites before death, but relatives, friends and sometimes but rarely a Zoroastrian priest may say prayers (Boyce, 2002; Hartz, 2009).

Care after death

Last offices are appropriate, particularly so as it is very important that the body be washed prior to being clothed in white garments. Generally families will supply a 'sadra' which is to be worn next to the skin under the shroud, with the sacred 'kusti', and may wish the head to be covered with a cap or scarf. Funerals should take place either on the same day of death or the day after. Orthodox Zoroastrians deem mutilation of the body is hostile to the will of God and so will be hostile to blood donation and transfusion, and organ transplantation. Autopsies are prohibited in religious law and would be declined. Zoroastrians believe that as soon as the body dies it becomes impure, death being the work of Angra Mainyu, the embodiment of all that is evil. In comparison Earth and all that is beautiful is considered to be the pure work of God. Hence contaminating the elements of earth, air, fire and water with decaying matter such as a corpse is considered sacrilege. Therefore, traditionally Zoroastrians lay out the deceased in purpose-built towers known as the Tower of Silence, enabling exposure to the sun and to be eaten by birds of prey such as vultures. In many countries outside India, though, this practice is either impractical or illegal and so Zoroastrians will opt for cremation rather than burial.

Conclusion

Apart from when an autopsy is required under the authority of HM Coroner, the consent will always remain with the next of kin. As this chapter has demonstrated, everyone holds personal beliefs and values about how we should live our lives and what is meant by death. Such beliefs and values can be similar, very different or even in opposition to our own. It is essential, therefore, to embrace knowledge about other religions and cultures so as to not only explain other people's beliefs and consequent behaviours, but to ensure that unintentional misinterpretation does not take place as this in turn will only portray the healthcare practitioner as someone the family has no faith or confidence in. Instead knowledgeable empathy on the part of the healthcare practitioner will provide families with trust and assurance in medicolegal processes.

Finally, Box 5.2 lists some useful contacts for helping with bereavement and coping with grief.

Box 5.2 Useful contacts for bereavement and coping with grief

- British Association for Counselling and Psychotherapy: www.bacp.co.uk
- Cruse Bereavement Care: www.crusebereavementcare.org.uk
- Depression Alliance: www.depressionalliance.org
- RoadPeace: www.roadpeace.org
- If I Should Die.co.uk: www.ifishoulddie.co.uk
- Jewish Bereavement Counselling Service: www.jvisit.org.uk
- National Association of Widows: www.nawidows.org.uk
- Samaritans: www.samaritans.org
- Support After Murder and Manslaughter: www.samm.org.uk
- The WAY Foundation: www.wayfoundation.org.uk

All sites accessed September 2009.

References

Bauer-Wu S, Barrett R, Yeager K (2007). Spiritual perspectives and practices at the end-of-life: a review of the major world religions and application to palliative care. *Ind J Palliative Care* **13**(2):53–8.

Boyce M (2002). *Zoroastrian Faith and Philosophy.* Available at www.religion-info.net (accessed September 2009).

Breuilly E, Palmer M (1999). *Religions of the World.* London: Collins.

Coogan MD (ed.) (2005). *Eastern Religions: Hinduism, Buddhism, Taoism, Confucianism, Shinto.* London: Duncan Baird Publishers.

Cracknell K, White SJ (2005). *An Introduction to World Methodism.* Cambridge: Cambridge University Press.

Cytron BD (1993). To honour the death and comfort the mourners: traditions in Judaism. In: Irish DP, Lundquist KF, Nelson VJ (eds) *Ethnic Variations in Dying, Death and Grief: Diversity in Universality*, pp. 113–24. London: Taylor & Francis.

Dandelion P (2008). *The Quakers: A Very Short Introduction.* Oxford: Oxford University Press.

Encyclopaedia Britannica (2006). *Encyclopaedia of World Religions.* London: Encyclopaedia Britannica UK.

Fisher MP (1997). *An Encyclopaedia of the World's Faiths: Living Religions.* London: IB Tauris.

Green J, Green M (2006). *Dealing with Death: Practices and Procedures*, 2nd edn. London: Jessica Kingsley Publishers.

Gudmundsdottir M, Martinson PV, Martinson IM (1996). Funeral rituals following the death of a child in Taiwan. *J Palliative Care* **12**(1):31–7.

Hartz PB (2009). *World Religions: Zorastrianism*, 3rd edn. New York: Chelsea House.

Kalsi SS (2007). *Simple Guides: Sikhism.* London: Bravo.

Kemp C (2002). Cultural perspectives in healthcare. Culture and the end of life: a review of major world religions. *J Hospice Palliative Nurs* **4**:235–42.

Klostermaier KK (2007). *Hinduism.* Oxford: Oneworld Publications.

Kramer K (2003). *The Sacred Art of Dying: How World Religions Understand Death.* Mahwah, NJ: Paulist Press International.

Long JD (2009). *Jainism: An Introduction to Religion.* London: IB Tauris.

Matthews M (2009). *World Religions*, 3rd edn. Florence, KY: Wadsworth Publishing.

McQuay JE (1995). Cross-cultural customs and beliefs related to health crisis, death and organ donation/transplantation. *Crit Care Nurs Clin N Amer* **7**:581–91.

Migration Statistics Unit (2007). *International Migration: Migrants Entering or Leaving the United Kingdom and England and Wales.* London: HMSO.

Momen M (2008). *The Bahá'í Faith.* Oxford: Oneworld Publications.

Nazarko L (2006). As death approaches: cultural issues. *Nurs Resid Care* **8**:441–4.

O'Collins G (2008). *Catholicism: A Very Short Introduction.* Oxford: Oxford University Press.

Office for National Statistics (2001). *Census 2001: Ethnicity and Religion in England and Wales.* Available at www.statistics.gov.uk/census2001 (accessed September 2009).

Partridge C (2004). *New Religious Movements, Sects and Alternative Spiritualities.* Oxford: Oxford University Press.

Reader I (2007). *Simple Guides: Shinto.* Simple Guides Series. London: Bravo.

Rees D (2001). *Death and Bereavement: The Psychological, Religious and Cultural Interfaces*, 2nd edn. London: Wiley Blackwell.

Religious Tolerance (2009). *Non-theistic Belief Systems.* Available at www.religioustolerance.org (accessed September 2009).

Rinpoche S (2008). *The Tibetan Book of Living and Dying.* San Francisco: Rider and Co.

Rutty JE (2001) Religious attitudes to death: what every pathologist needs to know. In: Rutty GN (ed.) *Essentials of Autopsy Practice*, vol. 1, pp. 1–22. London: Springer.

Rutty JE (2004) Religious attitudes to death: what every pathologist needs to know, part 2. In: Rutty GN (ed.) *Essentials of Autopsy Practice*, vol. 2, pp. 1–16. London: Springer.

Sarhill N, Mahmoud F, Walsh D (2003). Muslim beliefs regarding death, dying and bereavement. *Eur J Palliative Care* **10**:34–7.

Smith P (2008). *An Introduction to the Bahá'í Faith.* Cambridge: Cambridge University Press.

Solomon N (2000). *Judaism: A Very Short Introduction*. Oxford: Oxford University Press.

Toropov B (2004). *The Complete Idiot's Guide to the World's Religions*, 3rd edn. New York: Alpha Books.

Truitner K, Truitner N (1993). Death and dying in Buddhism. In: Irish DP, Lundquist KF, Nelson VJ (eds) *Ethnic Variations in Dying, Death and Grief: Diversity in Universality*, pp. 125–36. London: Taylor & Francis.

Wilson J (2004). *Funerals without God: A Practical Guide to Non-religious Funerals*. Buffalo, NY: Prometheus Books.

Woo KT (1992). Social and cultural aspects of organ donation in Asia. *Ann Acad Med* **21**:421–7.

Yao X (2000). *An Introduction to Confucianism*. Cambridge: Cambridge University Press.

Chapter 6

THE SAFE AND HEALTHY AUTOPSY

Julian L Burton

Introduction

The post-mortem room poses several potential threats to the health and safety of those working there. Greatest among these is the individual who is not aware of safe working practices, the hazards and risks present, and the methods and personal protective equipment which must be employed to minimise these risks. All staff who work in the post-mortem room have a duty to familiarise themselves with and to undertake safe working practices and to follow the department's standard operating procedures relating to health and safety.

Before the introduction of effective antimicrobial therapy and the routine use of personal protective equipment, it was not uncommon for those performing autopsies to develop potentially life-threatening infections, including streptococcal septicaemia and pulmonary tuberculosis. Prosectors' warts (cutaneous tuberculosis, 'verruca necrogenica') were also common. Infections still pose a threat to those working in the mortuary; the infections of greatest concern include human immunodeficiency virus (HIV), the viral hepatitides, group A haemolytic *Streptococcus* and tuberculosis.

Hazards and risks

The terms 'hazard' and 'risk' are often used as if they were synonyms when in fact they have quite different meanings in the context of health and safety. The danger of injury posed by a slippery floor, the sharp corner of a table, the blade of a knife or saw, or the point of a needle represents a hazard. In contrast, the chance of acquiring a blood-borne infection such as hepatitis B or HIV from a sharps injury represents a risk (Burton, 2003).

Within the post-mortem room, hazards are presented by the body, by the equipment used to perform the autopsy and reconstruct the body, and by the room itself (Table 6.1).

Hazards posed by the body being autopsied

Infections

The hazards posed by infectious agents can be stratified into groups depending on the likelihood of acquisition, the severity of the disease caused by the pathogen, the availability and efficacy of treatment, and the risk of transmission from the healthcare or mortuary worker to the general public. This stratification by the Health and Safety Executive Advisory Committee on Dangerous Pathogens (2005) has given rise to the system of hazard groups (HGs) (Table 6.2).

The autopsies of patients known or suspected to have an HG3 or HG4 infection are discussed in detail in Chapter 7, and these agents are not therefore considered further here. While pathologists and anatomical pathology technologists will principally be concerned with the avoidance of HG3 and HG4 pathogens, it should be remembered that at autopsy

Table 6.1 Hazards in the post-mortem room

Potential hazard	Comments
The body	
Infection	Hazard group 2, 3 or 4 pathogens. These may be acquired by inoculation, aerosol inhalation, contamination of mucous membranes or ingestion
Sharps injury	The cut ends of ribs, some implanted medical devices, needle fragments, bullets and other projectiles may pose a sharps injury hazard
Ionising radiation	This is a hazard present in people who have received radioactive implants and in bodies contaminated during a nuclear incident
Chemical agents	Bodies may contain or be contaminated by toxic chemicals such as cyanide or organophosphates
Electrocution	Implanted cardioverter defibrillators may cause electrocution if not deactivated prior to the autopsy
Back injury	This can result from poor movement and handling technique when positioning the body
Autopsy equipment	
Sharps injury	PM40 blades, scalpel blades, brain knife blades, hypodermic needles and suture needles may all cause a sharps injury
Electrocution	Improperly maintained electrical equipment such as oscillating saws may cause electrocution when used in the wet post-mortem room
Post-mortem room	
Physical injury	There is a trip hazard posed by water hoses and electrical cables on the floor, and a slip hazard posed by water on the floor
Infection	A hazard is present if the mortuary is not properly decontaminated

Table 6.2 Infectious disease hazard groups

Hazard group	Definition
1	Unlikely to cause human disease
2	Can cause human disease and may be a hazard to employees; it is unlikely to spread to the community and there is usually effective prophylaxis or treatment available
3	Can cause severe human disease and may be a serious hazard to employees; it may spread to the community, but there is usually effective prophylaxis or treatment available
4	Causes severe human disease and is a serious hazard to employees; it is likely to spread to the community and there is usually no effective prophylaxis or treatment available

Health and Satety Executive (2005).

the cadaver is a potential source of infection with other organisms, notably *Streptococcus pyogenes* (Hawke *et al.*, 1980), gastrointestinal organisms (including hepatitis A) and potentially *Neisseria meningitidis* (Healing *et al.*, 1995). Such pathogens give rise to potentially curable disease but nonetheless may result in significant morbidity (Hawke *et al.*, 1980; Burton, 2003).

Sharps injuries

It is possible to readily encounter sharp objects during the autopsy evisceration and dissection and these pose a hazard. Those most frequently encountered are the cut ends of the ribs when the anterior rib shield is removed. There are three methods available for the removal of the anterior rib shield, each of which has advantages and disadvantages.

The most traditional method is to cut through the ribs using rib shears. This is perhaps the most dangerous method as the ribs are crushed by the shears, producing jagged sharp edges. Although these cut edges can be covered by the skin of the chest wall or with towels, they pose a significant sharps hazard. An alternate method is to incise the ribs with an oscillating saw fitted with a fan-tailed blade. This produces smooth edges, removing the sharps hazard, but any underlying effusion will be aerosolised – potentially replacing one hazard with another. The author prefers the third method, in which a serrated long-bladed knife is used to incise the ribs, producing smooth cut ends without producing aerosols. Care must be taken to keep the blade of the knife almost parallel to the chest wall to avoid incising the underlying organs (Walker *et al.*, 2002). When the deceased has sustained fractures, the ends of these pose a similar sharps hazard. Care should especially be taken when eviscerating and examining the pelvis of individuals who have died following a road traffic collision or a fall from a height.

Individuals with a history of recurrent deep venous thrombosis and pulmonary thromboembolism may have a Greenfield inferior vena caval filter inserted. This is a roughly conical spoked wire device that is anchored to the wall of the inferior vena cava by sharp hooks on the ends of the spokes. Because the clinical history available at the time of autopsy is often vague or incomplete, and because there is no surgical scar to indicate the presence of the device, its presence may come as a surprise to the pathologist (Abraham and Greenfield, 1995). The author has injured himself on two such devices. Care must be taken in all cases when examining the retroperitoneal structures and the inferior vena cava.

Sharp objects within the body may alternatively be a consequence of the patient's lifestyle. Hutchins *et al.* (2001) reported a series of four patients with seropositive HIV infection who came to autopsy and were found to have retained fragments of needles in the subcutaneous tissues of the neck. Such needle fragments (which were between 10 and 45 mm long) were the legacy of long-term intravenous drug use in patients who resorted to deep cervico-clavicular injection when peripheral access became difficult. These cases were not associated with needlestick injury, but staff performing autopsies on those with a history of intravenous drug use must be aware of this potential (albeit rare) hazard. Radiographic screening has been suggested for cases where retained needle fragments are suspected (Nosher and Seigel, 1993; Hutchins *et al.*, 2001) but this is unlikely to be practicable in all autopsies performed on intravenous drug users. Needle fragments have also been discovered in the myocardium of intravenous drug users (Thorne and Collins, 1998; Burton, 2003).

The bodies of individuals who have been shot or suffered blast injuries pose a potential sharps hazard. Bullets may shatter bones, producing sharp frag-

ments, or may themselves fragment. The Winchester 'Black Talon' bullet is designed so that its jacket expands by peeling back to form 'petals' that slow its path through tissue, thus imparting more of its kinetic energy to the tissues. These petals are sharp and may cause glove puncture (McCormick *et al.*, 1996; Burton, 2003).

Sharp fragments of glass, metal or other debris may be projected into the bodies of individuals killed by an explosion. Such bodies should always be examined radiographically and the fragments recovered.

Radiation

On occasion, bodies that pose an ionising radiation hazard will present for autopsy. They may contain radioactive substances as a result of medical intervention or, less commonly, as a result of a nuclear incident such as an accident in a nuclear power plant. Victims of so-called 'dirty' bombs would also present such a hazard. Cases in which pathologists have received a significant radiation dose have been reported (Sharma and Reader, 2005). Autopsies on radioactive bodies that had been recently dosed with strontium-89 chloride prior to death have also been reported (Schraml *et al.*, 1997). In the reported case, the whole body and hand exposures were recorded as 0.000 for all personnel involved (although this is unsurprising – strontium is concentrated in the bones) (Burton, 2003).

Factors determining the risk to the autopsy pathologist and other attendant staff are summarised in Box 6.1. Owing to the variability in these factors it is not possible to give detailed advice that covers every eventuality. In general, the clinical history should include details of the therapy that was

---

Box 6.1 Factors affecting the risk posed by a radioactive body

- Radioactive isotope used
  - half-life
  - type of particle emitted (α, β or γ)
- Time since isotope was administered
- Personal protective equipment worn by staff
- Duration of exposure

administered (isotope, dose, date of administration) and the local hospital's medical physics department should be contacted for advice before starting the autopsy.

A case has been reported where brachytherapy pellets were identified in the prostate gland of a man at autopsy, in which there were no details of the therapy in the clinical records (Start *et al.*, 2007). Such pellets are identified as thin metallic silver-grey rod-shaped pellets approximately 5 mm in length and 1 mm in diameter. In such circumstances the pathologist should immediately halt the autopsy and evacuate the post-mortem room until advice can be sought from the local medical physics department (Burton, 2003).

Chemical agents

Although it is now relatively uncommon, some individuals commit suicide (or are murdered) using chemicals that are potentially hazardous to the pathologist performing the subsequent autopsy.

When metallic salts of cyanide are ingested, the action of gastric acid liberates hydrogen cyanide gas, which is toxic. The risk is therefore greatest in these autopsies when the stomach is opened and it is recommended the stomach be tied closed at the cardia and pylorus and then subsequently opened in a fume cupboard or on a down-draught table if cyanide poisoning is suspected (Sharma and Reader, 2005). However, the risk to health is small. In two reported cases of cyanide poisoning there was no increase in blood cyanide levels in the pathologists performing the examination, although headaches, light-headedness and a burning sensation in the throat have been reported (Forrest *et al.*, 1992; Nolte and Dasgupta, 1996). Hydrogen cyanide smells of burnt almonds but many people are anosmic to this (Fernando, 1992; Burton, 2003).

Aluminium phosphide is present in some pesticides and reports of suicidal ingestion exist (Anger *et al.*, 2000). When aluminium phosphide comes into contact with water it liberates copious volumes of hydrogen phosphide (phosphine, PH_3), an odourless and colourless gas (Sharma and Reader, 2005). This gas is toxic at concentrations of 2 ppm (Anger *et al.*, 2000). Once again the risk is greatest on opening the stomach and this should be performed in a fume cupboard.

Formaldehyde may be encountered at toxic concentrations if the formalin used to fix tissue samples for histopathology is spilt and when performing autopsies on bodies that have been embalmed. In the UK the latter is generally the case in bodies that have been repatriated prior to the examination, when phenol may also be present. Formaldehyde is highly volatile and exposure causes irritation to the eyes, mucous membranes and skin. In addition, it is sensitising and may cause pulmonary fibrosis and lung cancers. The legal safe limit for exposure is 2 ppm for 15 minutes. The odour of formaldehyde is detectable at concentrations of 0.1–1.0 ppm, so as a general rule if one can smell formaldehyde it is present at dangerous concentrations (Sharma and Reader, 2005). The hazard is combated by ensuring that there is adequate down-draught ventilation.

To the writer's knowledge there have been no reported cases of secondary toxicity due to organophosphates among autopsy staff, but there is a theoretical risk (e.g. deaths following industrial accidents or terrorist attacks). Organophosphates such as malathion and parathion may be consumed as part of a suicide attempt and pose a hazard when the stomach is opened (Sharma and Reader, 2005). Occupationally acquired organophosphate toxicity has been reported among healthcare workers who failed to take appropriare precautions when treating organophosphate poisoning (Geller *et al.*, 2002). Organophosphates that may be encountered as a result of terrorist attacks include sarin and tabun (Sharma and Reader, 2005). Organophosphates are readily absorbed through the skin. Healthcare workers handling the bodies of those contaminated by organophosphates should use chemical barrier protection (latex gloves and aprons afford little protection) and the body should be thoroughly washed with water or 5% hypochlorite solution prior to the examination (Geller *et al.*, 2002; Burton, 2003; Sharma and Reader, 2005).

Electrocution

The use of automated implanted cardioverter defibrillators (ICDs) to treat malignant tachyarrhythmias has become increasingly common in the last decade. The typical ICD is a titanium-covered box approximately $70 \times 51 \times 14$ mm and therefore is readily distinguished from implanted cardiac pacemakers by its larger size (Weitzman, 2003). When removed at autopsy and analysed, these devices can provide information that is valuable in determining the cause and mode of death (Dolinak and Guileyardo, 2001). However, these devices pose a potential electrocution hazard to the unwary pathologist and should be permanently set into a non-shock delivery mode prior to handling and removal (Prahlow *et al.*, 1997; Weitzman, 2003). This is typically achieved with the aid of a strong doughnut-shaped magnet, but the advice of the local ECG department or the patient's follow-up centre should be sought. As with cardiac pacemakers, the batteries within such devices can detonate when heated, so implantable defibrillators must be removed from bodies that are to be cremated and must not be disposed of by incineration (Burton, 2003). Further guidance from the Northern Ireland Adverse Incident Centre is available at www.dhsspsni.gov.uk/niaic_sn(ni)2002_40.pdf.

Other physical injury

The cadaver is, literally, a dead weight. Care must be taken when moving and handling bodies to use appropriate equipment if back injuries are to be avoided. Workstations must also be set at an appropriate height so that the evisceration and dissection can be performed without having to spend hours in a stooped position.

Hazards posed by the equipment used at autopsy

Safe sharps practice

Many of the instruments used to perform an autopsy constitute a sharps hazard, and safe sharps practice must be followed at all times. The basic autopsy tool set comprises a PM40 knife, a scalpel, a long-bladed non-serrated 'brain' knife and a pair of blunt-nosed scissors along with a steel ruler, a probe and a set of toothed forceps (Fig. 6.1). In addition, hypodermic needles may be needed to collect samples for further

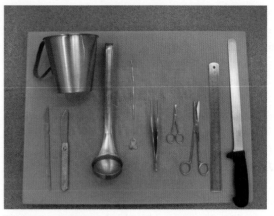

Figure 6.1 Equipment needed to perform an autopsy.

investigation, and a long suture needle is used when the body is reconstructed.

The following practices must be observed at all times (Burton, 2003):

1. Keep the number of sharp objects being used to a minimum. There is no need to have more than one of each blade present at an autopsy station at any time.
2. Scissors, PM40s and scalpels should have blunt-nosed blades. Pointed blades should never be used (Lucas, 1993; Patel, 1997).
3. Only one person should use sharp instruments on or in a body at any time. On occasion it is necessary to seek the help of the anatomical pathology technologist to reflect or hold structures during the evisceration, but their hands should be kept well clear of the area of dissection.
4. Sharps should be kept and used under direct vision at all times. Blind dissection, particularly during the evisceration of the neck and pelvis, should be avoided whenever possible. When not in use, sharps are kept away from the dissection. It is not safe to allow sharps to become hidden from view by organs or tissues. Some mortuary stations have a small shelf specifically designed to hold sharps. Where this is not available they may be placed safely in a jug.
5. Sharps are never to be passed hand-to-hand. Instead, sharps are passed from one individual to another either by placing them on the bench

in clear view, or in a tray to be picked up by the prosector.

6. Do not walk with sharps. It is necessary to move from one side of the body to the other during various stages of the evisceration. The prosector should not carry sharps while walking around the body. Instead, the knife is set down in clear view and picked up again once the prosector has moved.

7. Sharps should be used only if they are sharp. Injuries are more likely when using blunted blades as these require a greater force to be applied. Moreover, blunt blades are less easy to control and have a tendency to skip and jump during use. The pathologist should not feel afraid to ask the technologist for a new PM40, scalpel or brain knife when the one in use becomes blunt. On average the author requires at least two PM40s per autopsy.

8. When using a knife, always cut away from one's own body.

9. Needles are never resheathed. Once used, the needle is to be immediately disposed of into an appropriate sharps container (Fig. 6.2). Sharps containers must not be over-filled.

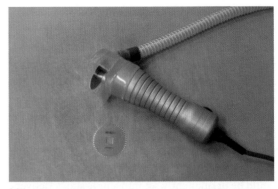

(a)

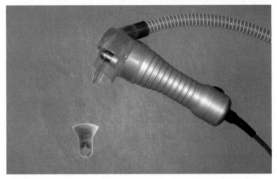

(b)

Figure 6.3 Oscillating saw fitted with (a) circular blade and (b) fantailed blade. The former is used for incising the cranial vault and the latter for incising ribs or the spine.

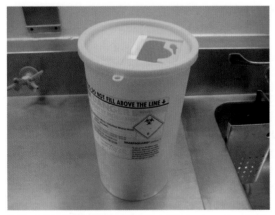

Figure 6.2 Appropriate sharps containers must be used for safe disposal. These must never be over-filled.

Oscillating saws

The oscillating saws (Fig. 6.3) used to open the cranial vault are potentially hazardous for three reasons. First, these pieces of electrical equipment are used in an environment that is wet. Improperly maintained and used oscillating saws pose a risk of electrocution. Second, the saws produce an aerosol of bone dust and body fluids. They must therefore be used with an exhaust system that collects this aerosol into a sealed container. Third, it has been suggested that the repeated prolonged use of these devices may be a cause of vibration white finger in anatomical pathology technologists (Toren and Jonsson, 1996). Curiously, while these saws are very effective at cutting bone, they pose little danger of cutting the operator.

Specimen containers

Blood and other body fluids, as well as tissue samples, may be collected into glass or plastic universal containers for subsequent toxicological, microbiological or other analyses. The pathologist must ensure that the outside of the container is not contaminated with the specimen before passing it to a technologist for labelling. If necessary the sample is transferred from the receptacle used to collect the specimen into a clean container.

Hazards posed by the post-mortem room

Even when all of the above factors are taken into consideration, the post-mortem room itself can still present a number of hazards. It is not uncommon for water or body fluids to be spilt onto the floor during the autopsy and this increases the risk of slipping on the floor and suffering an injury. Such spillages should be cleaned up promptly. Water hoses and electrical power cables present a trip hazard and whenever possible should not be left on the floor. It can be difficult to see these obstacles when carrying a heavy container of eviscerated organs to a dissection table.

Barriers

The design of the mortuary and the standard operating procedures that regulate working practices within it must impose a number of barriers between the various hazards contained therein and the workers within and visitors to the mortuary. These must have sufficient provision to care for professional visitors and the relatives of the deceased, and take into account also any potentially dangerous materials that leave the mortuary (Table 6.3).

Mortuary facilities

The mortuary must be of a sufficient size that it allows safe working and is able to accommodate the expected workload. In addition to one or more rooms in which autopsies are performed, facilities must exist for office work, staff recreation, changing rooms, body reception, discharge and storage, equipment storage, the viewing of bodies by relatives, and the viewing of autopsies by appropriately interested parties.

Each of these areas should be designated as 'clean', 'intermediate' or 'dirty' and physical barriers should be present between dirty/intermediate areas and the clean areas within the mortuary (Box 6.2). Such barriers may take the form of a glass screen (separating visitors to the autopsy room from the autopsy room floor), a water/disinfectant bath (between the autopsy room and the changing room), or lines painted on the floor. Handwashing facilities must be readily available in the clean and intermediate areas. The design of the mortuary will, ideally, reflect the working practices within it and facilitate its smooth day-to-day running while at the same time separating clean from dirty areas.

Box 6.2 Areas within the mortuary

Clean
- Office space
- Staff recreation room
- Toilet facilities
- Conference room
- Autopsy viewing gallery
- Relatives' room(s)
- Body viewing room for relatives
- Equipment storage
- Body reception

Intermediate
- Staff changing and showering rooms
- Body storage

Dirty
- Autopsy room(s)
- Equipment room
- Specimen room

Table 6.3 Barriers within the mortuary

Barrier level and definition	Examples
Primary: placed around perceived hazards	Physical facilities; safe working practices; disinfectant
Secondary: placed around the worker	Personal protective equipment; personal hygiene; occupational health services
Tertiary: placed around the autopsy room	Care of visitors; waste disposal procedures; specimen transport; disposal of the body

Safe working practices

Individuals who work within the mortuary should do so in such a way as to minimise hazards and their associated risks. The safe handling of sharps has already been discussed. In addition, care should be taken to minimise the formation of aerosols. Rough handling and squeezing of organs is eschewed, and high pressure water sprays are to be avoided. The intestines should be opened under water but not with the aid of a running tap.

Care is needed to avoid the contamination of clean surfaces by body fluids within the autopsy room. Telephones in the autopsy room should ideally by of a design that can be operated 'hands free', but if these are not available then on no account should the pathologist or technologist touch the telephone without first removing gloves and washing his or her hands. Photographic equipment must be similarly protected from contamination.

A circulator should be present who remains 'clean' while the autopsy is in progress. This is especially important when autopsies are performed on individuals known or suspected to have an HG3 infection (see Chapter 7). The roles of the circulator include labelling of specimens, completing paperwork associated with specimens, recording contemporaneous notes, adjusting overhead lighting if necessary, and observing the practice of the 'dirty' pathologist and technologist to ensure that standard operating procedures relating to autopsy room health and safety are being adhered to. The circulator can also liaise between the pathologist and other clinicians, avoiding contamination of clean surfaces such as telephones (Burton, 2003).

When autopsies are being performed, the number of people present within the autopsy room is limited to those with a legitimate reason for being present. However, at least two people should be present at all times – the pathologist and a technologist or circulator. Because of the risk of injury, neither the pathologist nor the technologist should work alone. A member of staff with up-to-date training in basic first aid should always be available within the mortuary to assist not only if a pathologist or technologist is injured but also if a visitor to the autopsy room faints (a not infrequent occurrence).

The care of equipment within the mortuary, and the cleaning-down and disinfection of the autopsy room at the end of the day's autopsies, is typically the duty of the anatomical pathology technologist. Tables, scales, dissection areas, boots and non-disposable equipment must be first cleaned with water and then with an appropriate disinfectant. The appropriate preparation and use of disinfectants is beyond the scope of this book. Pathologists should assist by keeping their station tidy and by wiping down their work area before leaving the dirty area. Disposable gloves, gauntlets, aprons, masks and caps are to be removed before leaving the dirty area of the mortuary and disposed of into an appropriately labelled clinical waste bin.

Personal hygiene

All staff and visitors in the autopsy room must ensure that their personal hygiene does not pose a hazard. Eating, drinking, smoking and the application of cosmetics is strictly forbidden within the autopsy room. This applies not only to the dirty area where autopsies are performed but also to any clean associated viewing gallery. Staff are required to wash their hands before leaving the autopsy room.

Occupational health services

All staff working in the autopsy room must, as a part of their contract, have a duty to attend occupational health services as appropriate. This will include pre-employment screening and vaccination. All staff working in the autopsy room must be immuno-competent. Individuals who are significantly immunocompromised for any reason (e.g. immunosuppressive therapy following receipt of an organ transplant or acquired immunodeficiency syndrome) should not enter the autopsy room or its viewing gallery. In addition, pathologists and anatomical pathology technologists must have completed a course of immunisation against hepatitis B, tuberculosis, tetanus and poliomyelitis. Local guidelines should be in place to deal with staff who refuse hepatitis B vaccination or who fail to develop antibodies to it. It must always be remembered that, while seroconversion following hepatitis B vaccination confers protection

Box 6.3 Standard operating procedure in the event of a needlestick or other contaminated injury

1. Call for appropriate help.
2. Wash the wound with copious amounts of soap and water (irrigate the eye with water).
3. Encourage free bleeding if a visible wound is present.
4. Apply an appropriate dressing to the wound.
5. Complete an incident form/accident report.
6. Contact occupational health services for further advice.

against hepatitis B, it offers no protection against human immunodeficiency virus or hepatitis C.

If an autopsy room worker sustains an incised wound, laceration or needlestick injury, a standard operating procedure should be followed (Box 6.3).

Visitors to the autopsy room and its viewing gallery

A number of different individuals may have a valid reason to visit the autopsy room or its viewing gallery when an autopsy is in progress. These include clinicians, medical students, paramedics, police officers, scene-of-crime officers and photographers. Such visitors may not be as aware of the dangers present within the autopsy room as the pathologists and technologists who work there on a day-to-day basis. Those who enter the dirty area of the autopsy room must have received vaccination to hepatitis B and tuberculosis and must be instructed to wear appropriate personal protective equipment.

As discussed in Chapter 3, the autopsy has a valuable educational role. However, requests by students and police officers to be present in an educational capacity should be politely but firmly declined when the body is known or suspected to be infected with an HG3 pathogen.

It is common for relatives to wish to view the body of the deceased either before or after the autopsy examination. On occasion they will be required to do so to assist in the identification of the deceased. Typically the relative will want to see the face of the deceased and perhaps hold their hand. Some religions will require the relatives to wash the body of the deceased (see Chapter 5). The author has encoun-

tered one relative who wished to see the genitalia of a severely decomposed body ('so I'll know it's him'). These practices should not be discouraged; once the body has been autopsied, washed and enshrouded there is no reason why relatives should not be permitted to touch the body. After all, they most likely frequently came into close contact with the body when the deceased was alive. A quiet area where bereaved relatives can sit, collect their thoughts and perhaps have a hot drink before or after seeing the body should be available. Toilet facilities should also be available for bereaved relatives, but it is advisable for the locks on these toilet doors to be of a type that can be opened from the outside in case a relative collapses.

Waste disposal

Waste from the autopsy room must be disposed of according to the relevant local and national guidelines. In general, all materials that are contaminated with body fluids or tissue fragments are disposed of as clinical waste in appropriately colour-coordinated strong plastic bags for incineration. Sharps bins are similarly disposed of by incineration. Once the fill line has been reached they are permanently sealed and labelled to indicate their origin.

Specimen transport

Specimens – be they for histopathology, microbiology, toxicology or other studies – should be transported in appropriately labelled and sealed containers. The key principle is that all of the specimen must be on the inside of the container. Sending containers to laboratories whose labels are contaminated with blood or other body fluids is not acceptable.

If the deceased is or could be infected with an HG3 pathogen, this should be indicated by the presence of a warning label on the container. In England and Wales these are typically yellow adhesive labels bearing the words 'Category 3 risk' in black text. It must be possible for all those who may come into contact with the specimen container in its journey to, and through, the laboratory to identify that there is an increased risk.

The specimen will be accompanied by a request form, and this too must bear a warning label. It is not sufficient, in the absence of such labels, simply to write 'Retrovirus positive' or 'HBsAg positive' on the request form. While the doctors in the laboratory will know what these terms mean, the porters transporting the specimens and the other laboratory workers may not. The pathologist sending specimens has a legal duty of care to warn all those who may come into contact with the specimen and its container of the potential risk. Risk stickers achieve this purpose and also can be used to preserve the confidentiality of the deceased.

Body disposal

When bodies are released from the mortuary after an autopsy they should leave in a condition that minimises the risk to the funeral workers and/or embalmers who will subsequently handle them. Wounds should be closed and all medical devices (excepting artificial joints) should have been removed. When there is a possibility that the deceased is infected with an HG3 pathogen, the funeral director should be made aware of this, and the potential routes of infection, but it is not necessary or even desirable to disclose the name of the infection itself. The deceased's confidentiality should be maintained. Bodies infected with an HG3 pathogen should be released sealed into a plastic body bag.

Personal protective equipment

The days when pathologists would perform autopsies while wearing their street clothes and smoking a cigarette have passed. Pathologists, anatomical pathology technologists and any others present on the post-mortem room floor (such as scene-of-crime officers or photographers) must wear the appropriate personal protective equipment (PPE). Whereas in surgery this equipment serves primarily to protect the patient from diseases that may be carried by the staff, in the mortuary it serves the opposite purpose. Employers have a duty to provide appropriate PPE and employees have a duty to wear it. Autopsies should not be performed if the appropriate equipment is unavailable.

Before entering the post-mortem room, staff should change out of their street clothes into a set of surgical scrubs. If it is the practice of the mortuary for staff in clean areas also to wear scrubs, these should be of a different colour from those worn in the dirty areas.

Next, the staff member should don rubber boots. Ideally these will have steel toecaps to protect the feet in the event that a sharp or heavy object is dropped. Although it takes practice to overcome the reflex, if equipment is dropped it should be allowed to fall to the floor. Broken equipment is preferable to catching a knife by the blade.

The forearms should be protected against splashes. Some pathologists prefer to wear a non-sterile surgical gown over their scrubs. Whether or not this is worn, plastic or plastic-coated paper forearm gauntlets should be worn. A plastic disposable apron is also worn. This must be long enough to reach below the tops of the rubber boots. Aprons that are too short allow blood and other bodily fluids to drip inside the boots.

Injuries to the hands are especially common, especially on the palmar surfaces of the thumb, index finger and middle finger of the non-dominant hand. Among pathologists, O'Briain (1991) found that cuts are twice as common as needlestick injuries. The frequency of injury is inversely related to one's clinical experience (Burton, 2003).

The hands are protected by a pair of surgical gloves, and these should be of the correct size. Gloves that are too tight will rapidly become uncomfortable, while gloves that are too large are easily damaged. Mast et al. (1993) have shown that wearing surgical gloves significantly reduces the volume of blood transferred during a needlestick injury by 63 per cent and 86 per cent for suture and hollow needles, respectively. Weston and Locker (1992) have shown that gloves, especially those of mortuary technicians, are frequently punctured at autopsy and that 31.8 per cent of such punctures go unnoticed (Burton, 2003). Rings must be removed before donning this pair of gloves, because studies in surgery have demonstrated that wearing rings increases the risk of glove puncture. Multiple perforations are often found at the base of the ring finger (Nicolai et al., 1997).

In every case the glove on the non-dominant hand should be protected with some form of cut-resistant glove. Several varieties are available, made of either Kevlar or chain mail. It must be remembered that these are cut-resistant, and not cut-proof (Bickel and Diaz-Arias, 1990; Zugibe and Costello, 1995). The author has cut his non-dominant hand while wearing a Kevlar glove while attempting to dissect heavily calcified coronary arteries. Kevlar gloves are often considered to be more comfortable and less cumbersome than those made of chain mail, but both types will reduce the dexterity and appreciation of fine touch of the hand on which they are worn. Neither type offers protection from needlestick injuries.

With a cut-resistant glove in place, a second pair of surgical gloves is worn on top. Double-gloving and frequent changing of gloves during the autopsy (whether or not they appear damaged) is recommended by some (Lucas, 1992) and felt to be an unnecessary expense by others (Dunn, 1992). Double-gloving helps to reduce the risk of injury, and has the added benefit of reducing the transmission of the odour of intestinal contents on to the hands. The second pair of surgical gloves must also be of an appropriate size. Gloves should be changed immediately if they become damaged (Burton, 2003).

The mucous membranes of the face require protection from splashes. A standard disposable surgical mask worn with goggles or a Perspex visor is usual, and masks with an attached visor are also available. Vision-correcting spectacles do not provide adequate eye protection. Moreover, a standard surgical mask does not provide adequate protection against *Mycobacterium tuberculosis*. If there is reason to suspect that this pathogen is present, additional protection is required (see Chapter 7). Finally, the hair is protected with a disposable surgical cap.

Some pathologists also elect to wear a disposable water-repellent suit over their scrubs, taping the sleeves to their gloves. Whether or not this is worn is a matter of personal preference but the author finds them cumbersome.

Ultimately the use of PPE is a balance between having appropriate protection against the hazards present in the mortuary and being overly encumbered. Cumbersome equipment may itself present a hazard by reducing dexterity or impairing communication (Burton, 2003). The combined use of PPE and the safe sharps handling practices discussed earlier in this chapter effectively form what are known as 'universal precautions'. Universal precautions should be adopted as a matter of routine in every case ('universal precautions, applied universally'). This allows staff to become familiar with the techniques in cases where the risks are low, so that their use is second nature in cases where the risks are high. Such high-risk autopsies are the subject of Chapter 7.

References

Abraham JL, Greenfield LJ (1995). Hazards to pathologists and anatomists from vena-caval (Greenfield) filters. *Lancet* **346**:1100.

Anger F, Paysant F, Brousse F et al. (2000). Fatal aluminum phosphide poisoning. *J Anal Toxicol* **24**:90–2.

Bickel JT, Diaz-Arias AA (1990). Metal mesh gloves for autopsy use. *J Forens Sci* **35**:12–13.

Burton JL (2003). Health and safety at autopsy. *J Clin Pathol* **56**:254–60.

Dolinak D, Guileyardo J (2001). Automatic implantable cardioverter defibrillator rhythm strip data as used in interpretation of a motor vehicle accident. *Am J Forensic Med Pathol* **22**:256–60.

Dunn PJ (1992). Glove puncture in the post mortem room (letter). *J Clin Pathol* **45**:548.

Fernando GCA (1992). Risk of inhalation of cyanide during necropsy. *J Clin Pathol* **45**:942.t

Forrest ARW, Galloway JH, Slater DN (1992). The cyanide poisoning necropsy: an appraisal of risk factors. *J Clin Pathol* **45**:544–5.

Geller RJ, Singleton KL, Tarantino ML, Drenzek CL, Toomey KE (2002). Nosocomial poisoning associated with emergency department treatment of organophosphate toxicity: Georgia, 2000. *MMWR Morb Mortal Wkly Rep* **49**:1156–76.

Hawke PM, Pedler SJ, Southall PJ (1980). *Streptococcus pyogenes*: a forgotten occupational hazard in the mortuary. *Br Med J* **281**:1058.

Healing T, Hoffman P, Young S (1995). The infection hazards of human cadavers. *CDR Review* **5**:R61–8

Health and Safety Executive (2005). *Biological Agents: Managing the Risks in Laboratories and Healthcare Premises*. Available at www.advisorybodies.doh.gov.uk/acdp/managingtherisks.pdf (July 2009).

Hutchins KD, Williams AW, Natarajan GA (2001). Neck needle foreign bodies: an added risk for autopsy pathologists. *Arch Pathol Lab Med* **125**:790–2.

Lucas S (1992). Glove puncture in the post mortem room [letter]. *J Clin Pathol* **45**:548.

Lucas SB (1993). HIV and the necropsy. *J Clin Pathol* **46**:1071–5.

Mast ST, Woolwine JD, Gerberding JL (1993). Efficacy of gloves in reducing blood volumes transferred during simulated needlestick injury. *J Infect Dis* **168**:1589–92.

McCormick GM, Young DB, Stewart JC (1996). Wounding effects of the Winchester Black Talon bullet. *Am J Forensic Med Pathol* **17**:124–9.

Nicolai P, Aldam CH, Allen PW (1997). Increased awareness of glove perforation in major joint replacement: a prospective, randomised study of Regent Biogel Reveal gloves. *J Bone Joint Surg (Br)* **79**:371–3.

Nolte KB, Dasgupta A (1996). Prevention of occupational cyanide exposure in autopsy prosectors. *J Forensic Sci* **41**:146–7.

Nosher JL, Siegel R (1993). Percutaneous retrieval of nonvascular foreign bodies. *Radiology* **187**:649–51.

O'Briain DS (1991). Patterns of occupational hand injury in pathology: the interaction of blades, needles, and the dissector's digits. *Arch Pathol Lab Med* **115**:610–13.

Patel F (1997). HIV serophobia in the mortuary: an algorithm system for handling high-risk forensic cases. *Med Sci Law* **37**:296–301.

Prahlow JA, Guileyardo JM, Barnard JJ (1997). The implantable cardioverter–defibrillator: a potential hazard for autopsy pathologists. *Arch Pathol Lab Med* **121**:1076–80.

Schraml FV, Parr LF, Ghurani S, Silverman D (1997). Autopsy of a cadaver containing strontium-89-chloride. *J Nucl Med* **38**:380–2.

Sharma BR, Reader MD (2005). Autopsy room: a potential source of infection at work place in developing countries. *Am J Infect Dis* **1**:25–33.

Start RD, Tindale W, Singleton M, Conway M, Richardson C (2007). Radioactive prostatic implants: a potential autopsy hazard. *Histopathology* **51**:246–8.

Thorne LB, Collins KA (1998). Speedballing with needle embolisation: case study and review of the literature. *J Forensic Sci* **43**:1074–6.

Toren K, Jonsson P (1996). Is skull sawing by autopsy assistants overlooked as a cause of vibration-induced white fingers? *Scand J Work Environ Health* **22**:227–9.

Walker JEC, Rutty GN, Rodgers B, Woodford NWF (2002). How should the chest wall be opened at necropsy? *J Clin Pathol* **55**:72–5.

Weston J, Locker G (1992). Frequency of glove puncture in the post mortem room. *J Clin Pathol* **45**:177–8.

Weitzman JR (2003). Electronic medical devices: a primer for pathologists. *Arch Pathol Lab Med* **127**:814–25.

Zugibe FT, Costello J (1995). Protective gloves for high-risk autopsies. *Am J Forensic Med Pathol* **16**:182.

Chapter 7

AUTOPSIES OF PEOPLE WITH HIGH-RISK INFECTIONS

Sebastian Lucas

Introduction

As with most of medicine, the risk for healthcare workers (HCWs) of acquiring a disease from a patient in mortuaries is small. Those workers – which includes mainly pathologists (senior and trainee) and anatomical pathology technologists (APTs), but also students and others who attend autopsies – need to know the potential hazards within and around the bodies they deal with. Tuberculosis, a classic high-risk infection, still infects healthcare workers in many settings.

Infection, radiation and chemical hazards need to be considered in advance of examining a dead person (i.e. risk assessment). There need to be protocols on what to do (and when to ask for advice in unusual cases). In addition, there must be systems for checking that the procedures used follow the protocols (governance) and for modifying the protocols if and when better and safer alternatives arise.

Performing autopsies on people with known or suspected high-risk infections (HRIs) is a divisive issue of great concern to the directly interested parties. Some mortuaries and their staff will not examine anyone with hepatitis B (HBV) infection on the grounds that it is dangerous, even though it is mandatory to be vaccinated against HBV in order to

work within the health services. At the other extreme, other mortuaries appear to operate without any real risk assessment process before autopsy, and so run the risk of significant infection to prosectors (pathologists and APTs).

This chapter is written for pathologists (senior and trainees) and APTs who work in mortuaries in the UK. Guidelines and legislation concerning autopsy practice, human tissue usage, safe practice under conditions of serious infections, testing for infectious agents, and consent issues are increasingly complex and intertwined, and vary considerably in different countries. Thus, although basic good and safe practice should be universal, it would be cumbersome and unhelpful to detail national variations. The principles and practices described here are applicable to all types of autopsies – adult, paediatric and perinatal, hospital/consented and medicolegal – without distinction. They also reflect the body of knowledge that examining boards such as the Royal College of Pathologists expect of successful candidates in their diploma examinations.

Much detail on body handling, mortuary building regulations, ventilation and lighting, cleaning and decontamination schedules is omitted; but this is available from many government and non-government sources. Some lower risk, but important, aspects of infectious disease autopsy practice are considered.

What follows reflects the author's extensive experience of examining deceased patients with serious communicable diseases (SCDs) – i.e. high-risk infections. The basic message is that when performing such autopsies there is, in nearly all cases, zero to minimal risk (much less than that of many sports, or simply travelling to and from home) provided the following precepts are followed:

1. have a routine practice of risk assessment for each and every autopsy;
2. know about the diseases that may be encountered;
3. use universal standard precautions;
4. have agreed protocols (or standard operating procedures) on how to manage the specific high-risk infection scenarios;
5. ensure that all involved parties are signed up to, and familiar with, the protocols;
6. follow the protocols, or be clear why one is deviating in specific cases;
7. audit how case management actually happens, and seek always to improve the procedures.

The governance of hospitals, pathology departments and mortuaries is increasingly complicated. A mortuary that is both effective (i.e. gets the right diagnoses in difficult cases) and safe has to have a clinical and experienced pathologist in ultimate charge and as the accountable leader. He or she must work in partnership with a similarly experienced technical operational manager, such as a senior APT.

Sources of information

There are few recent standard autopsy book texts that include infections and biosafety aspects (Finkbeiner et al., 2009). Nearly all the important information concerning infectious disease epidemiology and management is available on websites, which are easier to access than most journals and textbooks. Thus references here are kept to a minimum, but website addresses are indicated as sources – and for readers' personal updates as information changes.

The single most important generic practical source is the HSE/Health Services Advisory Committee book *Safe Working and the Prevention of Infection in the Mortuary and Post-mortem Room*, 2nd edition (Health Services Advisory Committee, 2003). This covers, in addition to autopsy practice, mortuary facilities, body viewing, cleaning and decontamination, hospital porter and funeral director issues, and embalming. It should be available in every pathology department and mortuary. Unfortunately it is not currently available on-line but has to be purchased from the HSE.

The most comprehensive background to biosafety, incorporating all the complex and sometimes contradictory statutory requirements – for example, the Management of Health & Safety at Work Regulations 1999 (MHSWR) and guidance principles – is the HSE Advisory Committee on Dangerous Pathogens (ACDP) manual *Biological Agents: Managing the Risks in Laboratories and Healthcare Premises*. It is available on-line at www.hse.gov.uk/biosafety/biologagents.pdf.

Useful general websites concerning the characterisation, epidemiology, disease clinical pathology, risks, and management of serious communicable diseases in the mortuary are given in Box 7.1. Under circumstances of unusual and unexpected deaths from infections, including potential bioterrorism (Lucas, 2008), urgent advice may be obtained via the HPA website.

Categorisation of high-risk infections

Most diagnostic histopathology concerns cancer or specific organ-based pathology. Hence there is less emphasis on understanding and managing suspected infectious diseases. Since 1976, numerous 'new and emerging infections' have been identified (Box 7.2). With the exception of new variants of pandemic influenza, it does not mean that they are genuinely 'new'; they are all zoonoses transferred to man, and have been causing human disease for decades-to-thousands of years before being formally identified.

Box 7.1 Websites for information on infections and their management in the mortuary

Health Protection Agency (HPA)	www.hpa.org.uk
Health and Safety Executive (HSE) and its various subcommittees	www.hse.gov.uk
Advisory Committee on Dangerous Pathogens	www.advisorybodies.doh.gov.uk/acdp/publications.htm
Royal College of Pathologists (RCPath) and its *Guidelines for Autopsy Practice*, 2002	www.rcpath.org/index.asp?PageID=240
Association of Anatomical Pathology Technologists (AAPT)	www.aaptuk.org
Human Tissue Authority (HTA) – in its revised Codes of Practice includes some guidance on autopsy infections	www.hta.gov.uk
General Medical Council (GMC) – published guidance on Serious Communicable Diseases (1997) which has since been withdrawn without comparably helpful replacement; this applied particularly to consent for testing for suspected HRIs	www.gmc-uk.org/guidance/good_medical_practice/good_doctors.asp
Clinical Pathology Accreditation (UK) Ltd – has basic requirements for mortuary biosafety	www.cpa-uk.co.uk
US Centers for Disease Control and Prevention (CDC) – has extensive resources available on infectious disease and cadaveric handling	www.cdc.gov
World Health Organization (WHO) – has constantly updated information on the global epidemiology of infectious diseases, to be consulted when considering returning travellers who have died	www.who.int

Hazard groups (HGs)

The categorisation of HRIs is based on the categorisation of biological agents by (in the UK) the Advisory Committee for Dangerous Pathogens (ACDP), under the umbrella of the HSE and of the Health and Safety Commission (HSC), and similar bodies in other countries. All infectious agents are placed in one of four hazard groups, HG1 being relatively innocuous and HG4 including the most lethal agents known. Broadly, HRIs are those agents in groups HG3 and HG4. The criteria for categorisation are:

- infectiousness and virulence;
- morbidity and mortality;
- capacity for epidemic spread;
- preventability;
- treatability.

It should be noted that the management guidelines for these agents were primarily aimed at microbiology departments and levels of containment – open benches, extractor cabinets etc. They have been transferred to mortuary procedures with varying degrees of success and relevance, owing to the different biosafety and logistical aspects of autopsy versus laboratory practice.

The latest HG categorisation, Approved List 2004, is available at www.hse.gov.uk/pubns/misc208.pdf.

HG3 and HG4 infections

Most UK mortuary infection problems arise in the HG3 group, which includes the human immunodeficiency virus (HIV), hepatitis C virus (HCV) and tuberculosis (TB). That said, HG2 includes *Neisseria meningitidis* and group A *Streptococcus pyogenes*, which do carry certain risks (see below).

HG3 agents have the following features (Health Services Advisory Committee, 2003):

- a biological agent that can cause severe human disease and presents a serious hazard to employees;

Box 7.2 Some of the newly recognised infectious diseases in humans and when they were identified (the list contains many HG3 and HG4 infections that cause the most concern in mortuaries)

1976	Ebola virus
1976	*Legionella* spp
1977	Rift Valley haemorrhagic fever
1977	Delta hepatitis
1977	Hantaan hantavirus
1980	Human T-cell lymphotrophic virus type 1 (HTLV-1)
1980	Marburg virus
1982	*Escherichia coli* 0157
1983	Lyme disease
1983	*Helicobacter*
1983	HIV-1
1985	*Enterocytozoon* and other microsporidia
1985	HIV-2
1989	Hepatitis C virus
1991	*Erlichia* spp
1992	*Bartonella* spp
1993	Sin Nombre hantavirus pulmonary syndrome
1993	*Cyclospora* spp
1994	HHV8 (Kaposi sarcoma virus)
1999	Nipah virus
2000	West Nile virus
2003	SARS coronavirus
2005	Pandemic influenza H5N1

- a possible risk of spreading to the community;
- usually the availability of effective prophylaxis or treatment.

Cadavers with these infections can be autopsied safely in most modern mortuaries when sensible risk-prevention measures are instituted.

HG4 infections are agents of severe infections with high mortality rates, likely to spread to the community, and there is usually no effective prophylaxis or treatment available. They include the many filoviruses and arenaviruses that cause viral haemorrhagic fevers. If these infections are suspected or known and an autopsy is required, then they have to be performed under conditions of greater safety than for HG3 cases, and the basic recommendation is not to autopsy unless absolutely necessary.

For the concern of mortuaries in the UK, Box 7.3 lists the most likely HG3 agents. These may be acquired in the UK or brought back by travellers.

Box 7.3 Hazard group 3 infections, classified by main type (omitting detailed virus classes); not all known HG3 agents are included

Viruses	Avian flu
	Human immunodeficiency viruses (HIV) types 1 and 2
	HTLV types 1 and 2
	Hepatitis B, C, D(delta), G and E and not-yet-identified hepatitis viruses
	Dengue viruses types 1–4
	Most hantaviruses
	Japanese B encephalitis
	Lymphocytic choriomeningitis
	West Nile fever
	Yellow fever
	Rabies
	Severe acute respiratory syndrome (SARS) coronavirus
	Chikungunya and Rift Valley fever viruses
Bacteria	*Bacillus anthracis*
	Brucella spp
	Burkholderia mallei
	Chlamydia psittaci
	Coxiella burnettii
	Escherichia coli verocytotoxigenic strains O157, O103
	Mycobacterium tuberculosis
	Mycobacterium leprae
	Rickettsia spp.
	Salmonella typhi and *paratyphi*
	Shigella dysenteriae
	Yersinia pestis
Parasites	*Echinococcus granulosus* and *multilocularis*
	Leishmania donovani and *brasiliensis*
	Naegleria fowleri
	Plasmodium falciparum
	Taenia solium
	Trypanosoma brucei rhodesiense
Fungi	*Blastomyces dermatitidis*
	Cladosporium spp
	Coccidioides immitis
	Histoplasma capsulatum
	Paracociccidioides brasiliensis
	Penicillium marneffei
Prions	The agents of Creutzfeldt–Jakob disease, variant CJD, and the inheritable transmissible spongiform encephalopathies (TSE)

Box 7.3 includes a large number of infective agents where one may query the stringency of precautions that are actually needed for safe practice in the mortuary (e.g. *Mycobacterium leprae*). Annex 1 in Approved List 2004 in fact lists many HG3 agents where not all the measures normally applicable need be so applied for laboratory and scientific work, according to the nature of the work and/or the nature of the agent. These include not only, for example, *E. coli* O157, *Echinococcus* spp and *Plasmodium falciparum*, but also HIV and HCV.

This emphasises that mortuary work is not necessarily comparable to laboratory work with infectious agents. Similarly, with universal effective vaccination against HBV for mortuary HCWs, it is pointless further to consider HBV as a high-risk infection. While histoplasmosis is on the HG3 list, the life-cycle form present in infected cadavers is not the form that is infective to prosectors by inhalation. In practice then, the real UK concerns are more focused on a smaller list – to be discussed below alongside appropriate practices – with the reminder that, if and when other listed agents come up for consideration, common sense is applied and one reviews the potential diseases from sources of information.

HG4 infections, however, are all real risks to mortuary prosectors and body handlers, and all must be managed with great care and stringency (Box 7.4).

Acquisition of infection in a mortuary

The routes of infection that may occur in the mortuary are given in Box 7.5. With now-standard personal protection for mortuary HCWs, ingestion and contamination of skin and mucosal surfaces really should not occur. Inoculation and inhalation are the important issues for risk reduction. Table 7.1 provides simple data on the likelihood of some HG3 infections, if breaches through personal protective clothing and apparatus do occur.

Principles and practice of risk reduction in the mortuary

As has been stated already, the key to satisfactory and safe performance of HRI autopsies is routine risk assessment, knowledge of the diseases that may be encountered, the use universal standard precau-

Box 7.4 Hazard group 4 infections; not all known agents are listed, but all HG4 agents are viruses

- Hendra
- Nipah
- Smallpox
- Russian spring/summer encephalitis and Omsk tick-borne viruses
- Ebola, Lassa, Marburg and Crimean/Congo haemorrhagic fever viruses

Box 7.5 Routes of acquisition of infection in a mortuary

- Percutaneous inoculation
- Inhalation
- Ingestion
- Skin contamination without inoculation through the epidermis
- Contamination of mucosal surfaces (eye, mouth, nose)

Table 7.1 Risks of acquiring a specific infection after significant exposure

Route of infection	TB	HIV	HCV	HBV	CJD	Fungi	Anthrax
Inhalation	++	–	–	–	?	–[a]	+[b]
Mucosa	+	0.03%	–	–	?	–	+[b]
Normal skin surface	?	–	–	–	–	–	–
Inoculation	+	0.3%	3%	30%	?	+	+[b]

? = insufficient data to be confident; the real risks of tuberculosis (TB) infection are not quantifiable, but are significant.
[a] For fungal infections, the life-cycle phase in cadavers is not infectious by inhalation, but may be by inoculation.
[b] For anthrax, the bacillus form in cadavers is not infectious, but the bacilli may convert to infectious inhalable spores when exposed to air.

tions, and having agreed protocols (or standard operating procedures) on managing specific HRI scenarios. In fact, the adoption of universal precautions (see below) might be regarded as rendering much pre-autopsy risk assessment redundant in practice, since it effectively protects the wearers against most risks. Similarly, several clinically severe diseases such as salmonellosis, staphylococcal infection and vancomycin-resistant enterococci (VRE) are protected against in the mortuary by universal precautions. However, it is important to consider the risks in each case because, if something goes wrong, the management is made clear.

The 'Safe Working' guidance (Health Services Advisory Committee, 2003) contains the necessary information on these procedures, and this section summarises and elaborates on the main points.

Risk assessment

One of the key duties under COSHH is risk assessment of a case before acting in a manner that might put workers in danger. The modes of pre-autopsy risk assessment are indicated in Box 7.6.

Box 7.6 Risk assessment of a case for autopsy: sources of information about known or possible HRIs

- The clinical history on a consent form
- The history as provided by a coroner
- Direct information from the treating clinicians
- Looking up the patient on a hospital laboratory database for positive serologies, bacterial isolates etc.
- Information from hospital infection control
- Information on an infection notice pro forma that should accompany each cadaver to the mortuary
- External examination of the body (e.g. if emaciated and/or unusual skin rash, ?HIV; if skin injection marks, ?IVDU)

The autopsy suite

Does one need a separate autopsy high-risk suite to perform such autopsies? The 'Safe Working' document (Health Services Advisory Committee, 2003) indicates that this is 'ideal' but not mandatory. What is more important is the provision of good ventilation in the working areas (autopsy table and dissec-

tion bench) and sufficient space and distance away from other activities.

Whole-room ventilation with the draught passing from ceiling height down and across the tables, exiting at floor level, is satisfactory. Alternatively, down-draft tables work well also.

Having all the necessary equipment to hand is important, to obviate having to leave the area to find more material.

The NHS Estates regulations on mortuary facilities are published in *HBN 20: Facilities for Mortuary and Post-mortem Room Services* (3rd edition, 2005). These are not available on-line, but from The Stationery Office (www.tso.co.uk/bookshop).

Behaviour and technique

Knowing the hazards determines how one operates, in conjunction with colleagues, doing an HRI autopsy. Training and demonstration of good safe practice is critical. Trainee pathologists may find it hard to get experience if their seniors consider HRI work too dangerous for them. Trainee APTs are usually inducted into such work in a more planned manner, led in part by the specific requirements of curriculum and Royal Society for Public Health (RSPH) diploma examinations. It is all common sense:

- round-ended scissors and PM40s are safer than sharp-pointed ones;
- restrict the number of sharps in the working area, and always know where they are;
- only one prosector operates within the body cavity at a time;
- always slice unfixed organs with a sponge holding the organ firm and protecting that hand;
- on sawing the skull, use an oscillator saw with suction extraction of the bone aerosol into a removable chamber, or a hand saw with a chain-mail glove;
- do not sheath needles after fluid sampling, but place the needle and syringe into a sharps bucket.

Staff in attendance

As the 'Safe Working' document states, for known high-risk autopsies, it is 'ideal' (but not mandatory) that the team on the case involves not only the necessary APT and pathologist, but another, circulator, assistant (Health Services Advisory Committee, 2003). This person undertakes ancillary tasks (sample labelling, communications). In practice, we find this to be unnecessary in most high-risk scenarios; frequent HRI autopsies enables one to know what will happen in nearly all cases, and have all the requisite bottles, containers, fixatives, forms etc. already prepared and labelled. In a suspected HG4 death scenario, however, such an assistant is crucial; how she or he would be attired depends on the nature of the expected pathogen.

Universal precautions and personal protective equipment

It has taken several decades of sloppy practice to arrive at the position where nearly all autopsy work in the UK is undertaken under conditions of standard (and effective) safety. While some mortuaries (lacking clinical governance) may be defective, hospital mortuaries are obliged to insist on good practice. In fact, all employers have to protect the health and safety of their employees under the Health and Safety at Work etc. Act 1974.

The key to this is personal protective equipment (PPE). For clothing of pathologists and APTs, it is standard for all autopsies that prosectors wear the following, which are either disposable or cleanable and reused:

- surgical scrub suit;
- hat to protect hair;
- clear visor to protect the face, eyes and mouth;
- respiratory protection, either as a standard surgical mask or a FFP3 mask which more effectively excludes small particles of infective material (Fig. 7.1);
- waterproof gown that covers the entire body, including the forearms;
- plastic apron over the gown;
- rubber boots with metal-protected toecaps and dorsal reinforcement;
- latex gloves (or other equivalent material);
- under these gloves, protective gloves made of Kevlar or neoprene that is cut-resistant (Fig. 7.2).

With this protection, most of the HG3 agents are as well protected against as is reasonably possible. Blood-borne viral agents are effectively excluded. Only agents that are transmitted by inhalation are not optimally (i.e. 100 per cent) protected against.

Additional personal protection

Tuberculosis has ever been a risk to mortuary staff (see below). Surgical masks do not adequately prevent infective aerosols getting into the respiratory tract. FFP3 masks are intended to be at least 95 per cent effective (hence they are also termed N95 masks in the USA). For those who want essentially 100 per cent protection, then prosectors can employ a whole-body suit with a powered air-purifying respirator with high-efficiency particulate air (HEPA; Fig. 7.3) filters, or the modified version that retains the head gear without having the whole body being so protected. These suits are not currently standard issue in UK mortuaries, but it is not impossible that they will be so for TB cases in the future. They are expensive to purchase and maintain. In the writer's unit, they are used mainly for examining chemical toxic deaths such as cyanide poisoning.

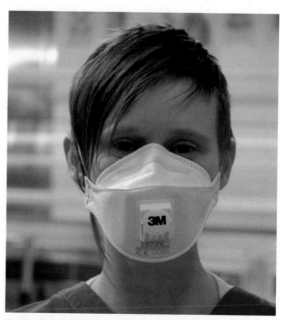

Figure 7.1 FFP3 mask – becoming the norm for all autopsies.

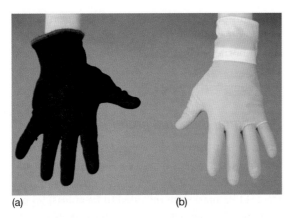

(a)   (b)

Figure 7.2 Gloves: Kevlar protective layer (a) under latex (b).

When bones are being sawn and the skull opened, some prosectors wish for additional hand protection and replace the fibre under-glove with a fine-mesh metal glove. This is satisfactory although manipulation is impeded, and it takes getting used to.

What to do in case of injury in the mortuary

Most mortuaries have standard procedures that dictate what happens when there is an accident. These will mostly be penetrating cuts through gloves with puncture of the skin. Encouraging bleeding with washing and cleaning of the wound comes first, followed by consideration of the case and the possible infective risk incurred.

Hospital occupational health (OH) units are familiar with the problem, and their advice should be sought. The incident has to be logged and reported locally. If the infection in the cadaver is already known, then appropriate action follows. For HIV infection, it is standard that exposed HCWs are offered a 1-month course of multi-drug therapy; for needlestick injuries, this has been shown to reduce the risk of HIV infection by 80 per cent (Expert Advisory Group on AIDS, 2008). For HCV, unfortunately there is no prophylaxis currently offered – just monitoring to detect infection if it occurs, with later appropriate treatment.

If the type of infection in the cadaver is not known but is suspected to be a blood-borne virus, then the procedures indicated below in 'Pre-mortem and peri-autopsy testing for HRIs' should be followed.

Under the Reporting of Injuries, Diseases and Dangerous Occurrences Regulations 1995 (RIDDOR), the Incident Contact Centre (ICC) in Caerphilly is to be notified if a HCW, through work:

- is infected with a pathogen on the list (mainly HG3 and HG4 agents); or
- suffers a 'dangerous occurrence' such that the incident could have resulted in such infection.

How assiduous mortuaries are in such reporting is unclear. The critical thing is to have prepared protocols on what to do in case of injury.

Trimming sampled HRI autopsy material

The optimum histopathology is always obtained from well-fixed and well-orientated tissue blocks. This entails fixation for 24 hours before trimming, and is the author's practice. The advent of the Human Tissue Act 2004 has made the bureaucracy of tissue retention significant, to the extent that mortuary and other staff are less willing to have pathologists take tissue samples (particularly in medicolegal cases). When tissue is retained it is preferred that it be cassetted at the time of autopsy, so that there is no residual tissue to manage.

For HRI work, this approach must be resisted, as diagnostic optimisation is the main concern. A second, practical, aspect that supports pre-fixation is that trimming thin slices of tissue frequently causes glove puncture and may result in inoculation of infective agents.

Vaccination schedules

Under standard conditions of employment in exposure-prone professions, it is mandatory that all mortuary HCWs be successfully vaccinated against HBV (i.e. produce an antibody response) and have had BCG vaccination against tuberculosis.

Although it is not mandatory, several mortuaries sensibly further protect APTs and some medical staff with hepatitis A vaccine and top-up vaccinations against diphtheria, poliomyelitis and tetanus. If and when an effective meningococcal vaccine

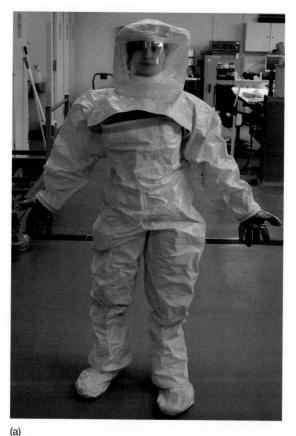

(a)

Figure 7.3 Whole-body ventilated suit: (a) shows the front, (b) shows HEPA filter providing clean air on the back. Might this be the future for all autopsies? It is safe, but communication is not easy.

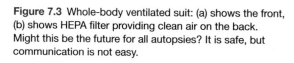

(b)

against the strains that cause most deaths is available, this should also be on the list.

Further vaccination than this is arbitrary and depends on location and case mix. If the mortuary is co-located with an infectious disease clinical centre and/or near an international airport, then yellow fever and rabies vaccines are seriously to be considered. If the mortuary is likely to receive casualties of suspected bioterrorist attack, then smallpox and anthrax vaccine may also be considered – see 'Bioterrorism' below (currently no mortuary staff in the UK have been offered these prophylactically).

Post-autopsy practices: viewing, information for funeral directors, and repatriation

The viewing of bodies with known or suspected HRI causes much grief if mortuaries or funeral directors refuse relatives this right because of concern over transmission of an infection. This is, essentially, nonsense: the relatives have been closely contacting the deceased up to the time of death, so what has changed? With a very few exceptions (HG4 agents), viewing of a properly cleaned post-autopsy body is safe.

Funeral directors rightly expect some information on the likely risk entailed in handling a cadaver, including embalming. 'Safe Working' addresses this. In order not to break patient confidentiality, it is best just to indicate the HG category of infection on the Infection Control Notification form, and state whether it is blood-borne or not. The HSE publishes *Controlling the Risks of Infection at Work from Human Remains*. This guide for those involved in the funeral services (including embalmers) and those involved in exhumation is available on the HSE website.

For repatriating bodies by air cargo, most handlers require a 'Freedom from Infection' or similar document signed by a pathologist. If there is an HG3 or HG4 infection in the body, the writer's unit practice is to state (for example) that: 'there is a Hazard Group 3 blood-borne virus infection that poses no risk when the body is placed in a hermetically sealed coffin' – using a Notification of Infection form.

Specific high-risk infections

This chapter is *not* a summary text of high-risk infection (HG3 and 4) pathology. It is worth noting some particular points that pathologists in the mortuary may find useful in discharging their obligation of identifying the clinical pathology in the deceased. Also, epidemiological changes in certain HG3 infections in the UK are important.

HIV disease

The acquired immunodeficiency syndrome (AIDS) was first identified clinico-pathologically in 1981. Autopsy examinations provided a large quantum of the information that was rapidly gained about this 'new' disease. The main virus, HIV-1, was identified in 1983, then the West African HIV-2 in 1985. Currently some 45 million people globally are living with HIV. A standard source of information on the epidemiology and clinical aspects is from UNAIDS (www.unaids.org).

Transmission of HIV is by sexual contact, from mother to fetus, by injection of contaminated fluids (intravenous drug users; IVDUs), by receiving infected blood products (haemophiliacs etc.), and, occasionally, by inoculation of infected material into healthcare workers.

In the UK, the demography of HIV has changed markedly. Initially it was confined to men who had sex with men (MSM), haemophiliacs and some IVDUs. Since the mid-1990s, immigrants from Africa – men, women and children – who bring HIV with them have dominated newly identified infections, which currently run at about 7300 per year (see www.hpa.org.uk for quarterly updates on the UK epidemiology). With the advent of effective multi-drug chemotherapy for HIV after 1996, most HIV-infected people who present to health centres and are diagnosed in time will expect to live a nearly normal life span. That said, the single most common scenario of death from HIV in the UK currently is late presentation: patients with advanced HIV disease who present for healthcare but are too ill to be saved, and were not previously known to be infected (Lucas *et al.*, 2008). This emphasises the need for more widespread HIV testing before clinical symptoms commence. About 500 HIV-infected people die each year in the UK.

Thus the pathologist may be in the position of diagnosing HIV disease for the first time in such a patient. It must be emphasised that this is a small minority of the HIV patients who may come to autopsy. Most are already known to be infected, and the writer's personal UK experience is that fewer than 10 per cent of HIV autopsies are diagnosed as HIV-positive this late (see 'Pre-mortem and peri-autopsy testing for HRI' below).

Risk of acquiring HIV infection at autopsy

Nearly all the information on infection risk to HCWs derives from phlebotomists' experiences, and the standard risk is approximately 0.3 per cent (1 in 300). One pathologist is known to be infected, having cut his hand during scalp removal (Johnson *et al.*, 1997), but there presumably have been others. There are two important principles to bear in mind:

- A cadaver that contains HIV will continue to be potentially infective despite refrigeration and the passage of time. Thus delaying such an autopsy is pointless with regard to risk reduction, and only blurs its diagnostic utility through autolysis (Lucas, 1993).

- Modern therapy renders many HIV-infected people effectively non-infectious at autopsy. The risk of infection depends on the HIV viral load in the tissues and blood, and therapy aims to reduce this to undetectable levels. While this may be reassuring to prosectors, it does not remove the need to pursue the normal relevant safety protocols.

While there is not likely to be an effective prophylactic HIV vaccine in the foreseeable future, post-exposure prophylaxis is available and effective (see above).

Specific pathological aspects of HIV autopsies

The range of HIV-associated infections, tumours and degenerative conditions is large and continues to expand as patients live longer. Numerous sources of information are available in books, journals and websites on these clinicopathological aspects. Some aspects are less well known or are particularly difficult, and these are summarised in Box 7.7.

Tuberculosis

Against expectations 30 years ago, TB has not been eradicated as a public health problem in any country. In fact the incidence and prevalence rates of infection increase almost everywhere, driven by four factors: increasing global population, poverty, migration from poor to rich countries, and immunodeficiency (particularly HIV infection).

In the UK, an overall annual incidence for newly diagnosed pulmonary plus extra-pulmonary TB of 14 per 100 000 hides wide geographical variations: in London it is 43/100 000, while in Northern Ireland it is below 5/100 000. This reflects demography, immigration and HIV (data from the Office for National Statistics and the HPA (2008): www.hpa.org.uk).

Much of the TB identified at autopsy is not diagnosed pre-mortem; and conversely (personal observations), there is much clinical over-diagnosis of TB which turns out to be other diseases at autopsy (particularly autoimmune disease, vasculitis and lymphoma).

Traditionally, autopsies on known or suspected TB

Box 7.7 Specific points about HIV autopsies in the UK

1. About a half of deaths of HIV-positive individuals are from standard HIV-associated conditions (opportunistic infections, lymphoma etc.). The others include accidents, drug overdose and suicide; and an increasing number of HCV-related liver disease as HCV–HIV co-infection is increasingly common. Further, as the HIV-infected population ages and lives longer, cardiac ischaemic disease and chronic obstructive pulmonary disease are more commonly seen as final events. HIV and its therapy have complex interactions with these pathologies.

2. The number of anti-HIV therapies expands and brings with it toxicity. Few deaths are directly related to HIV therapy (e.g. liver toxicity or Stevens–Johnson syndrome), but these complex aspects need to be considered carefully in the final evaluation of a case. Second, there is the immune reconstitution inflammatory syndrome (IRIS) that frequently occurs early after initiating HIV therapy. This can kill through inflammatory expansion of lesions (e.g. tuberculosis in the brain) or enhanced local tissue damage (e.g. ARDS in the lung, or HIV encephalitis in the brain).

3. The neuropathology of HIV disease is more complicated than the standard texts indicate. Thus if the case is specifically brain/cord-focused, ensure that adequate sampling is done (fixed and fresh tissue, for combined histopathology and microbiological investigations) to solve the problem.

4. Many puzzling deaths in HIV patients revolve around multi-organ failure (MOF) '?cause'. The aetiopathogenesis can be difficult to determine, even at autopsy, and the following entities should be considered when more obvious causes are eliminated:
   - haemophagocytic syndrome (HPS), primary or secondary to sepsis;
   - HHV8 infection and multi-centric Castleman's disease (MCCD);
   - lymphoproliferative disorders (LPDs), including B- and T-cell lymphomas, Hodgkin's disease, and EBV-driven LPD.

   Thus, sampling of lymph nodes, spleen, liver and bone marrow is critical.

---

patients have been two-stage processes, whereby formalin is tipped via the upper airways into the lungs, and the body is only dissected the next day, nominally to reduce the risk of infection to HCWs in the mortuary. There is no positive evidence to substantiate this practice, and there are four other facts against it:

- It wastes time and resources.
- The formalin will not gain access to extra-pulmonary TB loci.
- It might destroy the chance to obtain cultures for TB, which may be critical for diagnosis in uncertain cases, and important for drug-sensitivity testing, strain profiling, and contact tracing.
- Mycobacteria may remain viable in formalin-fixed (and embalmed) tissues for days (Gerston *et al.*, 2004).

Thus best practice is to get on with the autopsy using the standard protective measures.

What can happen in unprotected circumstances was well evidenced by a small outbreak in the USA, where one previously unknown TB cadaver was autopsied. All five attendant HCWs acquired the infection, and two of them became sputum-positive – i.e. developed disease (Templeton *et al.*, 1995). BCG vaccination does not convey immunity to infection. However, TB is a very treatable condition.

Tissue sampling is very important for microbiological diagnostics (culture and molecular techniques such as PCR) for species identification and drug sensitivities. In the twenty-first century, it is not adequate for a pathologist to say that TB is present on the basis only of acid-fast bacilli and granulomatous inflammation, with or without necrosis – if and when the pathologist could have gone further with microbiological sampling. Drug-resistant TB is fortunately uncommon in the UK (1.2 per cent of new diagnoses; see the HPA website). Box 7.8 indicates some practical points about suspected TB autopsies.

Hepatitis C virus (HCV)

HCV was identified only in 1989, but it is already one of the fastest growing infectious diseases epidemiologically. It causes chronic liver disease in about 80 per cent of those infected, which results in end-stage liver diseases (cirrhosis, carcinoma, liver failure) over a period of 20 or more years. Although HCV

Box 7.8 Some points about tuberculosis autopsies

1. Tuberculosis may be grossly evident or occult, so a low threshold of suspicion is essential, with histological and microbiological confirmation undertaken.
2. Drug-resistant TB is no more (or less) infectious at autopsy than drug-sensitive TB.
3. Unusual patterns occur in the absence of typical coexistent sentinel lung pathology; e.g. in the brain, heart, bones.
4. 'Miliary TB' may be mimicked by a large number of other pathologies, particularly in the lungs (Fig. 7.4), such as:
   - carcinoma and lymphoma;
   - herpes simplex and varicella zoster pneumonitis;
   - nocardiosis;
   - histoplasmosis, aspergillosis, and other fungal infections;
   - toxoplasmosis;
   - pneumocystosis;
   - chalk nodules from chronic intravenous drug use.

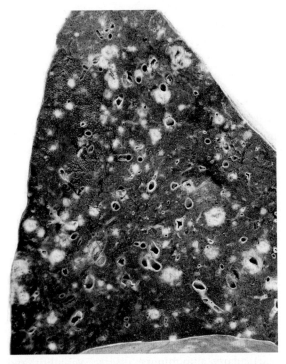

Figure 7.4 Gross lung slice showing miliary necroses. It could be one of many aetiologies including tuberculosis (it is actually toxoplasmosis).

1. In the mortuary setting, only a minority of HCV-infected patients have cirrhosis or grossly advanced liver disease.
2. Because of the associations, HCV-infected persons may have many other co-morbidities, such as illicit drug toxicity and HIV disease.
3. HCV does cause disease in organs other than the liver. Cryo-globulinaemia (skin lesions) and glomerular disease are well documented. Cerebral disease, with an undetermined morphological counterpart, is also of increasing interest.

infection is treatable, the cure rate is not impressive, and there is no prophylactic vaccination.

In the UK, about 0.5 per cent of the population is now infected, again with regional differences (see the HPA website). The main routes of infection are: intravenous drug use, contaminated blood products, liver and renal dialysis (though these routes have been nearly eliminated in industrialised countries), and some sexual transmission. For HCWs in the mortuary, the risk is entirely through accidental inoculation of blood and tissues through the skin. Box 7.9 indicates some HCV-related autopsy aspects.

Prion diseases

Classical Creutzfeldt–Jakob disease (CJD) has an annual incidence of about 1 per million in most populations; thus it is rare in the average mortuary. The recent epidemic of variant CJD (vCJD), derived from consuming contaminated beef, may well have passed the peak, and may or may not be a threat to UK citizens through iatrogenic contamination. The inherited transmissible spongiform encephalopathies (TSEs) are even rarer.

Nonetheless, suspected TSE cases come for autopsy and require evaluation; pre-mortem tests, such as measuring protein 14.3.3 in the cerebrospinal fluid (CSF), imaging and EEGs do not have very high sensitivity and specificity rates. Personal observations suggest that about one in three cases submitted for autopsy as clinically '?CJD' has that disease; the rest have Alzheimer, Lewy body or vascular dementias.

Box 7.10 Suggested procedures for suspected prion disease autopsy and histopathology

1. The autopsy procedure is undertaken by a pathologist and two APTs, wearing standard protective clothing plus FFP3 mask.
2. The body bag containing the cadaver is opened and draped by absorbent material all around. These are incinerated later.
3. The dissection of the organs after evisceration is performed on a small covered table placed over the body; fluid spillage is thus minimal or absent.
4. There is a dedicated set of basic instruments (scissors, forceps, hand saw for the skull) which are only used for ?TSE cases, and are returned to a labelled box after cleaning.
5. Disposable instruments – scalpel, organ cutting blade, suturing needle – are disposed of by incineration after the autopsy.
6. The brain is removed by a stryker hand saw – not by an electric saw, nor with the head encased within a clear plastic protective bag.
7. The extent of the rest of the autopsy is dictated by the clinical information, and usually does not involve wholesale removal of organs, but only sampling, to confirm, for example, terminal pneumonia. If vCJD is suspected, samples of spleen, lymph nodes and tonsil are always taken.
8. The brain is fixed in 10% formalin for 2 weeks, then cut with a disposable brain knife. The trimmed blocks are post-treated in 96% formic acid, then formalin, before processing alongside other histological material in the routine tissue processing machine.
9. The original fixing formalin, the 96% formic acid, and the post-formic acid formalin solutions are disposed of separately as clinical waste.
10. The wax block trimmings are not disposed of separately in a clinical waste bag.
11. To confirm or exclude the prion diagnosis, a minimum of three brain blocks – cerebellum, frontal lobe, hippocampus – are referred to the neuropathology centre where the appropriate panel of immunostains for prions and markers of other dementia conditions can be performed. This is considerably cheaper than a full neuropathological autopsy, and will capture all prion +ve cases, even if it may not confidently confirm alternative diagnoses.
12. If a case of TSE is identified when not previously suspected, then the tissue wax blocks are processed back to alcohol and water, post-fixed in formic acid, and reprocessed to paraffin wax. (This procedure will become standard in UK laboratories for such autopsy and surgical biopsy material.)

The risk to HCWs of infection is historically zero. No mortuary or histopathology laboratory worker has contracted CJD in the course of his or her work. However, a large body of protocols has been developed to ensure that HCWs do not become infected (Bell and Ironside, 1993; Finkbeiner *et al.*, 2009). All are agreed that such autopsies should be done with a separate dedicated set of (ideally disposable) dissection instruments, with as little contamination beyond the body or autopsy table as possible. The brain must be immersed in formalin and fixed for at least 2 weeks before cutting; and all histopathology sample tissues are to be post-fixed in 96% formic acid for 1 hour to minimise prion infection in the tissue wax blocks, followed by formalin. Thereafter it is safe to cut histopathological sections, and to file the slides and blocks in the main archives.

Where there are disagreements is over the number attending the autopsy; the level of pathologist and APT personal protection; how the brain is removed; the appropriate extent of the extracerebral autopsy examination; and whether the debris from wax block cutting requires separate disposal procedures.

Thus each unit will develop its own procedures. Box 7.10 indicates the procedures at the author's department. The government information site for managing suspected TSE in laboratories and mortuaries is www.advisorybodies.doh.gov.uk/acdp/tse guidance/index.htm.

Rabies

Rabies occurs infrequently in the UK and is virtually always imported. There has been one recent case acquired from bats within the British Isles. Rabies is nearly always fatal. If suspected, the diagnosis can in fact be made by skin biopsy of the neck and appropriate immunohistochemistry (IHC), in life or post-mortem.

If an autopsy is required, then the most important aspect is that all HCWs who eviscerate, examine or sew up the cadaver have had previous successful rabies vaccination. This established, a standard autopsy is done; fresh brain tissue is usually taken to the appropriate research laboratory for diagnostic confirmation by rapid IHC. The fixed brain (and

other organ) tissue can be safely trimmed and processed for light microscopy etc. Identification of the typical Negri bodies in neurons confirms the diagnosis. See the HPA and CDC websites for more information.

HG2 high-risk infections

HG2 infections are not normally, by definition, of particular safety concern in the mortuary. However, three specific bacterial infections should be noted, evaluated proportionately, and appropriate precautions taken; that is, standard universal precautions will be sufficient.

Meticillin-resistant *Staphylococcus aureus* (MRSA) infection is now notorious as a major hospital-care-acquired infection (HCAI). Like any other staphylococcal infection, it can be acquired in the mortuary through inoculation, and may be more difficult to treat. It is important that the pathologist places its contribution to a death in the context of the whole case, and neither over- nor under-emphasises its significance. In practice, MRSA surface or nasal colonisation *per se* is unimportant, while MRSA bacteraemia or visceral sepsis usually is important.

Clostridium difficile-associated colitis (Cdif) is another HCAI. It is not infectious to prosectors from a diseased cadaver. In suspected cases, it is important to confirm or exclude this disease because of its importance in hospital hygiene. Faeces should be sent to the microbiology department for evaluation of the Cdif toxin; the differential diagnosis of pseudo-membranous colitis (PMC) includes ischaemia and cytomegalovirus infection, which are evaluated histologically.

Group A *Streptococcus pyogenes* infection (GAS) is a classical severe infectious disease that has killed and will continue to kill large numbers of humans in all regions. It is known as the main agent of necrotising fasciitis, and it is still a significant cause of UK maternal mortality (e.g. puerperal sepsis) (Confidential Enquiry into Maternal and Child Health, 2007). One reason for performing blood cultures on cadavers in the unexplained sudden-death scenario is to identify GAS infection. It is important to mortuary HCWs, since accidental inoculation can result in significant local or systemic disease.

HG4 high-risk infections

These are rarely encountered in the UK; none are endemic and all suspected cases are imported by returning travellers or nationals from endemic zones. One case of a viral haemorrhagic fever infection (VHF) is diagnosed every year or so in the UK. In contrast, many suspected cases arrive in mortuaries to be resolved by a mixture of pre- and post-mortem testing of appropriate blood and other fluid samples. In the writer's experience, the main simulators of VHF infections are streptococcal infection, chemical toxicity, haemophagocytic syndrome, and meningococcal sepsis.

The Health Protection Agency (HPA) has laboratories in Colindale (London NW10) and Porton Down (Wiltshire) where all the appropriate tests are performed within 24 hours of receipt. The HPA website provides the contact details.

Box 7.11 What to do if a dead person is suspected of harbouring a HG4 infection

1. Courier pre-mortem blood samples (ideally) or post-mortem blood to the HPA laboratory.
2. This will be tested for the range of VHF infections appropriate to the patient's likely provenance (i.e. travel history).
3. It will also be tested for dengue, yellow fever, malaria and leptospirosis.
4. If positive for any of these, with the exception of VHF, then the autopsy is safe to proceed with under the standard conditions for blood-borne HG3 infections such as HIV; if malaria, then less stringent conditions are appropriate.
5. If no infection is identified, then examine the cadaver with the many differential diagnoses in mind.
6. If it is a true VHF, then serious consideration is needed as to whether an autopsy is necessary at all. If it is done, it has to be under strict conditions of personal protection, including a full body suit with a powered air-purifying respirator with high-efficiency particulate air (HEPA) filters. There are few mortuaries in the UK that function at this level, and thus further description is unnecessary here.

The procedure recommended in the Royal College of Pathologists' 2002 guidelines is reiterated in Box 7.11. Smallpox is considered under 'Bioterrorism' below.

Pre-mortem and peri-autopsy testing for HRIs

The General Medical Council's 1994 guidance on SCDs stated:

Where a post-mortem examination is to be carried out, doctors may undertake testing of a deceased patient for communicable diseases in order to establish the cause of death. Where there is a reasonable suspicion that the patient may have been at high risk of an infectious disease, suitable precautions should be taken to protect the healthcare workers concerned, but prior laboratory testing for communicable disease is not essential to the process and should not be considered routinely. Disclosure of positive test results may take place in confidence to healthcare workers directly involved in post-mortem procedures and to known sexual partners and other contacts considered to be at risk.

This GMC guidance has been withdrawn, but without any definitive statements regarding the legal position.

The Human Tissue Authority (HTA) has not (yet) produced guidance, so the author's unit practice is presented here:

1. There is no justification for universal pre-autopsy testing of body fluids for SCDs. 'Safe Working' concurs.
2. Peri-autopsy testing for SCDs that are not already known pre-mortem can and should be done if the clinical and pathological evidence suggests the possibility, and knowing the results will influence the consideration of cause and circumstances of the death.
3. If a healthcare worker is accidentally exposed to a SCD through inoculation, then the cadaver should be tested promptly, while the HCW attends the occupational health clinic for baseline screening, post-exposure prophylaxis if

appropriate, and arrangement of follow-up visits. Information that the cadaver is or is not so infected must be passed promptly to the OH clinic. If there is any hesitation about testing a cadaver for a high-risk infection when a HCW is injured, remember that the health and safety of our staff is more important than the ethical, legal and tissue retention niceties of consent.

4. If a significant infection is so discovered in a cadaver that was not hitherto known (and this is mainly HIV, HCV and HBV), then the next of kin or partners have to be informed (duty of care). This can be done via the general practitioner, hospital clinician or the local authority consultant in communicable disease control (CCDC); as a last resort, the pathologist is obliged to communicate directly.

Bioterrorism and pandemic influenza

These are included in this chapter because of perceived threats to public health, and an immense amount of preparation that most industrialised countries' health departments and local government planners have put in place.

Bioterrorism

Bioterrorism is an area of ignorance among UK medical staff, including pathologists. This is paradoxical since it is pathologists and APTs in the mortuary who are more likely to be involved closely than many other medical and paramedical staff. It is defined as:

> ... the use or threatened use of biologic agents against a person, group, or larger population to create fear or illnesses for purposes of intimidation, gaining an advantage, interruption of normal activities, or ideologic activities. The resultant reaction is dependent upon the actual event and the population involved and can vary from a minimal effect to disruption of ongoing activities and emotional reaction, illness, or death.
>
> (Nolte *et al.*, 2004)

In the late 1990s, the Centers for Disease Control and Prevention (CDC), the federal public health institute in the USA, consulted experts and drew up a consensus list of the most likely and dangerous agents that bioterrorists might use. They comprise the so-called category A list (Centers for Disease Control and Prevention, 2000; Nolte *et al.*, 2004):

- smallpox (variola);
- anthrax (*Bacillus anthracis*);
- plague (*Yersinia pestis*);
- tularaemia (*Francisella tularensis*);
- botulism toxin (*Clostridium botulinum*);
- viral haemorrhagic fevers (Ebola, Lassa, Marburg viruses).

Following the anthrax attack in 2001 in the USA, these were consolidated. Two further categories of infective agents were then considered that might be used in a bioterrorism attack, but carried a lower mortality than the category A list agents. One stimulus to including these was the perception at the CDC that the diagnostic capabilities for these agents needed to be improved and expanded nationally. They can be studied on the CDC website.

Detailed consideration of how a bioterrorism threat will be managed in theory and practice, and how mortuaries will function, is beyond the remit of this chapter, but information is available in textbooks (Lucas, 2008) and online from the HPA (www.hpa.org.uk/infections/topics_az/deliberate_release/menu.htm).

Pandemic influenza

Every few decades, a new strain of influenza virus emerges from avian influenza viruses. If it can infect man and combine with an existing human strain that makes it easy to transmit to other humans, then the potential for pandemic influenza (PF) exists. The potential for significant morbidity and mortality, and great disruption to social and hospital services, is evident. Recently a new avian strain, H5N1, has caused hundreds of deaths already, mainly in the Far East, and has yet to acquire the property of easy human-to-human transfer. At the time of writing there is a pandemic of H1N1 influenza, with a slowly rising death toll in the UK, particularly among those with co-morbidities and pregnant women.

If there is a serious epidemic of pandemic influenza in the UK, then pathologists and APTs will be at the front line for making the first diagnoses, in cadavers. Once the clinical pathology of the disease has become familiar, then the need to autopsy those with suspected PF will fall, and only those cases of medicolegal importance will be pursued.

The infectious agents are not (unlike bioterrorism agents) in the HG3 and HG4 categories once the initial phase of the epidemic has passed. Nonetheless, it is likely that there will be reluctance among mortuary HCWs to perform such autopsies. Standard protection (as for TB autopsies) is sufficient, and there will be provision of the antiviral chemotherapy (oseltamivir) for those exposed.

It will be important that a standard tissue sampling protocol is followed so as to optimise the diagnosis of suspected PF in a cadaver. This has been posted, along with health and safety guidance, on the Royal College of Pathologists website: http://www.rcpath.org/resources/pdf/g020 adviceautopsy-influenzaaoct09.pdf

The latest government plans for managing a PF epidemic can be found at www.dh.gov.uk/en/Public health/Flu/PandemicFlu/.

Notifiable infections

Most pathologists are unaware that there are many specific diseases, including infections, that are statutorily notifiable by law to the local authority. The notifier is usually the clinician diagnosing the disease; but if a pathologist is making the diagnosis for the first time, it is his or her duty. The list of such infections is given by the Health Protection Agency (see Box 7.12 and data source: www.hpa.org.uk).

Leprosy is notifiable, but directly to the HPA. Note that HIV infection is not currently a notifiable disease. *Clostridium difficile*-associated colitis (Cdif) and MRSA bacteraemia or sepsis are also, in practice, notifiable infections.

Of these listed notifiable infections, it is likely that only leprosy, malaria, some viral meningo-encephalitides, Cdif and tuberculosis will be diagnosed by an autopsy pathologist, without the necessary direct diagnostic help of a microbiology department. Such departments are well used to reporting these infections to the local authorities, and will normally report the other cases that pass through their diagnostic hands. If the pathologist has to notify a case, the contact is the local CCDC (consultant in communicable disease control), whose contact details are available on-line.

While HIV infection is not a notifiable infection, for historical reasons, it is reported to the HPA for national statistics, by the diagnosing virology departments. The current list of notifiable illnesses is in the process of reformulation as part of secondary legislation for the Public Health Act 2008.

Box 7.12 Diseases notifiable to Local Authority Proper Officers under the Public Health (Infectious Diseases) Regulations 1988

Acute encephalitis	– *Haemophilus influenzae*	Scarlet fever
Acute poliomyelitis	– viral	Smallpox
Anthrax	– other specified	Tetanus
Cholera	– unspecified	Tuberculosis
Diphtheria	Meningococcal septicaemia	Typhoid fever
Dysentery	(without meningitis)	Typhus fever
Food poisoning	Mumps	Viral haemorrhagic fever
Leptospirosis	Ophthalmia neonatorum	Viral hepatitis
Malaria	Paratyphoid fever	Hepatitis A, B and C
Measles	Plague	Whooping cough
Meningitis	Rabies	Yellow fever
– meningococcal	Relapsing fever	
– pneumococcal	Rubella	

Post-vaccination fatality

Immunisation is undoubtedly a public health success story in preventing disease, and – in the case of smallpox – eradicating a disease with a high fatality rate. However, it is not 100 per cent safe, and morbidity and some deaths inevitably follow. It is important that such deaths be evaluated with the utmost rigour in order to determine, as far as is possible, the contribution of the recent vaccination to death. Otherwise, political and public confidence in vaccination programmes may be lost, and herd immunity decline such that the disease that is intended to be reduced in incidence actually increases and causes many more deaths than the vaccine. Apart from the UK public loss of confidence in MMR vaccine through spurious association with autism, there has been concern over the safety of hexavalent immunisation and a possible association with unexpected deaths in infancy. Much criticism over the lack of proper autopsy protocol and investigative rigour has attended reports of such deaths in Germany (Schmidt *et al.*, 2006).

For high-risk infections, the infections of concern are tuberculosis, rabies, yellow fever and smallpox. BCG vaccine for tuberculosis causes disseminated infection in immunocompromised subjects; rabies vaccine has no apparent association with post-vaccine mortality; yellow fever vaccine (YFV) complications have become more important as more groups of people outside the standard epidemic zones are vaccinated (e.g. the military) (www.vaccinesafety.edu/cc-yellowfever.htm).

Smallpox now exists in only two national reference laboratories, and, under normal circumstances, few relevant workers would be prophylactically vaccinated. However, the threat of bioterrorism and the Gulf Wars have resulted in many tens of thousands of doses administered, mainly to young armed services personnel, and a cadre of HCWs (including small numbers of pathologists and APTs) with attendant morbidity and some mortality (Advisory Committee on Immunization Practices, 2001).

Protocol for performing a post-vaccination fatality

As with any autopsy, a clear appraisal of the question(s) being asked concerning the death is required. Is the person seriously considered to have died of a vaccine-related complication, specifically dissemination of the infective vaccine? What is the pattern of clinical pathology produced by that vaccine? Is the time period since vaccination and reported clinical scenario consistent with a vaccine effect? What co-morbidities might or does the patient have? What other diseases are likely to have killed the patient?

A protocol for addressing such deaths depends, obviously, on the nature of the vaccine and target organs. The autopsy should be addressed according to the hazard group of the infective agent. Full organ sampling is essential, and – critically – retention of frozen tissue samples and frozen spun autopsy blood, so that biological investigations can be pursued later if required. Thus for a suspected YFV fatality, a sample of liver must be retained frozen.

Postscript

Throughout this chapter there has been much reference to tiers of statute, governance and guidance from government and non-government agencies with bewildering acronyms – i.e. the increasingly complex bureaucracy concerning how mortuaries, pathologists and APTs deal with HRIs. As if all this were not enough, note the requirement in *The Control of Substances Hazardous to Health Regulations 2002* (COSSH) to keep a list of employees exposed to HG3 or HG4 biological agents for at least 40 years (sic) after the last exposure. This requirement also extends to employees exposed to HHV8 (in HG2). A note in the autopsy register of which APT assisted in a case suffices. It is likely that the bureaucracy surrounding how we address such infections in the dead can only increase in the future.

Keep a clear view of the essentials: What is the actual risk? Are the protocols proportionate and effective? And, finally, infections are both important for public health and interesting pathologically, so do not be deterred from pursuing them.

References

Advisory Committee on Immunization Practices (2001). *Vaccinia* (smallpox) vaccine: recommendation of the ACIP. *MMWR* **50**(RR10):1–25.

Bell JE, Ironside JW (1993). How to tackle a possible Creutzfeldt–Jacob disease necropsy. *J Clin Pathol* **46**:193–7.

Centers for Disease Control and Prevention (2000). Biological and chemical terrorism: strategic plan for preparedness and response. *MMWR* **49**:1–14.

Confidential Enquiry into Maternal and Child Health (2007). *Saving Mothers' Lives: Reviewing Maternal Deaths to Make Motherhood Safer: 2003–2005*. London: CEMACH.

Expert Advisory Group on AIDS (2008). HIV Post-exposure Prophylaxis: Guidance. Available at www.dh.gov.uk/en/Publicationsandstatistics/Publications/PublicationsPolicyAndGuidance/DH_088185 (1 July 2009).

Finkbeiner W, Ursell PC, Davis RL (2009). Autopsy biosafety. In: *Autopsy Pathology: Manual and Atlas*. Philadelphia: Saunders Elsevier, pp. 25–34.

Gerston KF, Blumberg L, Tshabala VA, Murray J (2004). Viability of mycobacteria in formalin-fixed lungs. *Hum Pathol* **35**:571–5.

Health Services Advisory Committee (2003). *Safe Working and the Prevention of Infection in the Mortuary and Post-mortem Room*, 2nd edn. London: HSE Books.

Johnson MD, Schaffner W, Atkinson J, Pierce MA (1997). Autopsy risk and acquisition of HIV infection: case report and reappraisal. *Arch Pathol Lab Med* **121**:64–6.

Lucas SB (1993). HIV and the necropsy (editorial). *J Clin Pathol* **46**:1071–5.

Lucas SB (2008). Bioterrorism. In: Rutty GN (ed.) *Essentials of Autopsy Practice*. London: Springer-Verlag, pp. 135–66.

Lucas SB, Curtis H, Johnson MA (2008). National review of deaths among HIV-infected adults. *Clin Med* **8**:250–2.

Nolte KB, Hanzlick RL, Payne DC *et al.* (2004). *Medical Examiners, Coroners, and Biologic Terrorism*: a guidebook for surveillance and case management. *MMWR* **53**(RR08):1–27.

Royal College of Pathologists (2002). *Guidelines for Autopsy Practice*. London: RCP.

Schmidt H-J, Siegrist C-A, Salmaso S *et al.* (2006). B. Zinka *et al.*: unexplained cases of sudden infant death shortly after hexavalent vaccination. *Vaccine* **24**:5781–2.

Templeton GL, Illing LA, Young L *et al.* (1995). The risk of transmission of *Mycobacterium tuberculosis* at the bedside and during autopsy. *Ann Intern Med* **122**:922–5.

Chapter 8

THE EXTERNAL EXAMINATION

Guy N Rutty

Introduction

This chapter is a synopsis of the external examination with a worked example of a basic examination as could appear in a report. To present all the changes and findings that could occur at an external examination is beyond the scope of this book. Specialist texts must be considered by the reader as highlighted within the text. In this book, consideration of the external examination of injuries is found in Chapter 9.

External examination

Prior to undertaking the evisceration and internal examination, be it a 'hospital' (clinical) or a medicolegal autopsy, it is essential that the pathologist personally performs a systematic external examination. The National Confidential Enquiry into Patient Outcome and Death (2006) severely criticised the practice of delegating this task to anatomical pathology technologists. This may form the extent of the 'autopsy' examination procedure in those jurisdictions where so-called 'view and grant' and 'scan, view and grant' examinations are permissible. Many pathologists are unfortunately under the impression that, in cases other than 'forensic' autopsies, the external examination is of less importance than the internal examination. This often results in cursory and poorly documented external examinations being performed by themselves or, even worse, by the anatomical pathology technologist (APT, mortician). Such an impression could not be further from

the truth. Despite the fact that the body may have been examined by doctors, police or paramedical staff, these examinations may be undertaken by persons with little if any formal training in this field of expertise and thus are often poorly documented and full of mistakes – for example, lacerations described as incised wounds or natural skin lesions described as bruises.

The first reason to undertake an external examination is to satisfy oneself that the person is in fact dead. Patients in deep coma may appear 'dead' and thus the pathologist must never make the presumption that the person is deceased even if they have been previously refrigerated within the mortuary.

The external examination not only yields information about the natural diseases that the deceased suffered from in life, but also contributes towards the identification of the deceased, the time of death, the place of death, the cause of death and the manner of death, i.e. the principal questions to be answered in any autopsy examination. This must start prior to cleaning the body as critical evidence can be lost at this point. It is unfortunate that on occasion autopsies are started by APTs prior to the arrival of the pathologist, who then realises once the body has already been opened and even eviscerated that the death is suspicious and that a criminal investigation is required. There is only one chance to get this right, and retracing one's steps or interpreting, for example, bruising in the previously eviscerated neck (using a midline larynx-to-pubic incision) is fraught with difficulty. Thus, pathologists should perform a full external examination on every single case that they deal with prior to the cleaning and opening of the body (Madea, 1999; Royal College of Pathologists, 2002, 2004, 2007; Knight, 2004; Burton, 2007).

It is worth emphasising that the external examination should include both the front and the back of the body. Although this may be done while the APT holds the body on its side, best practice is for this to be performed by turning the body completely over so that it is lying prone. The position facilitates examination of the deep soft tissues of the back and limbs, removal of the spinal cord, examination of the rectum and en-bloc dissection of the external genitalia (if required), as well as examination of the posterior neck compartment and posterior aspect of the skull. Fingerprinting of a body is more easily undertaken in this position.

This examination must be documented. Common to both the autopsy examination and report one should, wherever possible, use lay words to record descriptions. Many pathologists make the mistake of using medical terms in autopsy reports. As most reports are nowadays read by non-medical personnel, this may lead to the production of a report that is unintelligible to most of its readers. Using simple terms – for example, collar bone not clavicle, breast bone not sternum, and knuckle not metacarpophalangeal joint – will assist this process. Ideally this should be done in writing, preferably on to an autopsy examination pro forma, although one must take care not to transfer body tissues or fluid to the recording medium. This is particularly important in high-risk cases where the transference of chemical, biological or radiological material must be avoided. A scribe can be used to avoid transfer but, if used, shorthand and abbreviations specific to an individual or a medical discipline must be avoided. The scribe can be present in the mortuary itself or in a remote clean area with the examination being transferred directly to a word processor by means, for example, of a secure radio network. When an individual has external marks these should be drawn onto the pro forma or onto separate anatomical diagram sheets (Fig. 8.1). With unidentified people or victims of mass fatalities, the pro forma may take the form of the Interpol disaster victim identification

(DVI) forms or an electronic system such as Plass-Data (PlassData Software, Germany) or the UK Fimag system (Fig. 8.2) (Interpol, 2002; Rutty et al., 2009).

The use of an analogue tape recorder to dictate findings in the mortuary is to be avoided. A tape does not form a permanent record of the examination (as it will degrade over time), may fail to record in the first place, and can be easily erased. In cases of medicolegal interest a brand-new tape would have to be used each time. As original autopsy records have to be kept and disclosed – so that, if requested, they can be examined by the defence or produced in court – this leads to problems as to how to store and subsequently produce the tapes (Crown Prosecution Service:, 2006).

Modern alternative systems for recording the findings at autopsy include digital recorders, digital pens, video recorders (head-mounted, ceiling-mounted, static), and laser keyboards with Bluetooth laptop or palmtop connections. The findings on the body can be recorded by digital photography and surface body scanners. The use of digital technology must follow local and national protocols for handling of digital media, and may require the saving of raw data files or image/data CDs at the end of the examination while still in the mortuary.

Identification

Before starting an autopsy the pathologist must be satisfied that the body about to be examined is that of the deceased. This may be a requirement or recommendation of the legislation or licensing authority pertinent to the jurisdiction of practice – for example, in England and Wales, the Human Tissue Authority (www.hta.gov.uk).

Known individuals

In the majority of cases the identity of the deceased will be known. The body will have been booked into the mortuary under this name and often allocated a unique identifying number, the details of which will be recorded on at least one identification band usually secured to the wrist or ankle area. The use of several bands at multiple sites is encouraged. Wherever pos-

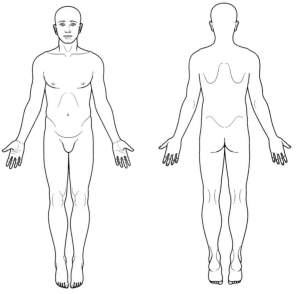

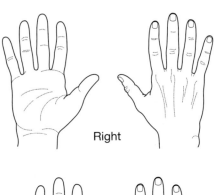

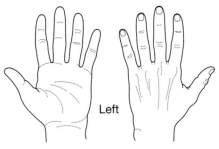

Right

Left

(c)

(a)

(b)

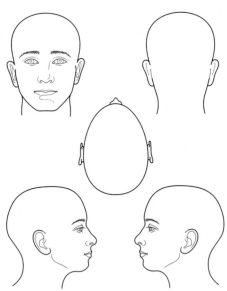

(d)

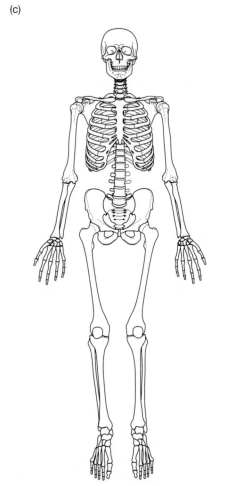

(e)

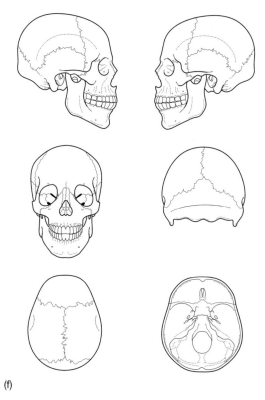

(f)

Figure 8.1 General body diagrams.

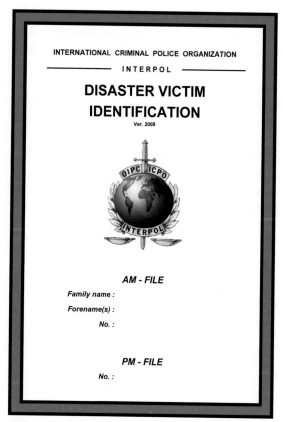

Figure 8.2 Interpol disaster victim identification (DVI) form.

sible, toe tags should not be used as they may become detached from the body (with the potential for re-attachment to the wrong body). Some mortuaries will write the name and mortuary number on the body, usually on the leg, either in permanent marker pen or typist's correction fluid. The use of implanted electronic devices such as radio-frequency identification tags has gained little support in autopsy practice, although this forms a secure means of body labelling and global tracking (Meyer *et al.*, 2006; Thevissen *et al.*, 2006). In some cases an individual – for example, a nurse, coroner's officer or police officer – may identify the body directly to the pathologist.

No matter how the identification of the body is established, the means, location, time and date of the identification should be recorded within both the autopsy notes and report; for example:

Identification – an identification band bearing the name 'John Smith' and the number 123456AR was present to the right wrist. A second band bearing the same details was present to the left ankle.

Identification – the body was identified to me as John Smith of The Red House, Leicester, by PC 1234 Jones at the Leicester Royal Infirmary mortuary, at 0900 on 1 July 2009.

The autopsy examination should not proceed until the body has been identified in this way.

Unknown individuals

The pathologist may be faced with one or more individuals whose identification at the time of the autopsy is unknown. This can be made worse if the body is disrupted, decomposed, skeletonised or co-mingled with parts from other bodies. In these circumstances the pathologist assists in the gathering of information that will be used to identify the deceased. This may be done in conjunction with other experts from other fields of medicolegal practice, including forensic odontologists, and may employ international assistance and the use of the Interpol DVI forms.

A variety of means can be used to assist in the identification of an individual. These are traditionally split into:

- *primary* – a characteristic considered unique to the individual that can be used on its own to identify an individual;
- *secondary* – a characteristic that is not unique but can be used in combination with another secondary or primary characteristic to identify an individual;
- *assistance* – a characteristic that is not unique to an individual but can be used to assist identification in combination with a primary or secondary characteristic or only on its own as a matter of last resort.

A list of these identification characteristics is shown in Table 8.1. More specialist means can be engaged at times, including for example podiatry, pollen, anthropology, facial reconstruction and isotopic/elemental tracing . If these systems are unfamiliar, the pathologist should seek specialist advice or refer to specialist texts (Thompson and Black, 2006; Rutty, 2009).

Clothing

Most bodies will arrive from the hospital ward naked or in a shroud or hospital gown. This should be documented. If the body is within a body bag this should be documented, including the colour of the bag and whether the bag is sealed. If sealed, the nature of the seal and any unique identification number should all be recorded as this may form part of the continuity process from the scene to the mortuary. In the case of mass fatalities, a unique number and scene book should have been attached to the outside of the bag and should be removed and checked prior to the opening of the bag.

Dressed bodies

If the body arrives dressed in the deceased's own clothing, each article of clothing should be examined before and after its removal from the body. The type, make and size of a piece of clothing should be recorded, as should any abnormality (e.g. if the shirt has been cut open during resuscitation attempts). Pockets should be examined and any personal effects documented. The possibility that pockets may contain needles and other sharps must be remembered: they should never be examined with fingers until they have been examined with forceps if a sharps injury is to be avoided (Fig. 8.3). Cutting of pockets is permitted provided a record is kept that this has been done.

In police cases, clothing should be photographed and handed to an exhibits officer who will attribute

Table 8.1 Identification criteria

Primary	Secondary	Assistance
Fingerprints	Jewellery	Photographs
Odontology	Personal effects	Body location
DNA	Distinctive marks	Clothing
Unique characteristic (e.g. prosthesis)	Distinctive scars	Descriptions
	X-rays	
	Physical disease	
	Blood grouping	
	Tissue identification	

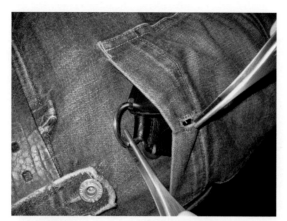
Figure 8.3 Examination of pockets with forceps.

an exhibits number to each item and place them into an appropriate exhibits bag. Blood-stained clothing may require packaging in brown paper to avoid movement of blood from one part of the article to another following removal from the body. In fire and explosive deaths, nylon bags should be used. With unidentified bodies, the temptation to examine and remove items from wallets must be avoided so as not to lose or contaminate potential evidence such as DNA or fingerprints which may be present on, for example, plastic credit cards.

Undressed bodies

If the body was undressed prior to the pathologist's arrival, consideration should always be given to obtaining the clothing and examining it. If the clothing is in a bag in the mortuary, and is not to be examined, then the fact of its presence and what is contained within should be recorded in the autopsy notes and report. This is of particular importance in cases of sudden infant death, as children are often redressed prior to going to the mortuary and the clothing they are presented in may not be the clothing they died in. Subtle marks left on baby-grows may be missed if not actively sought, and thus an unnatural death might be missed. Soiled nappies should not be discarded. Most infants pass urine prior to or at the time of death, so it may not be possible to collect a urine sample for metabolic screening from the bladder. The nappy, however, may be saturated with urine and can be submitted for laboratory

analysis – be it toxicological or metabolic screening (Edwards *et al.*, 1997).

Jewellery

The presence or absence (e.g. a mark in an area of sun-tan), site and type of all jewellery should be carefully documented. This is particularly important if only to prove that it has not been removed by a member of staff for any purpose other than the autopsy examination. Simple descriptions should be used. Metal should be described by its colour rather than attempting to determine its composition (e.g. 'a yellow metal ring was present to the ring finger of the left hand'). In police cases, jewellery should be handed to the exhibits officer and processed as for clothing.

General examination

Once the deceased is naked the examination progresses with the documentation of a number of general observations. These will form the introduction to the external examination in one's report.

Cleanliness

This will start with the general state of cleanliness of the body – for example, whether it is unwashed, whether there has been faecal or urinary incontinence, or the presence of head lice. This is of particular importance when considering a case of neglect. The absence of scars or decubitus ulcers should equally be noted to illustrate good care in those presented as a case of possible maltreatment or neglect. A clean, well-nourished child without nappy rash is important if a question of abuse or neglect has been raised.

Fluids, blood and exogenous material

The distribution, colour and constituency of any fluid, such as gastric contents or pulmonary oedema (froth), should be recorded. The presence of blood should be recorded and in police cases should be sampled in consideration as to whether it is the victim's or the offender's blood. Other exogenous material, such as oil from motor vehicles or ink on the hands or limbs of psychiatric patients, should be noted and, if required, sampled as this may be relevant to the cause of death or the mental state of the decedent at the time of death. Other biological and non-biological evidential material – gunshot residue, paint, fibres, glass, semen, saliva (both human and animal) or third-party DNA – may be present to the external surface of the body.

Gender, age and race

The first major observations to be recorded are the race and gender of the individual. For race, the preferred terms are 'white' rather than Caucasian, 'Afro-Caribbean' rather than black, 'Indo-Pakistani' and 'Oriental'. The term 'Asian' should be avoided as in some parts of the world it refers to Indo-Pakistani individuals and in others to Oriental individuals. The colour of the skin may also offer clues to potential natural or unnatural diseases; for example the yellow discoloration of liver disease (jaundice), the cherry-pink change of carbon monoxide poisoning, the brick-red discoloration of cyanide poisoning, and the depigmentation of vitiligo. If the deceased has a sun-tan, its distribution should be recorded.

The gender of an individual may be obvious, but it should be remembered that a body that is phenotypically female could be genetically male and vice versa (Fig. 8.4). A careful examination of the external genitalia and anus should be performed. In males, the presence or absence of the foreskin is recorded, as is any change to the anus which may suggest regular anal penetration ('funnel' anus). It must be remembered, however, that so-called 'funnel' anus can be present as a normal anatomical variant and is not pathognomonic of repeated anal penetration. Similarly, the presence of shiny skin around the anus can be attributed to regular anal penetration but is also seen in patients suffering from pruritus ani of any cause. Both males and females may be the recipients of regular anal penetrative intercourse. Perianal tears, bruising and haemorrhoids should also be noted. Female circumcision is a rare finding but should be looked for. Sexual maturity should be noted using the Tanner stages (Marshall and Tanner, 1969, 1970).

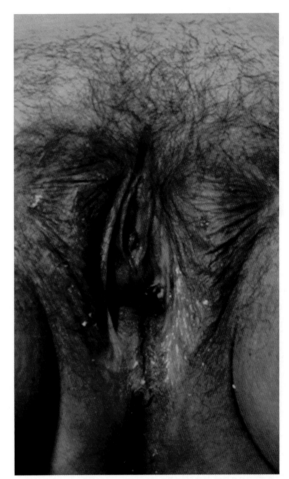

Figure 8.4 Transsexual genitalia.

It is difficult to estimate the age of an individual by external examination alone. However, a phrase such as 'in keeping with the stated age of 36 years' or 'appeared older than the stated age of 36 years' can be used. Individuals can be described in broad terms as fetuses, neonates, infants, children, young adults, middle-aged adults and elderly adults. Specialist examinations including radiology for dental eruption and epiphyseal fusion, as well as an anthropological examination of bones such as the ribs and pelvis, can assist in more precise ageing estimates, particularly in the young.

Congenital and dysmorphic features

Although more relevant to the paediatric autopsy, the presence of congenital or dysmorphic features is not confined to children and should be recorded. These could include anything from an extra digit and accessory nipples to spina bifida or syndromic facies.

Hair, eyes, teeth and ears

Common to each of these four parameters is an assessment of (a) whether they are present and (b) whether they are the body's own. The distribution of hair (male and female patterns) to the entire body should be noted. Hair may be lost from the body by natural disease or by shaving, for example from the legs, pubic area, armpits or chest. This may be done by the individual in preparation for their death. The presence or absence of head hair (male balding pattern), its colour (natural or dyed), length (measured) and style should be recorded. Natural hair can also be used for race determination, toxicology (for drug and poison analysis) and DNA testing (Mieczkowski, 1996). The presence and make of a wig should be noted. Injuries to natural or false hair should be recorded (Fig. 8.5).

The presence or absence of real or false eyes is sought. The colour of the irises and state and symmetry of the pupils should be noted, as should any natural or unnatural diseases such as cataracts, arcus senilis, Kayser–Fleischer rings, tache noir and petechial haemorrhages. Coloured dyes can be injected into the conjunctivae to produce tattoos. The diameter of the pupil may change after death as a result of rigor mortis affecting the iris. It should be remembered that the colour of the eyes is a less reliable identifying feature than the presence of eyes. The pathologist will look foolish if stating that both eyes were natural when in fact one was artificial! In individuals with blue, green or grey eyes the iris colour not uncommonly changes to brown in the post-mortem period, for reasons that are unexplained. This is the most common cause of complaint about autopsies to coroners and the pathologist should be prepared to explain any discrepancy in court. The individual may have worn contact lenses or glasses. If these have been removed prior to the autopsy the latter often leave indentations to the bridge of the nose or behind the ears.

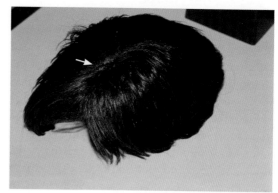

(a)

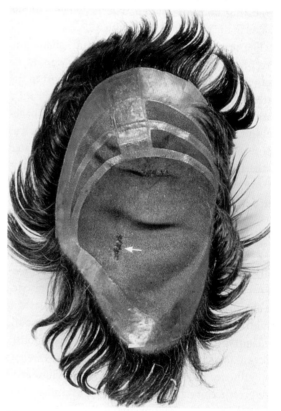

(b)

Figure 8.5 Injury to a hairpiece (a) external view, (b) underside of wig

Teeth can be present, absent, real, false or modified. The state of the dentition, lips, gums and oral cavity should be recorded within the limits of competence of the pathologist. A detailed dental examination is not within the remit or expertise of most autopsying pathologists and if required should be undertaken by a forensic odontologist. The presence or absence of dental restoration may be of importance in the identification of an individual. The absence of teeth or dentures at the time of the autopsy does not preclude a dental identification (Jacob and Shalla, 1987). If charting of the teeth is required, the assistance of a dental practitioner or forensic odontologist is advisable. As with the examination of clothing or any body orifice, the pathologist should not put fingers into the mouth except under direct vision as this is a sure way to receive a glove puncture injury from broken teeth, projecting bone or foreign objects which can be placed maliciously into the mouth.

The presence or absence, placement, shape and size of the ears can be recorded. They should be examined for local disease, such as blood within the external auditory process (which may indicate a basal skull fracture) and petechial haemorrhages behind the pinna, as well as systemic disease such as gouty tophi or lobar creases which are associated with cardiac disease. Ear morphology may be unique to individuals and can be used for identification purposes (Meijerman, 2006).

Hands and feet

The dorsal and volar surfaces of the hands, feet and, particularly, the digits should be examined for evidence of natural or unnatural disease. The presence or absence of normal creases is noted particularly in children. The state, length and colour of the nails (including the presence or absence of nail polish, decorations and extensions) are recorded as well as the presence of injuries. Nails may give clues as to the presence of natural disease – for example, clubbing, leuconychia, koilonychia, yellow nails, pitting or splinter haemorrhages. Digits can be used for identification purposes by their prints, and the nails can be used for toxicology, DNA, and geometric fingerprinting techniques. The assistance of a forensic podiatrist may be considered in mass fatality investigations (Vernon, 2006). In police cases, a careful inspection for the presence of trace evidence (e.g. fibres or hairs) must be undertaken. Any evidence should be photographed prior to lifting with adhesive tape. The interdigital webspaces may contain

needle puncture marks in individuals dying from drug overdoses.

Height and weight

All bodies should have their naked length and weight recorded. Length (height) should be measured from the heel to the vertex of the skull, not from the toe (coffin size). This should be recorded and reported in both imperial and SI (Systeme Internationale) units. It is unfortunate that many mortuaries do not have body-weighing facilities. A weight is important for the estimation of the time since death using temperature-based algorithms, the interpretation of toxicological results and the interpretation of apparently enlarged organs. If available, the weight should be recorded in kilograms, or the last known body weight recorded in life obtained from the hospital notes and reported again in both imperial and SI units. Finally, if both parameters are known, the body mass index (BMI) can be calculated using the formula

$$\text{body mass index (kg/m}^2) = \frac{\text{weight (kg)}}{\text{height (m}^2)}$$

and expressed within the report. This is of particular importance if the deceased appears to be malnourished or obese. It is the practice of one of the editors (JLB) to consider that death may have been in part due to morbid obesity only if the body mass index exceeds $40\,\text{kg/m}^2$.

Detailed examination

Once the general examination has been undertaken, the body is examined in detail for the presence of signs of natural disease, modifications, medical intervention, drug misuse and injuries (both fresh and historical). Evidence of medical/surgical intervention is discussed in Chapter 18.

Natural disease

Attempting to list all the natural diseases that can be identified on the external surface of a body may at times prove an overwhelming task. Needless to say, when evidence of natural disease is present (e.g. prominent naevi, port wine stains, or rashes) this should be recorded, stating the type of disease present and the area of the body affected. The presence or absence of oedema or swelling (e.g. unilateral swelling of a lower limb due to a deep venous thrombosis) should be recorded. The degree of calf swelling should be measured using a standardised point measured from above the ankle or below the knee (e.g. 100 mm below the lower border of the patella). Cardiac, hepatic or renal failure may cause peripheral oedema affecting the lower limbs, scrotum and presacral areas. Where a rash or area of infection (e.g. a pressure sore or decubitus ulcer) is present, skin can be sampled for histology and swabs for bacteriological and viral culture should be collected. In the case of pressure sores these should be recorded using a standardised clinical scale such as the Waterlow system.

Body modifications

A wide range of permanent and non-permanent modifications can be made to the body. They can be used for identification purposes or can on occasion result in disease and death due to the complications of the procedures (Swift, 2004).

Tattoos can be found anywhere on the skin and occasionally on the internal aspects of the body. They can be unintentional, related to the occupation of the individual – examples are coal miner's tattoos, amalgam tattoos related to dental restoration and ballistic tattooing from gunshot residue. Intentional tattoos can be split into artistic and therapeutic; the latter, for example, related to beam areas used in radiotherapy. Artistic ones may be expensive, complex, colourful, professional tattoos, or simple, monochrome, home-made or prison tattoos. Occasionally one will encounter tattoos made with inks that fluoresce under ultraviolet light but which are difficult to see under natural light.

Non-permanent henna tattoos are prevalent within some cultural groups. Non-permanent tattoos produced with black ink are not uncommonly associated with surrounding skin irritation. Their nature, size and site on the body should be recorded.

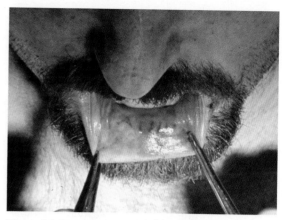

Figure 8.6 Tattoos may be present within the mouth.

Tattoos may be found inside the mouth (particularly the mucosa of the lips; Fig. 8.6). Tattoos may be altered or even removed; this can result in one or more tattoos at one site or a tattoo scar.

Piercings are not confined to the ear and may be seen at a multitude of sites on the body. The site and nature of the jewellery should be noted (Fig. 8.7). Specific names are associated with piercings at specific sites (Burton, 2007).

Brandings and scarification are encountered from time to time, although these tend to occur in specific countries – for example, in the college age group of the USA. They are, as yet, uncommon in the UK.

Modifications are split into non-surgical and surgical. Examples of the former include the use of cosmetics, hair treatments, nail extensions and dermabrasion. Surgical modifications include dental treatment and filing (to produce animal-like teeth), surgical implants, prostheses and gender reassignment (see below). Some individuals shave some or all of their body hair (particularly around the genitals) and this should be recorded. Apotemnophilia (amputation of healthy body parts) and trephination (non-surgical) are extreme forms of paraphilia that may be occasionally encountered either to the deceased or as the cause of death. Some individuals modify their body by having their tongue divided into two or their penis split (meatotomy). In some cultures, such as Aboriginal Australians, meatotomy is a cultural practice.

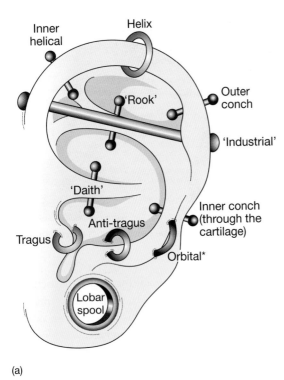

(a)

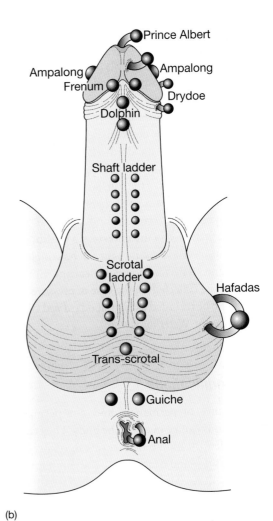

(b)

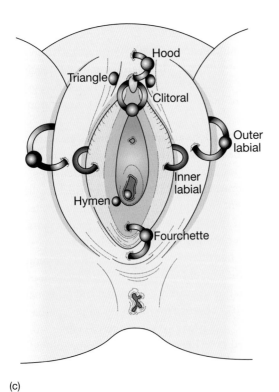

(c)

Figure 8.7 Examples of body piercings. (a) The ear. Common sites of piercings to the pinna. (b) The genitals, male. (c) The genitals, female. (Redrawn from Swift, 2004; with permission.)

* This refers to the style not the location with a complete loop, half of which sits posterior to the lobe, connected by two piercing holes

Medical intervention

Acts of medical intervention may have been performed on the deceased prior to death even if they have not died in hospital, for example by bystanders or a paramedic ambulance crew. The presence and location of all tubes, catheters and operation sites should be documented. Single or multi-tailed cannulae may be present. The phrase 'antecubital fossa', although anatomically correct, should be avoided and 'in front of the elbow', 'the bend of the arm' or 'bend of the elbow' are preferred terms. Craniotomy scars or intracranial pressure monitor sites may be present and may be sutured or stapled, closed with Steri-Strips or covered by dressings. Nasogastric and endotracheal tubes may be present. ECG monitor pads may be present, as may automated defibrillator pads, external pacing wires, tracheostomies, gastrostomies, colostomies or urinary catheters. The site and correct placement of automated defibrillation pads should be checked and noted. These may be associated with shaving of chest hair to ensure close contact of the pads with the skin.

All forms of medical intervention should have been left *in situ*, and not removed prior to the body arriving at the mortuary. This is essential if the pathologist is to check that each tube has been correctly inserted. When the body arrives in the mortuary accompanied by airways that have been removed this should be recorded. The evisceration and dissection should always be undertaken in a way that allows the internal siting to be confirmed. This may require an in-situ neck dissection to confirm the siting of endotracheal tubes and central venous catheters. Tubes and cannulae may be required also for histological examination or microbiological culture. If facial viewing is to be done prior to the autopsy, it is permissible for the external part of an endotracheal tube to be cut away leaving the internal portion in place.

Drug misuse

The observation of findings that could relate to misuse of drugs should alert the pathologist to the possibility of a toxicological death, so that additional precautions should be taken during the autopsy procedures. Needle marks, both fresh and old, of differing sizes depending on the calibre of needle used may be seen not only on the external surface of the body (e.g. arms, groins and lower leg areas) but also inside the mouth, under the tongue, between the fingers and toes, and on the genitalia. A thorough, detailed examination of the body is always

required. Knowledge of any medical intervention is essential for the interpretation of needle marks to the neck, bend of the arm, wrist and groin areas.

Consideration should be given to sampling of the needle site for histological or toxicological examination. If necessary, the puncture mark can be excised and submitted for toxicology – a higher concentration of an illicit drug than is present in venous blood would indicate that the site was used to inject illicit drugs.

Whether or not needle marks are associated with dressings should be noted. For example, an individual dying following an accidental heroin overdose may have needle marks due to the self-injection of heroin and needle marks as a result of medical resuscitation attempts.

The use of a ligature may leave a mark at a level above the needle mark. However, if hands have been used then the marks may be in the form of a grip mark and this should raise concerns regarding the possible involvement of a second party in the death. Such cases are best dealt with by a forensic pathologist.

Other signs of drug misuse may include a perforated nasal septum and sinuses in the groins. These latter changes may be associated with infection, lymphoedema or deep vein thrombosis. Tablet dye residue can sometimes be found on the palm of the hand in those that have taken a 'handful' of tablets. Small round scars are seen in 'skin-popping'. Scars resulting from self-inflicted injuries can be found in those who misuse drugs. A careful search of the mouth, foreskin, vagina and anus should be undertaken for concealed drugs (Fineron, 2001).

Decomposition

During the post-mortem period the body will undergo putrefaction. This results in external changes that include the onset of rigor mortis and hypostasis. The timing and sequence by which decomposition occurs is influenced by the environment, so an interpretation as to how long a body may have been dead based purely on its appearance remains no more than a generalised estimation. A detailed consideration of decompositional changes is presented in Chapter 20.

Box 8.1 Example of a concise report

The identification

The body was identified to me as that of Joan Jones of 1 The Street, Anytown, by the duty mortician at 0900 on the 1 July 2009 at the public mortuary, Anytown. This was in accordance with identification bands bearing the name and mortuary identification number 12345 which were present to the right and left wrist and right ankle areas.

The external examination

The body was that of a white adult female with an appearance in keeping with the stated age of 40 years. The hair was a natural brown in colour and straight, measuring on average 10 cm in length at randomly measured sites. The eyes were natural, with blue irises. The pupils were midpoint and equal. There was no evidence of petechial haemorrhages to the skin or mucosal surfaces of the face. Facial congestion or cyanosis was absent. The sclera were normal. There were no glasses or contact lenses present. Both ear lobes were free with single piercings to each lobe. The teeth were natural and showed dental restoration. There were no injuries or natural disease to the mouth. Both breasts were normal. The nipples were brown. The armpits and legs were shaved. Pubic hair was present in a 'Brazilian' distribution. The external genitalia and anus showed no evidence of injury. The fingernails where cut and extended 3 mm beyond the fingertips. Pink purlescent nail varnish was present to all fingernails. The index and middle fingers of the right hand showed cigarette tar staining. The toe nails were neatly cut and showed chipped red nail varnish.

The body was presented in a white body bag. The zip was sealed with a cable tie bearing the number 12345. The following article of clothing was present with the body:

- Nightdress, size 12, make unknown. Inspection showed no abnormality.

The following jewellery was present on the body:
- White metal band ring on the right index finger.
- Yellow metal band ring with a blue stone on the left ring finger.

The following tattoo was present on the body:
- A professional-looking multi-chromic pictorial tattoo to the right buttock, measuring 3 cm by 2 cm in maximum dimensions.

The following marks of medical intervention were present:
- A cannula secured with a transparent dressing to the anterior aspect of the bend of the right arm.
- Automated defibrillation pads to the right upper and left lateral chest areas. They were correctly sited and orientated.

The following old injuries were present:
- A 3 cm long, horizontally orientated well-healed scar to the anterior aspect of the right knee.
- A 9 cm long appendicectomy scar to the right lower quadrant of the abdomen.

The following fresh injury was present:
- A 2 cm diameter discoid blue bruise to the lateral aspect of the left upper arm, 12 cm above the crease in the bend of the arm.

Rigor was established throughout to both small and large muscle groups. Non-blanching post-mortem hypostasis was established in a posterior distribution.

Body weight was 52 kg (8st 3lb) and height 162 cm (5ft 4in). Using these measurements, the body mass index is calculated as 19.8 (WHO normal range: 18.5–25 kg/m^2).

Depending on the location of the body, it will then undergo skeletalisation, mummification or the formation of adipocere, either on their own or in combination. The mechanisms of these changes are beyond the scope of this chapter. Many changes that occur in the post-mortem period may also mimic ante-mortem disease or violence. These changes should be documented but interpreted with caution (Rutty, 2001). The body can also be altered by the action of predators, which may be mammals, birds, insects or aquatic life depending on the location of the body. Sampling of insects and arthropods can be used for estimating a time since death, and the former for DNA identification and toxicological investigations.

In all cases the presence or absence of rigor should be recorded. This can be assessed simply by opening and closing the jaw or flexing the limbs.

Hypostasis will, in general, be seen in the dependent areas of the body where blood within the skin has redistributed under the action of gravity. A more comprehensive review of the onset, distribution and duration of rigor mortis and hypostasis, as well as other post-mortem changes to the body and their use in the estimation of the time since death, should be sought from a specialist text (e.g. Henssge *et al.*, 2002).

Example of a basic external examination

Using the methodical approach to external examination outlined above and in Chapter 18, a clear and concise report can be constructed. An example is shown on page 102.

References

Burton J (2007). The external examination: an often neglected autopsy component. *Curr Diag Pathol* **13**:357–65.

Crown Prosecution Service (2006). *Disclosure: Expert's Evidence and Unused Material, Guidance Booklet for Experts.* CPS Corporate Communication Team, Bolton: Blackburns of Bolton.

Edwards A, Voort J, Newcombe R, Thayer H, Jones KV (1997). A urine analysis method suitable for children's nappies. *J Clin Pathol* **50**:569–72.

Fineron P (2001). Deaths due to drug and alcohol misuse. In: Rutty GN (ed.) *Essentials of Autopsy Practice*, Vol. 1. London: Springer, pp. 199–220

Henssge C, Knight B, Krompecher T, Madea B, Nokes L (2002). *Estimation of the Time Since Death in the Early Postmortem Period*, 2nd edn. London: Arnold.

Interpol (2002). Disaster vicitim identification forms, available from www.interpol.int/Public/DisasterVictim/Forms/Default.asp (1 May 2009).

Jacob RFK, Shalla CL (1987). Postmortem identification of the edentulous deceased: denture tissue surface anatomy. *J Forensic Sci* **32**:698–702.

Knight B (2004). The autopsy: external examination. In: *Forensic Pathology*, 3rd edn. London: Hodder Education.

Madea B (1999). *Die Arztliche Leichenschau.* London: Springer.

Marshall WA, Tanner JM (1969). Variation in the pattern of pubertal changes in girls. *Arch Dis Child* **44**:291.

Marshall WA, Tanner JM (1970). Variation in the pattern of pubertal changes in boys. *Arch Dis Child* **45**:13–23.

Meijerman L (2006). *Inter- and intra-individual Variation in Earprints.* Leiden: Barge's Anthropologica.

Meyer HJ, Chansue N, Monticelli F (2006). Implantation of radio frequency identification device (RFID) microchip in disaster victim identification (DVI). *Forensic Sci Int* **157**:168–71.

Mieczkowski T (1996). The use of hair analysis for the detection of drugs: an overview. *J Forensic Med Pathol* **3**:59–71.

National Confidential Enquiry into Patient Outcome and Death (2006). *The Coroner's Autopsy: Do we Deserve Better?* London: NCEPOD.

Royal College of Pathologists (2002). *Guidelines on Autopsy Practice.* London: RCP. Available at www.rcpath.org/index.asp?PageID=240 (1 May 2009).

Royal College of Pathologists (2004). *Code of Practice and Performance Standards for Forensic Pathologists.* London: RCP. Available at www.rcpath.org/resources/pdf/CodeOfPracForensicPath1104.pdf (1 May 2009).

Royal College of Pathologists (2007). *Code of Practice and Performance Standards for Forensic Pathologists Dealing with Suspicious Deaths in Scotland.* London: RCP. Available at www.rcpath.org/resources/pdf/cop_for_forensic_paths_scotnov07web.pdf (1 May 2009).

Rutty GN (2001). Post mortem changes and artefacts. In: Rutty GN (ed.) *Essentials of Autopsy Practice*, Vol. 1. London: Springer, pp. 63–95.

Rutty GN (2009). *Body Identification.* National Policing Improvement Agency, UK.

Rutty GN, Robinson C, Morgan B *et al.* (2009). Fimag: the UK disaster victim/forensic identification imaging system. *J Forensic Sci* **54**:1438–42.

Swift B (2004). Body art and modification. In: Rutty GN (ed.) *Essentials of Autopsy Practice: Recent Advances, Topics and Developments.* London: Springer, pp. 159–86.

Thevissen PW, Poelman G, De Cooman M, Puers R, Willems G (2006). Implantation of an RFID-tag into human molars to reduce hard forensic identification labor. I. Working principle. *Forensic Sci Int* **159**(suppl 1):S33–9.

Thompson T, Black S (2006). *Forensic Human Identification: An Introduction.* London: CRC.

Vernon W (2006). The development and practice of forensic podiatry. *J Clin Forensic Med* **13**:284–7.

Chapter 9

THE PATHOLOGY OF WOUNDS AND INJURIES

Guy N Rutty

Introduction

Often, by far the longest part of the external examination is the recording of the presence of injuries. It would be most unusual for an individual not to have suffered some form of injury during life which, depending on the nature of the injury, may have left a scar or deformity. In addition, many individuals will suffer an injury during their terminal collapse, especially to the scalp or face.

Although meticulous documentation of injuries is usually associated with the work of the forensic pathologist, the pathologist should undertake a careful external examination of the front and back of the body and document the presence of any fresh or old marks of injury even in those dying suddenly and unexpectedly at home, for example from a ruptured abdominal aneurysm. The absence of any comment within the external examination part of the report of the presence of injuries where old or fresh marks clearly existed may, if the findings of the examination are brought into question, be considered as an indication of the quality of the examination that was undertaken by the pathologist.

Legal definition

When one describes injuries – within the report/statement or in verbal evidence – one must be certain of the correct use of terminology. Milroy provides us with a concise summary of the case law and definitions within this area, which can be further summarised as follows: bodily injury is simply defined as physical injury to the body whereas the use of the term 'wound', in English law, should be reserved for those injuries where the full thickness of the skin (i.e. the epidermis and dermis) is breached (Milroy, 2005). This legal definition thus excludes abrasions, bruises, penetrating injuries of the eye, and closed internal injuries and fractures.

General comments

Injuries are traditionally divided into five groups: the bruise; the abrasion; the laceration; the incised wound; and the burn (Knight, 2004). Gunshot wounds can be considered as a specific form of laceration. The use of the correct terminology is essential as this will assist in the identification of the mechanism of causation. For example, abrasions, bruises and lacerations are caused by blunt trauma whereas incised wounds are caused by sharp-edge trauma. The use of phrases such as 'an incised laceration' is incorrect and meaningless (Milroy and Rutty, 1997).

The groups can then be subjectively subdivided into 'fresh' injuries (< 48 hours) and 'old' injuries (> 48 hours). The state of healing should be documented as this may become important in the timing of an injury in relation to its causation. Histological examination and the use of histochemical/immuno-histochemical stains can be considered for the dating of injuries (Van de Goot, 2008).

Injuries can occur anywhere on the body, in any age group, and each has a different mechanism of causation. When one considers causation one must remember that an injury can be ante-, peri- or post-mortem and arise due to medical intervention, resuscitation, violence, handling of the body, and embalming. An injury can alter after death owing to post-mortem decomposition or, for example, animal or insect predation. The position on the body can assist in determining whether the injury was accidental, self-inflicted or inflicted by a second party, which will have significant implications if an assault is alleged.

When one comes across an injury it should be recorded both in writing and in pictorial form. Injuries should be photographed, at right angles to the injury with a suitable scale, if a second party is involved (Fig. 9.1). It is important to be able to recognise the colour yellow – which can be produced in any paint processing program with the colours red (240), green (240) and blue (000). As there is wide variation in the general population's ability to perceive yellow, a standardised colour chart should be included when photographing bruises to ensure consistency in colour interpretation (Langlois, 2007). The use of alternative light sources for intra-dermal injuries should be considered.

The description of an injury should define the

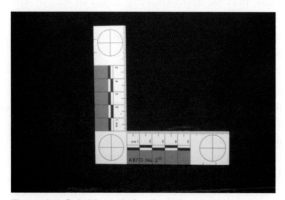

Figure 9.1 Suitable scale for photographing injuries.

type using one of the foregoing five groups (singularly or in combination) and then describe its shape, colour, age (old or fresh), dimension and position on the body related to an anatomical site, which should be recorded in lay terms. All of this should be recorded in the autopsy contemporaneous notes, in writing, diagrams and – where appropriate – photography. In some institutions, surface injuries can be captured using surface laser scanners or modern radiological imaging for subsequent computer image production and injury causation reconstruction (Thali *et al.* 2003) – although the author's experience of such technology is that the injury can be both visualised and described in far greater detail using naked eye examination and digital photography than by the use of this technology.

Blunt trauma injury

Abrasions

An abrasion, which can be referred to in lay terms as a graze or a scratch, is the most superficial of the blunt trauma injuries. Strictly speaking it is an injury that is confined to the epidermis; although, owing to the anatomy of the skin, abrasions may extend to involve the papillary dermis. As this latter site is where small blood vessels are found, abrasions may bleed. Unlike bruises, abrasions can occur both before or after death. Distinguishing between the two is important in cases, for example, where a body has been moved after death in an attempt to conceal it or simply remove it from the place of death. Abrasions also change character in the post-mortem period, becoming brown and leathery (parchmented) in appearance. Abrasions often ooze plasma, and may be coated with a 'scab'.

Abrasions can be formed by the application of a force in either a tangential direction (a 'brush' abrasion) or a vertical direction (a 'crush' abrasion). The force can be generated either by the body itself moving across or onto a static surface (e.g. a fall against a wall) or by the surface of an object moving across the static or moving body (e.g. being struck by a piece of wood).

Brush abrasions may be seen, for example, when a

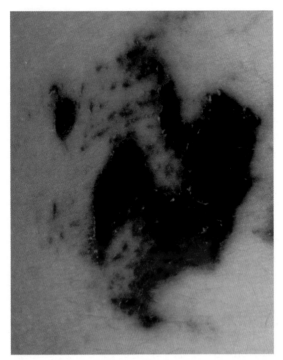

Figure 9.2 Brush abrasion with skin tags.

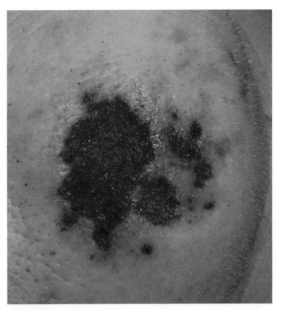

Figure 9.3 Crush abrasion.

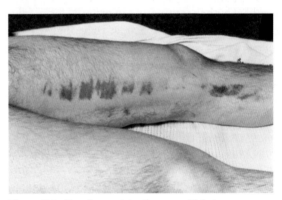

Figure 9.4 Abrasions arising from a vehicle tyre.

person has been dragged along the ground by a vehicle or if the subject was struck by a rough surface such as a glancing kick by a shod foot. The direction of the applied force may be determined by the presence of a terminal tag of skin at the point distal to the first point of impact (Fig. 9.2). A crush abrasion will have no such tag, as the vertically applied force will leave an impact impression (Fig 9.3). This can again be used to determine the causation of the wound, for example a stamping injury from a shod foot. Such marks may have patterns within them derived from the object. An example of this is a ligature mark.

Abrasions may be found in combination with other blunt trauma injuries such as lacerations or bruises. An example of this is the mark that may be generated when a person falls backwards onto a tarmacked road.

Abrasions may show characteristic shapes and patterns to assist with consideration of the mechanism of causation (Fig. 9.4). Two good examples of this are fingernail and bite marks. Fingernail marks can be seen, for example, in cases of strangulation where the victim has caused the marks to the neck while trying to remove a ligature or assailant's hand.

They may be approximately 5 mm in length and straight or curved. Caution must be expressed not to over-interpret the curve in relation to how the nail was applied to the skin, as the curve may be opposite to that of the applied nail. The most superficial form of a bite mark may be a semicircular collection of abraded skin marks. In both types of injury, consideration should be given to swabbing the injury in an attempt to retrieve the assailant's DNA, which may be present at the site by the process of secondary transfer (Rutty, 2002; Graham and Rutty, 2008).

Thus, in relation to the external examination, the abrasion should be described within the fresh or old injuries section of the report/statement, depending on its apparent subjective age. There should be a description of its appearance, size and anatomical location. An example is presented below:

The following fresh injury was present: a brush abrasion, 4.5 cm × 2.6 cm to the posterior aspect of the left lower arm (forearm), 7 cm above the wrist. Skin tags were present to the lower-most aspect (edge nearest the wrist).

Bruises

Bruises may also be known as contusions, although the former implies an injury that can be seen through the skin and the latter an injury to the deeper tissue or an internal organ. A bruise is a blunt trauma injury, which may occur on its own where the skin remains intact or in combination with other types of injury. Bruises are an extravascular collection of blood where blood has leaked from damaged arterioles, venules or veins but not capillaries. Bleeding from capillaries is not visible to the naked eye. Bruises can vary in size, which can be further used to aid their description.

When describing a bruise the pathologist usually refers to an injury that is present within the subcutaneous tissues. However, so-called intra-dermal bruises may occur where the blood accumulates in the sub-epidermal area. Such bruises occur when the skin is distorted by being forced between ridges or grooves of an object. Bruises related to tyre marks or shoe tread marks are examples of such bruises (Fig. 9.5).

The smallest form of a bruise is the petechial haemorrhage. The presence or absence of petechial haemorrhages should be sought at every autopsy. Although they can occur on any aspect of the external surface of the body, they are often found, case dependent, in the skin of the face, particularly around the eyes or behind the ears as well as to the mucosal surfaces of the eyelids and mouth. They can also be seen to the deeper tissues – for example the deep aspect of the scalp or to internal organs. Those to the scalp may be a pure post-mortem artefact, so caution must be expressed in their interpretation, if present. They can occur in approximately 20 per

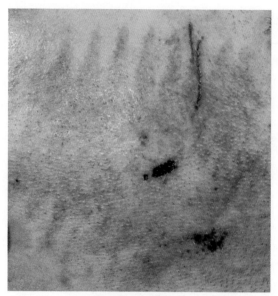

Figure 9.5 Bruise caused by the tread of the sole of a shoe.

cent of natural deaths such as heart attacks as well as in those dying of the various forms of asphyxia. The presence of petechial haemorrhages on the head and neck should be regarded as an indication to perform a layered anterior and posterior neck dissection in a bloodless field, to exclude unnatural causes of death. Petechial and larger, punctuate, haemorrhages may also be seen in the post-mortem period as part of the process of hypostasis.

As with other forms of injury, there are several factors that will affect the appearance of the bruise. The position of the bruise on the body itself will influence the appearance. Bruising occurs more easily to areas where the skin is lax (e.g. around the eye) as opposed to the palms where the skin is fibrous. Obese individuals bruise more readily than those with a normal or low body mass index. The laxity of the skin will also allow for blood to move from the site of injury to another site. An example of this is the black eye, which can arise by movement of blood from an injury to the forehead, nose or orbital parts of the frontal bone. If the skin is thin over a bone or bony prominence, then damage can be done more easily to the blood vessels than in fatty areas. The age of the patient, the fragility of the blood vessels, and the presence of any natural disease or drug

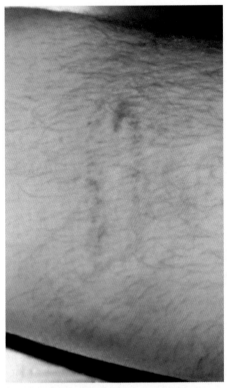

Figure 9.6 So-called 'tram track' bruise.

Figure 9.7 Fingertip bruises.

therapy that alters the coagulability of the blood are all factors that affect the appearance of a bruise (Vanezis, 2001).

Bruises may take hours to days to form and appear in the skin, although a deep bruise may never be seen on the external surface of the body. These larger collections of blood under the skin are known as haematomas. To find such injuries a more extensive dissection of the soft tissues of the body is required. Bruises change colour with time, the traditional sequence being red, blue, green, yellow and brown. Two bruises inflicted at the same point on the body at the same time may appear different in colour. A bruise in the elderly may retain one colour considerably longer than that of a child, or a bruise may miss out some steps of the sequence. The most important colour for ageing a bruise, as discussed above, is yellow – although the identification of yellow within a bruise is often not as easy as it may seem (Langlois, 2007).

The site of a bruise and its appearance, if correctly documented, may assist in identification of the cause of the injury. Examples are 'tram track' bruising (parallel linear bruises with a space between – Fig. 9.6) caused by a cylindrical or rectangular object; patterned bruises from the sole of a shoe, and discoid-shaped bruises of approximately 1 cm diameter suggestive of 'fingertip' bruises left by gripping or, if in pairs, pinching (Fig. 9.7).

As with abrasions, bite marks may cause pure bruises. Assistance should be sought from a forensic odontologist to consider whether the mark is caused by an animal or a human, be it a child or an adult (Fig. 9.8). Such bruises may be caused by the teeth or by the action of suction (the so-called 'love-bite').

Not all pink areas are bruises. The classic mistake is to see pink areas over the elbows, hip and knee regions which may in fact not be bruises but rather reflect the changes of hypothermia. Such changes are also seen in bodies that have been refrigerated for some time, perhaps over a weekend. If necessary, the lesion can be incised and sampled for histological examination.

Although bruises are traditionally considered to be an ante- or peri-mortem injury owing to the requirement for sufficient pressure to be present to force the blood out of the vessels into the surround-

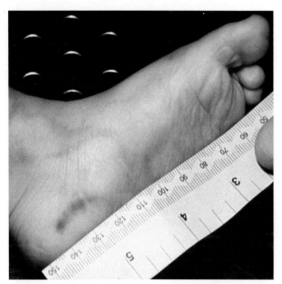

Figure 9.8 Bruising caused by a child biting a child.

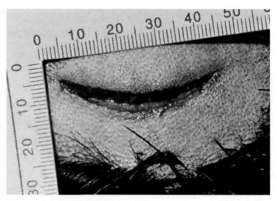

Figure 9.9 Laceration.

ing tissue, a few publications do suggest that bruising to a body may occur after death. However, it is generally accepted that for this to occur the force required is great. Polson *et al.* (1985) was able to produce bruises in the post-mortem period by striking the occiput with a mallet. It has also been reported that a body, devoid of bruises prior to burial, when exhumed showed a number of bruises that the author attributed to having occurred in the post-mortem period (Burke *et al.*, 1998). In addition to this it should be rememebered that deep contusions may take some time to become apparent as dermal bruises. Injuries that are not apparent at the time of the autopsy may be visible if the body is re-examined 24–48 hours later.

Lacerations

A laceration is a blunt trauma injury with a resulting tear to the involved tissue. As it is a tearing injury the wound has irregular margins, bruising and crushing to the edges, and may have persistent strands of tissue or hair across the wound. All these features can be used to distinguish a laceration from an incised wound (Fig. 9.9).

The causative force of the laceration may be vertical or tangential to the body, and this will affect the appearance of the wound. If a weapon is involved then this may cause a shape to the laceration that can assist in the subsequent identification of the injury's causation – for example the curved laceration associated with a blow from a hammer. Lacerations tend to occur on the body where the skin is supported by a rigid underlying structure (the body's skeleton). As a result, they are caused easily to the scalp, face, mouth and shin areas but are rarely seen on the abdomen. They can occur to the chest or abdomen but more force is required to cause an injury to this site.

A blow from a weapon may cause a laceration that has an appearance similar to that of an incised wound. A commonly quoted example of this is a blow from an axe where an examination of the underlying bone can assist in identifying a possible causation (Knight, 2004). Lacerations may also occur when broken bones protrude through the skin – for example broken nasal bones.

Extreme forms of lacerations are those associated with blunt penetrating injuries as can occur when a body is impaled on an object such as a railing. Flaying and degloving injuries where large areas of both the skin and subcutaneous tissues are torn from the body may be associated with injuries resulting from the rotating wheel of a vehicle. Degloving injuries may be open or closed. The open degloving injuries can be truly considered to be lacerations as there is a full-thickness split in the skin caused by blunt force trauma. Closed degloving injuries are more difficult to characterise. They are not uncommonly discovered in the victims of road traffic collisions, particularly pedestrians. In a closed degloving injury there is no tear in the skin, but evisceration reveals that the skin and superficial soft tissues have been sheared from the underlying structures.

Firearm injuries

Firearm injuries are a form of laceration. A detailed consideration of the pathology of firearm injuries is beyond the scope of this book, so the reader should refer to more specialised texts (DiMaio, 1999). However, all pathologists performing an autopsy must be able to recognise firearm injuries in order to know when to stop and refer deaths to a pathologist with forensic training. This section will thus be confined to a brief synopsis of the external appearances of the main two categories of firearms (rifled and non-rifled weapons) as well as a brief consideration of injuries caused by crossbows and explosives.

The external wound will provide an indication of the category of weapon as well as the angle at which the projectile entered the body and the distance of discharge of the weapon from the body. Prior to examination, radiological imaging should be performed. Discharge residue swabs, which often come in pre-packaged kits, can be sampled from the body prior to autopsy. Care must be taken with the use of such swabs/kits that the person undertaking the sampling is not carrying residue from other weapon sources.

Rifling is the process of adding grooves to the inner surface of the barrel of a firearm to apply a spin to the bullet to improve the accuracy of the shot. Rifled weapons fire a single projectile and include handguns and rifles. The appearance of the wound, as with non-rifled weapons, is dependent on the distance of discharge of the weapon from the body and the area of the body that the projectile passes through. Contact wounds can be discoloured owing to the effect of carbon monoxide within the muzzle gases. Those occurring over bone classically show stellate tearing of the wound edges due to the action of muzzle gas pressure. The muzzle itself can cause a patterned abrasion to the wound edges. Sooting and propellant tattooing are a feature of near contact and intermediate wounds (Fig. 9.10). The entrance wound can show burning to the edges, with the size dependent on the size of the projectile. Fragments of clothing may be drawn into the wound, and so-

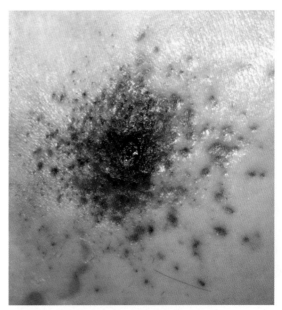

Figure 9.10 Near-contact rifled weapon injury.

called 'bullet wipe' may be seen to the edges of the wound or underlying bone. As the distance of discharge increases, the wound margin becomes devoid of sooting, burning and tattooing.

Injuries caused by crossbows and arrows can have a similar shape and size to those of, for example, handguns. A radiological examination will show the absence of a projectile in the body in a case with an entrance but no exit wound. This may cause initial confusion to those investigating the death until it is realised that they may be dealing with a crossbow- or arrow-related death (Fig. 9.11).

The shotgun is an example of a non-rifled weapon. Although it can discharge single projectiles,

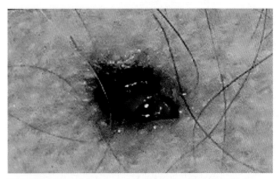

Figure 9.11 Crossbow injury mimicking a handgun entrance wound.

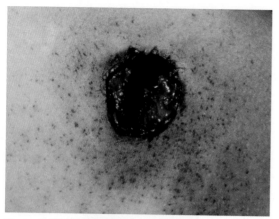

Figure 9.12 Shotgun injury.

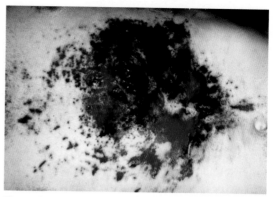

Figure 9.14 Injury as a result of an explosion.

more commonly multiple projectiles are fired. Thus, as for rifled weapons, the wound edge can show splitting, burning, sooting, pink change and tattooing depending on the distance of discharge. However, the entrance wound is larger and more irregular; and as the distance of discharge increases one sees multiple entrance wounds caused by multiple projectiles as well as injuries caused by the wadding striking the body (Fig. 9.12).

Shotgun injuries to the head tend to be extremely disruptive. Reconstruction of the skin and cranial bones may be required for the pathologist to examine the entrance wound.

Injuries caused by buckshot can show an appearance suggestive of an injury caused by a rifled

weapon. It may not be until the projectiles are recovered from the body that this type of shot is identified as the causation of the fatal wounds (Fig. 9.13).

Air-powered weapons and so-called humane killers can cause a fatal penetrating injury, the characteristics of the injury being determined by the type of weapon or projectile involved (Hunt and Kon, 1962; Milroy *et al.*, 1998).

Where the death has occurred in relation to an explosion, a variety of external and internal injuries may occur, including amputation and severe disruption of the body. Multiple projectile lacerations may be present of variable size as well as burning and dust tattooing (Fig. 9.14). A detailed examination of the body for device components may be required, and radiological examination of the body to assist in the recovery of these is essential.

Sharp-edge injuries: incised wounds

Incised wounds are caused by sharp objects, such as a knife, glass or pottery. They can be further subdivided into two types:

- the cut/slash where the length of the injury is longer than its depth;
- the stab wound where the depth is greater than the width.

Both types (unlike a laceration) will have clean, well-demarcated edges with minimal injury to the immediate surrounding tissues.

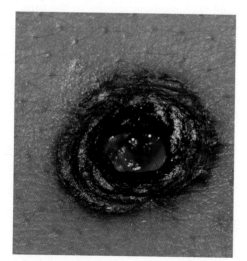

Figure 9.13 Buckshot injury mimicking a handgun injury.

Examination of an incised wound may yield a considerable amount of information, which can in turn be used to identify a causative weapon. In the case of a stab wound, the site on the body and the relationship to any adjacent wounds should be recorded, such as whether it has gone in and out through the arm and into the armpit. The dimensions of the wound should be recorded to estimate the possible width of the blade – although the length of the wound may underestimate the width of the blade owing to elastic recoil of the skin. The depth of penetration will not only identify what structures have been injured and whether these injuries were life-threatening, but also provides an estimate of the length of the blade. Again, this may under- or overestimate the true length of the blade. If the blade has passed all the way into the body, an area of bruising or abrasion may be present at one end of the wound where the hilt of the weapon or the hand of the assailant has impacted on the skin resulting in a blunt trauma injury.

Where multiple injuries are present the pathologist should consider whether or not the same weapon caused all the injuries, as this may indicate the possible involvement of a second assailant (Fig. 9.15).

The force used to inflict the injury should be estimated – although this is often a subjective assessment (Davidson, 2004; Hainsworth *et al.*, 2007). The skin provides the greatest resistance to the insertion of a blade and once penetrated a blade may be inserted into the body with minimal force.

The two types of incised wound commonly described are the self-inflicted injury and the defence injury. Self-inflicted injuries can occur on any part of the body that the deceased could reach with their own hand. In the case of incised wounds they are classically shallow cuts that occur as parallel groups of injuries, for example to the side of the neck or anterior aspect of the lower arms. There may be numerous shallow incised wounds ('intention incisions') associated with a deeper incision, produced as the deceased develops the courage to make the final incision.

Defence-type injuries occur as the defendant tries to ward off an attack. It is the position of the injury

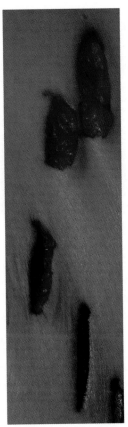

Figure 9.15 Stab wounds caused by the use of two knives wielded simultaneously.

on the body rather than the nature of the injury itself that enables use of the term 'defence injury'. In the case of incised wounds the blade may be grabbed in the hand with resultant injuries to the palms and fingers. If the hand is held up in front of the blade this may result in a penetrating hand injury. If the defendant tried to curl up into a ball, injuries may be seen to the legs and arms.

As indicated above, knives are not the only weapons to cause incised wounds. The wound shape may in fact be characteristic for another type of object; examples are the irregular 'Z' shape caused by scissors, the cruciform '+' shape of the screwdriver, and the small rhomboid marks of shattered glass.

Burns

A burn injury is an area of tissue damage caused by the effect of heat, cold, electricity, acid or alkali – as a result of either direct transfer of thermal energy or indirectly when another form of energy is converted to heat (e.g. electrical energy, chemical or friction injuries). Burn injuries can be caused by extremes of temperatures. In the case of heat they can be caused either by wet/moist heat (scalding) or by dry heat by conduction or radiation.

The resulting damage to the body can be charted using the 'rule of nines' to determine the total area burnt. The pathologist should also determine whether the burns are superficial or full-thickness (Cooper, 2006). The terms first-, second- and third-degree are no longer used to describe the severity of burns.

As with the other injuries (except the bruise), burns can occur before or after death. This is an important issue as one part of the investigation will be to determine at what point the person died. The distribution of burns is also important when considering whether an attempt has been made to dispose of the body by fire or, in the case of a living victim, whether it was an accident or abuse. In the latter case it is important to know the temperature of the material causing the burn, the surface area of contact and the time of heat exposure (Moritz and Henriques, 1947).

The severity of thermal burns is dependent on the temperature of the heat source causing the burn, the presence or absence of overlying clothing (which may protect from dry burns and exacerbate wet burns), and the duration of the exposure to the heat source. An object at 40°C may take several hours to produce a burn whereas an object at or exceeding 60°C may produce a burn within seconds.

Burns may present the shape of their causation. Examples are the contact burn of a cigarette lighter or the bars of an electric fire, and the blister on the finger of an electrical contact point. Those resulting from lightening may show a fern leaf pattern to the chest or limbs due to conduction of the electrical impulse through the small vessels of the skin, and may be associated with disruption of the clothing. The run patterns of scalds should be examined to determine whether they were accidental or inflicted by another party.

Old marks of injury

Healing injuries and scars

During the examination the pathologist should attempt to distinguish between fresh, recent and old/historical injuries. Healing injuries can be placed into the old injury description section, but it should be recorded that the injury is a healing injury rather than a scar. This is important as it may relate to an incident 1–2 weeks ago that could be related to the deceased's death. There may also be a pattern of injury to the body suggestive of poor medical care or neglect (e.g. healing pressure sores) or physical abuse (child, domestic or elder).

The state of healing and any complications to the wound should be noted. Consideration should be given to undertaking a microscopic or microbiological examination of such injuries should a complication such as wound infection or septicaemia be considered. Finally, the absence of scars to areas of the body such as the ears, elbows, buttocks and heels should be noted if the care of an individual comes under question.

All scars should be noted and their length, appearance and anatomical site documented. At times it is useful to subdivide scars into those arising as a result of an old injury and those occurring as a consequence of previous medical intervention. If there are a large number of scars (e.g. to the back of the upper limbs in old people or the limbs of those who self-harm) it is permissible to group scars of similar causation into one description, noting the number, site, state of healing, and the smallest and largest lengths present.

Although scars tend to be non-specific in appearance they can suggest their causation. A good example of this is the presence of multiple, linear scars to the fronts of the forearms in those who cause self-inflicted injuries. A special type of scar formation is that of keloid; usually seen in Afro-Caribbean people, this can form extensive disfiguring areas of scaring.

An example of how to record such marks is as follows:

The following old injuries were present: (1) a 3 cm horizontally orientated well-healed scar to the anterior aspect of the right knee; (2) a 9 cm appendicectomy scar to the right lower quadrant of the abdomen.

Amputations and contractures

The part of the body that has been amputated surgically and the condition of the scar is recorded as for any other surgical scar. Contractures may arise in association with neurological diseases or in those who have suffered extensive burns. Dupuytren's contractures are an example of deformities of the hands and may be idiopathic or associated with the use of phenytoin.

Fractures

Fractures are internal injuries that can cause external abnormalities. They can result in deformities, for example, of the limbs or rib cage, or false mobility/laxity of joints. Closed penetrating injuries of the pleural cavities may result in surgical emphysema, which may manifest as palpable crepitations or abnormal swelling of, for example, the neck or – in extreme cases – the scrotal sac. Identification of a long bone fracture either through external palpation and manipulation or radiography may be sufficient in some cases, although lower limb injuries as a result of road traffic incidents will require invasive exploration.

References

Burke MP, Olumbe AK, Opeskin K (1998). Postmortem extravasation of blood potentially simulating antemortem bruising. *Am J Forensic Med Pathol* 19:46–9.

Cooper PN (2006). Burn injury. In: Rutty GN (ed.) *Essentials of Autopsy Practice: New Advances, Trends and Developments*. London: Springer.

Davison AM (2004). The incised wound. In: Rutty GN (ed.) *Essentials of Autopsy Practice: New Advances, Trends and Developments*. London: Springer.

DiMaio VJM (1999). *Gunshot Wounds: Practical Aspects of Firearms, Ballistics and Forensic Techniques*, 2nd edn. London: CRC.

Graham EA, Rutty GN (2008). Investigation into 'normal' background DNA on adult necks: implications for DNA profiling of manual strangulation victims. *J Forensic Sci* 53:1074–82.

Hainsworth SV, Delaney RJ, Rutty GN (2007). How sharp is sharp? Methods for quantifying the sharpness and penetrability of kitchen knives used in stabbings. *Int J Legal Med* 122:281–91.

Hunt AC, Kon VM (1962). The pattern of injury in humane killers. *Med Sci Law* 37:139–44.

Knight B (2004). The pathology of wounds. In: *Forensic Pathology*, 3rd edn. London: Hodder Education.

Langlois NEI (2007). The science behind the quest to determine the age of bruises: a review of the English language literature. *Forensic Sci Med Pathol* 3:241–51.

Milroy CM (2005). Scalp, facial and gunshot injuries. In: Whitwell HL (ed.) *Forensic Neuropathology*. London: Hodder Arnold.

Milroy CM, Rutty GN (1997). If a wound is 'neatly incised' it is not a laceration. *Br Med J* 315:1312.

Milroy CM, Clark JC, Carter N, Rutty G (1998). Air weapon fatalities. *J Clin Pathol* 51:525–9.

Moritz AR, Henriques FC (1947). Studies of thermal injury. II. The relative importance of time and surface temperature in the causation of cutaneous burns. *Am J Pathol* 23:695–720.

Polson CJ, Gee DJ, Knight B (1985). *The Essentials of Forensic Medicine*, 4th edn. Oxford: Pergamon Press, pp. 102–4.

Rutty GN (2002). An investigation into the transference and survivability of human DNA following simulated manual strangulation with consideration of the problem of third party contamination. *Int J Legal Med* 116(3):170–3.

Thali MJ, Braun M, Dirnhofer R (2003). Optical 3D surface digitizing in forensic medicine: 3D documentation of skin and bone injuries. *Forensic Sci Int* 137(2/3):203–8.

Van de Goot FRW (2008). The chronological dating of injury. In: Rutty GN (ed.) *Essentials of Autopsy Practice: New Advances, Trends and Developments*. London: Springer.

Vanezis P (2001). Bruising: concepts of aging and interpretation. In: Rutty GN (ed.) *Essentials of Autopsy Practice*, Vol. 1. London: Springer.

Chapter 10

THE EVISCERATION

Guy N Rutty and Julian L Burton

Introduction

Once the pathologist has confirmed that authority has been given to undertake an invasive autopsy examination, has identified that the correct body is presented, and has personally undertaken a detailed external examination, the body may be opened and eviscerated to permit a detailed examination of the viscera. Before opening the body the pathologist should consider whether samples are needed for toxicological or microbiological purposes that could be contaminated during the evisceration process. If required, clean urine can be collected using a suprapubic stab, blood can be aspirated from the femoral vein, and vitreous humour can be aspirated from the eye. The techniques used to obtain such specimens are discussed in Chapter 15.

The techniques employed to eviscerate a body have apparently altered little in recent times, with the possible exception of a move away from the 'standard' midline incision used to open the body (Box, 1919; Wilson, 1972). Too often, this aspect of the autopsy examination is delegated to the anatomical pathology technologist (APT), and not infrequently is undertaken in the absence of the pathologist. The evisceration is a vital aspect of the autopsy and should ideally be performed by the pathologist. In a busy mortuary, the evisceration may be undertaken by the APT but the pathologist should be on hand to inspect the organs at each stage and prior to their removal. It is

strongly recommended that the evisceration be performed by the pathologist in investigations of postoperative deaths, otherwise vital information can be lost (Start and Cross, 1999). Similarly in cases of trauma, decomposition, or if there is an element of suspicion or homicide, the pathologist should undertake the process as he or she is required to observe findings within each body cavity as it is opened and examined. Under no circumstances should the APT be permitted to eviscerate a body before the pathologist has undertaken an external examination.

In this chapter, the techniques employed to open the body cavities and remove the contents of the thorax, abdomen and pelvis are described. These techniques require modification in certain circumstances, for example when examining the muscles of the rectus sheath, and such modifications are dealt with. The methods employed in removing the brain, spinal cord, eyes, middle ears and vertebral arteries are described in Chapter 12.

From time to time the pathologist may have to perform a procedure that is not routinely performed during a hospital or medicolegal autopsy. These are commonly referred to as 'special procedures', although in truth the pathologist should be fully proficient in any procedure that may be required during an autopsy. As with other aspects of the general examination, under the Human Tissue Act 2006 these procedures must be carried out at licensed premises by a registered medical practitioner or a

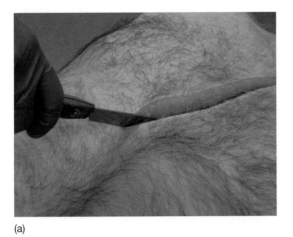

(a)

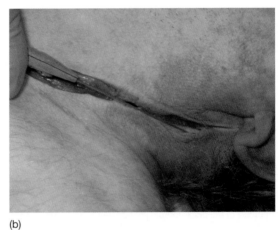

(b)

Figure 10.1 Making a skin incision. (a) The knife is held perpendicular to the skin. (b) The chamfered incision produced when the blade is not held perpendicular to the skin.

person in the employment of a health authority acting on the instructions of a registered medical practitioner (see Chapter 4 for more information on the Act). We have included within this chapter the so-called 'special procedures' that can be employed to enhance the examination. These techniques have been placed into the relevant cavity or organ system to provide a more logical layout. Those examinations related to organs rather than general evisceration have been incorporated into the chapter concerning dissection (Chapter 11)

Incisions

A variety of incisions can be used to open the body (Knight, 1996). These basically all involve a midline anterior approach and differ in respect of the neck dissection. Regardless of the method chosen, the body should be placed in the supine position with a block under the shoulders to extend the neck. The incision should be made with a sharp fresh blade held perpendicular to the skin. This produces a clean cut that is easy to close at the end of the autopsy (Fig. 10.1a). If the blade is held at an angle, a chamfered skin incision results, which can give rise to an unsatisfactory reconstruction (Fig. 10.1b).

The incision used needs to be safe for the operator. It should provide maximum exposure and at the same time permit a satisfactory reconstruction of the body. We recommend that a U-shaped or Y-shaped incision be used (Fig. 10.2a). The incision begins 1 cm behind the external auditory meatus, passes down the lateral aspect of the neck as posteriorly as possible, and crosses over the clavicle over the outer third (Fig. 10.2b). A similar incision is made on the opposite side and joined with a smooth curve meeting over the sternal angle. This produces a flap of skin that can be cleared from connective tissue back to the mandible (Fig. 10.2c). While reflecting the skin of the neck, the blade is angled away from the skin, so avoiding damage to the skin itself. This reveals the neck structures, submandibular glands and the parotid glands and makes the removal of the tongue a visible and safe process. The incision is then followed down the anterior body wall, skirting the umbilicus, to the mons pubis.

Other techniques widely practised include a T-shaped incision that is also known as a 'bucket handle' incision (Fig. 10.3a) and a single midline incision (Fig. 10.3b). With the former technique, the neck is opened with a transverse incision which runs from acromion process to acromion process along the line of the clavicles; in the latter a single incision is made from the laryngeal prominence to the mons pubis. Earlier texts have regarded the single midline incision as the 'standard' for opening the body, preferring it over the U-shaped or V-shaped incision described above (Box, 1919; Wilson, 1972). However, both the T-shaped and

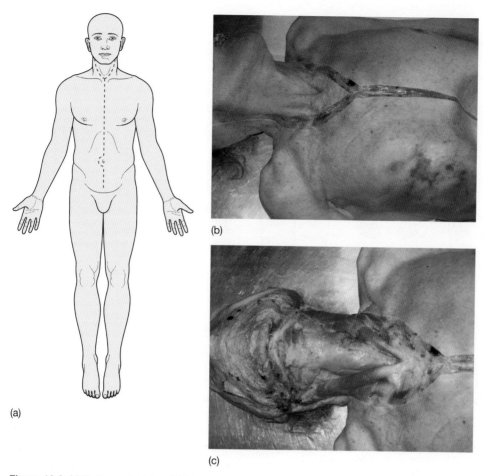

(a)

(b)

(c)

Figure 10.2 (a) Y-shaped incision. (b) Dissection of the Y-shaped neck incision. (c) Reflection of the neck skin flap.

the 'standard' incision are to be avoided as they do not allow adequate visualisation of the neck structures. Although popular with some APTs because it results in less sewing at the end of the autopsy, the use of a single midline incision is especially dangerous to the operator as it does not allow room for dissection of the tongue and neck under direct vision. In addition, single midline incisions disfigure the neck and result in a reconstruction that may be unacceptable to the relatives of the deceased. When viewed in a funeral home, a U or Y incision leads to a better presentation as the neck is not as distorted by the presence of midline sutures and the lateral neck sutures can be hidden by careful placement of the pillow or bed sheets. Thus the single midline incision should be vigorously avoided in autopsy practice.

In cases where the consent given for a hospital ('consent') autopsy to be performed is limited and forbids opening of the neck (or indeed of the thorax), the body may be opened via a T-shaped subcostal incision. An initial midline incision is made extending from the xiphisternum to the mons pubis. The skin and muscles of the abdomen can then be incised along the costochondral margins (Fig. 10.3c). The skin flaps so produced fall away to give safe and wide access to the abdominal and pelvic cavities.

Dissection of the neck

Whenever there is a possibility of trauma to the neck (as, for example, in hanging, strangulation, or where there is bruising in the anterior neck or petechial

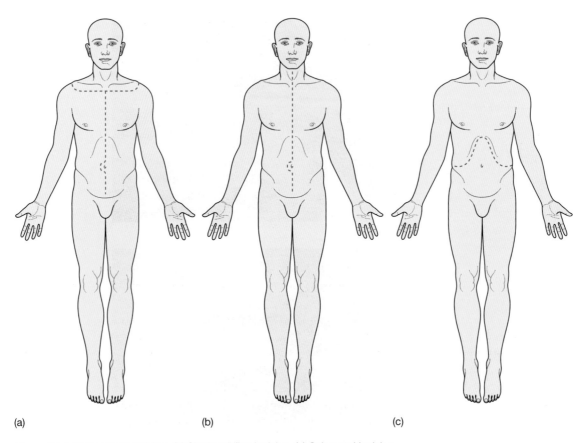

(a)   (b)   (c)

Figure 10.3 (a) T-shaped incision. (b) Single midline incision. (c) Subcostal incision.

haemorrhages in the eyes) the skull should be opened first and the brain removed. The chest and abdomen should then be opened and the thoracic contents removed utilising an incision across the thoracic inlet. This leaves the neck structures *in situ* for layered dissection. Removal of the cranial and thoracic contents decompresses the neck veins, which is done in an attempt to differentiate artefactual 'Prinsloo–Gordon' haemorrhages within the neck from traumatic bruises (Prinsloo and Gordon, 1951; Rutty *et al.*, 2005). If trauma is not suspected and there are no external marks or bruising to the strap muscles on reflection of the skin, then removal of the tongue and neck structures in continuity with the thoracic organs can proceed.

Dissection of the neck can be considered from two aspects, the front and the back. The former is the more often performed although the latter may be of more importance – for example in a case involving the application of force to the neck (e.g. in manual strangulation where there may be more bruising found in the posterior neck compartment than in the anterior one) or in cases of hyper-extension or flexion of the neck as may occur in the shaken baby syndrome or road traffic incidents.

Anterior approach to neck dissection

The anterior approach starts with a Y-shaped incision to the skin of the neck, which is reflected back to the level of the jaw (Fig. 10.4a). The immediate subcutaneous tissue and platysma muscles are inspected (Fig. 10.4b). An in-situ layered dissection of the structures is then performed. The insertion of each sternocleidomastoid muscle into the clavicle is identified and incised. Each muscle in turn is then dissected to the level of the jaw (Fig. 10.4c). The lesser belly of each omohyoid is then identified (Fig. 10.4d) and dissected off to the attachment on the hyoid bone. In a similar manner, the sternohyoid and sternothyroid muscles are dissected away (Fig. 10.4e and f). Finally the thyrohyoid muscles are lifted away from the thyroid cartilage (Fig. 10.4g). At this stage the hyoid bone, thyroid and cricoid cartilages are examined *in situ*. The thyroid gland is incised and can be removed and weighed. The tongue is detached and the central neck structures are removed. Each carotid sheath is then examined (Fig. 10.4h). The internal jugular vein and carotid artery and its branches are identified, examined and opened *in situ* with blunt-nosed scissors (Fig. 10.4i). The vagus nerve is also examined *in situ*. The oesophagus is opened on the back of the neck pluck. An incision is made to the lateral aspect of the hyoid bone and laryngeal cartilage to examine the greater horns and the hyoid bone is separated from the base of the tongue. The tongue is cut in half with an incision starting at the base and running transversely to the tip. Finally the larynyx and trachea are opened from behind (Vanezis, 1989; Adams, 1990, 1991). Histological examination of hyoid bone, laryngeal and cricoid fractures can be performed in order to assess vitality and injury age.

An alternative method of dissection of the larynx has been described by Maxeiner (1998). This provides a method to assist with the examination for incomplete fractures of the dorsal surfaces of the thyroid laminae and incomplete or non-dislocated fractures of the cricoid cartilage. It requires the complete resection of the thyroid cartilage and a horizontal incision through the cricoid cartilage before opening the larynx dorsally.

Posterior approach to neck dissection

The body must be completely turned over to examine the neck from behind. The usual scalp incision is extended down along each side of the neck to the level of the shoulders and the skin reflected downwards. As this examination should be undertaken in conjunction with the anterior inspection, a single Y incision to the neck allows both compartments to be examined. As with the anterior approach, a layered dissection is performed with each muscle being examined in turn. The muscles are detached from their superior attachment to the skull and reflected downwards towards the back. Exposure of the posterior aspect of the cervical spine allows for inspection of the ligaments, bones and upper aspect of the vertebral arteries. This approach also allows for the posterior periosteum to be removed from the skull to allow for inspection of, for example, lambdoid wormian bones or posterior skull fractures.

The thorax and abdomen

The skin and muscles of the chest wall are freed from the rib-cage taking care not to disrupt the intercostal muscles. Bruising that may be the result of cardiopulmonary resuscitation or other trauma to the soft tissues of the anterior chest wall is noted if present. Tears may occur to the anterior and posterior chest muscles in bodies that have been dragged by their arms or have hung by their arms from a height – for example a person dangling by the arms from a window or balcony.

Demonstration of a pneumothorax

The possibility of the presence of a pneumothorax should always be considered before starting the autopsy, since procedures for demonstrating one must be performed prior to opening the thoracic cavity. Three methods of demonstrating a pneumothorax are described, one being a more refined version of another which requires more equipment. Prior to any procedure the need to perform or review any radiological imaging must be considered. Putrefactive decomposition may result in a false–positive test, whichever method is chosen.

Direct inspection

In the first method the usual midline incision is made to the anterior chest skin. A layered dissection

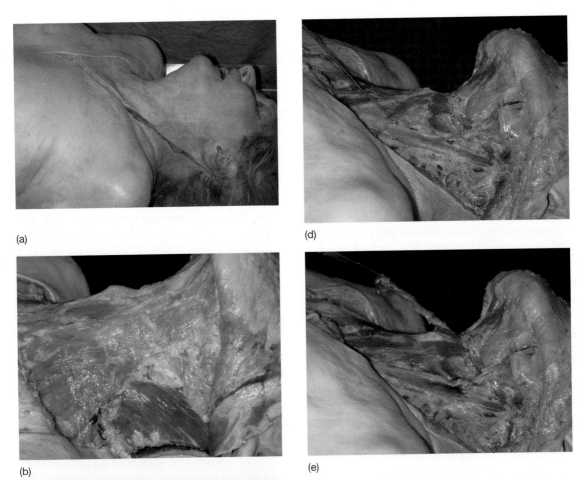

(a)

(b)

(c)

(d)

(e)

Figure 10.4 (a) A Y-shaped incision is made to the neck. (b) The skin is reflected and the platysma is inspected. (c) The sternomastoid muscle is exposed. (d) The omohyoid is exposed. (e) The sternohyoid muscle is dissected free.

of the subcutaneous fat and anterior chest wall muscles is undertaken, taking care not to puncture the intercostal muscles. With the rib-cage exposed, an anterior intercostal muscle is carefully removed with a scalpel making sure not to penetrate the parietal pleura. On removal of the muscle, direct visual inspection through the pleura will reveal whether or not the underlying lung is normally sited beneath it. If one can see lung then the deceased does not have a tension pneumothorax. This can be repeated at several sites on both sides. Once assured that no pneumothorax is visible then the chest is opened in the usual way.

Underwater technique

The APT can be requested to hold the reflected tissue away from the chest and the intervening space

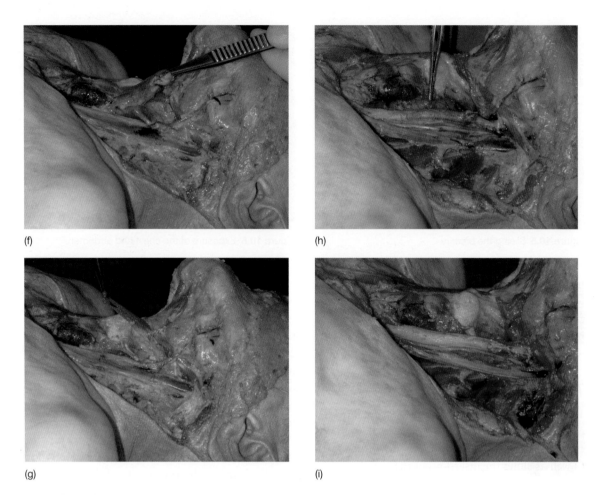

(f)

(h)

(g)

(i)

Figure 10.4 *continued* (f) The sternothyroid muscle is dissected free. (g) The thyrohyoid muscle is dissected free. (h) The contents of the carotid sheath are examined. (i) The carotid artery and internal jugular vein are opened.

is filled with water. One of the intercostal spaces is then punctured, under water, with a blunt instrument and careful observation for bubbles is made. A blade should not be used as this may puncture an underlying bulla and give a false–positive result. Compression of the chest may be required in the case of a non-tension pneumothorax. The procedure is repeated to the other side of the chest.

Quantifiable underwater technique

In the third method a wide-bore hypodermic needle (approximately 18 gauge) is connected to a 20 or 50 mL syringe from which the plunger has been removed. The needle is then pushed just into the subcutaneous tissue above an intercostal space over the anterior chest without entering the chest cavity. The syringe is then filled with water and the needle is advanced into the pleural space, making observation of any bubbles. The procedure is repeated to the other side of the chest.

The breasts

The breasts can be examined when the soft tissues have been freed from the rib-cage. These are first palpated, with the advantage that at autopsy one can palpate from the external and internal aspects simultaneously. The breast tissue can then be sliced at no greater than 10 mm intervals internally, making sure to follow the axillary tails out to the axillae (Fig. 10.5). The breast should be supported with a sponge and delicate stokes of the blade are needed to avoid incis-

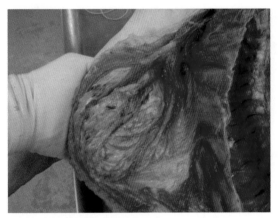

Figure 10.5 Slicing the breasts.

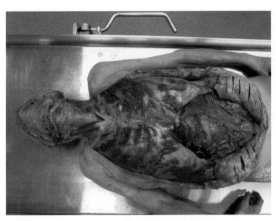

Figure 10.6 Exposure of the chest and abdomen.

ing the skin. The breasts should be examined in this way in every female autopsy. If the body is being eviscerated by an APT the pathologist must remember to return to the body to carry out this examination, which is frequently overlooked.

The abdominal wall

The abdominal skin and underlying fat are reflected off the abdominal musculature (Fig. 10.6). Incisions can then be made to the midline of the rectus sheath as well as along the insertions of the muscles to the right and left side of the lower aspect of the rib-cage. This allows for the abdominal wall to be flapped open. If the skin is intractable owing to significant obesity or cold, firm adipose tissue, a midline abdominal incision can be used to open straight into the abdominal cavity to display the abdominal contents. A series of anterior–posterior cuts on the inner surface will generally allow the skin to be folded back without risk of it flopping into the dissection (Fig. 10.6). In mortuaries lacking scales to weigh the body, the thickness of the abdominal panniculus can be measured in lieu of a body mass index determination. The presence, nature and volume of any fluid within the abdominal cavity is best recorded at this point, prior to opening the chest cavities.

The rectus sheath can be examined in detail in cases where there has been abdominal surgery or blunt trauma. It may be necessary to identify the site of an abscess within the sheath or the location and size of a bruise.

Starting with the midline incision, the skin is reflected laterally, separating the subcutaneous tissue from the underlying muscle (Fig. 10.7a). At this stage a finger can be placed in each inguinal canal to retrieve and examine the testis. The proximal insertion of the rectus sheath into the rib-cage is identified and incised. Each muscle is then dissected off the underlying structures working towards the symphysis pubis (Fig. 10.7b). In a similar manner, without entering the abdominal cavity, the external and internal oblique muscles (Fig. 10.7c and d) as well as the transversus abdominus muscles are identified on each side and dissected free. Finally, the midline incision enters the abdominal cavity and goes to the symphysis pubis. Finally, as described above, incisions are then made along each insertion of the abdominal fascia into the coastal margin, working laterally to allow the abdominal wall to open with two flaps (Fig. 10.7e). This allows maximum access to the abdominal cavity without the need to further incise the muscles.

The chest cavity

The chest cavity can now be opened. The muscles of the right and left side of the chest wall should be reflected in layers to assess for injuries or natural pathology. This permits a greater exposure of the rib-cage, allowing for the assessment of a pneumothorax as described above, and makes the process of opening the rib-cage easier.

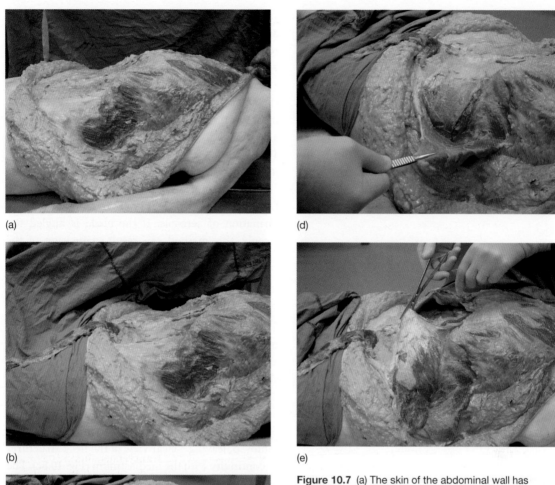

(a)

(b)

(c)

(d)

(e)

Figure 10.7 (a) The skin of the abdominal wall has been reflected. (b) The rectus muscles are reflected to the symphysis pubis. (c) The external oblique muscle is reflected. (d) The internal oblique muscle is reflected. (e) The abdominal cavity is exposed.

The sternoclavicular joints are identified and disarticulated with a PM40 blade. There are several alternative methods of incising the chest wall. Some pathologists prefer to cut through the ribs at the costochondral cartilages; this can often be achieved with a PM40 blade or a sharp bread knife, but when this is difficult, rib shears can be used (Wilson, 1972). The ribs are separated up to the first rib, which is left intact. This permits inspection of the chest contents without significant leakage of blood from adjacent large vessels, which inevitably occurs when cutting the first rib. Alternatively, the thorax can be opened with a more lateral incision which runs from the sternoclavicular joint to the anterior axillary line. This method has the advantage of offering a wide field of view of the thoracic contents and provides greater access for the subsequent removal of the spinal cord. Such an incision can be

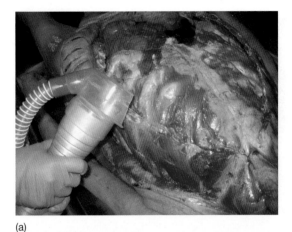

(a)

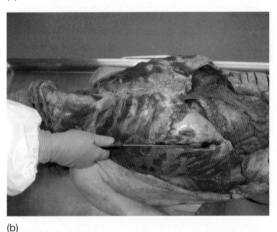

(b)

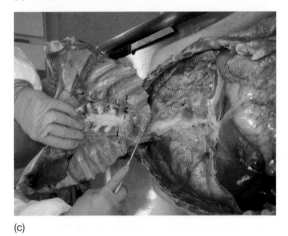

(c)

Figure 10.8 (a) Division of ribs with a saw. (b) Division of ribs with a breadknife. (c) Rib shield removed.

made using rib shears, an oscillating saw or a bread knife. Reflection of the muscles of the chest wall as described above makes the passage of the shears or

saw easier. Rib shears are the least preferred method as they leave sharp edges which pose a hazard when removing the thoracic contents. An oscillating saw with a fan-shaped blade leaves smooth edges (Fig. 10.8a) but will create aerosols if there is fluid within the pleural cavity. A bread knife is the cheapest and most acceptable option. The knife should be held almost horizontal – at an angle of approximately 10–15 degrees from the chest wall (Fig. 10.8b) – and used with firm downward pressure. The result is a rib incision with smooth edges, without the need to first incise the chest wall muscles, and without the formation of aerosols. If the blade is angled too steeply, this method can result in incision of the underlying organs (Walker *et al.*, 2002).

The anterior rib shield can be reflected, taking care not to damage the structures underneath. Special care is needed where coronary artery bypass grafts have been performed using the internal mammary arteries. When the cavity has been examined and the gross disposition of the organs regarding situs and pathology has been determined (e.g. hyperinflation of the lungs in asthmatics), the first rib is cut and the medial attachments of the clavicles are severed. The sternum and rib segments are then removed, leaving a clear view of the neck structures in continuity with the mediastinum (Fig. 10.8c). The muscles of the rib shield are incised, to facilitate the detection of anterior rib fractures. Returning to the body, the cut ends of the ribs should be covered either with the skin flaps or with towels to prevent sharps injuries. This is especially important when the ribs have been divided with shears. The risk of sharps injuries during the evisceration, and particularly from the cut surfaces of bones, cannot be over-emphasised (Weston and Locker, 1992; Burton, 2003).

Removal of the neck, thorax and abdominal organs

The choice of method used to remove the internal organs will depend on the individual case and the personal preference of the pathologist undertaking the examination. The organs may be removed in a single block (Letulle technique), which includes the neck structures, thoracic, abdominal and pelvic viscera in continuity, or in two blocks, separating the neck and thoracic organs from the abdominal and pelvic viscera. The removal of the organs one by one following the technique advocated by Virchow and propounded by some authors (Gresham and Turner, 1979) is not recommended as it prevents examination of the viscera in anatomical continuity. One-block and two-block eviscerations are described here.

Removal of the neck structures and thoracic contents

The following procedure should be undertaken only if a layered neck dissection is not required (see above).

Once the chest cavity has been opened the tongue and neck structures can be freed. The neck flap is lifted and the tip of a PM40 blade inserted submentally. The tongue is cleared by an incision which follows the inner surface of the mandible, taking care not to damage the skin of the lips and face. If the pathologist inserts the fingers of their non-dominant hand into the buccal cavity from below, the tongue can then be retracted inferiorly, allowing the structures within the mouth to be freed of their lateral and posterior attachments under direct vision (Fig. 10.9a and b). In this way, the tongue and the upper limits of the pharynx and oesophagus are

removed intact in direct continuity with the neck structures. The presence or absence of foreign bodies in the laryngeal opening should be sought at this point. If the clinical history suggests that death was due to choking, the larynx and trachea can be opened *in situ* using a PM40 blade and scissors. This will allow foreign objects lodged at the level of the vocal cords to be visualised *in situ*.

All of the neck structures can now be cleared from the anterior aspect of the cervical vertebrae, severing the carotid arteries as high as possible above the bifurcation. Alternatively, the carotid artery, jugular vein and vagus nerve can be dissected free and examined *in situ*. The soft tissue connections and vessels at the thoracic inlet can then be cut following the line of the upper ribs backwards to the cervical bodies. The neck structures and thoracic organs can now be freed in continuity with blunt dissection from the anterior aspect of the thoracic vertebrae down to the level of the diaphragm. This can be facilitated by an incision made into the parietal pleura bilaterally along the vertebral pedicles. The organs are then replaced in the chest and neck and attention is turned to the abdomen.

The presence of pleural adhesions may hamper removal of the lungs. Where only a few are present, they may be incised with a knife. In cases where the pleural cavity is obliterated by adhesions, a cleavage plane may be made with the hand before pulling the lungs free. Where dense adhesions or tumour prevents this, the lung can be removed by running a

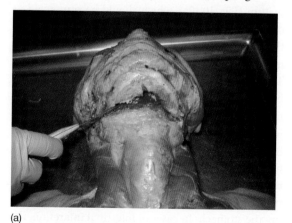
(a)

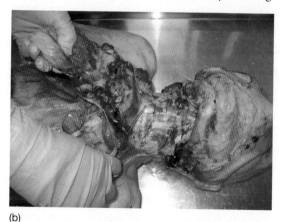
(b)

Figure 10.9 (a) Tongue being freed from the mandible. (b) Neck structures freed from the vertebral bodies, taking care not to apply pressure to the larynx.

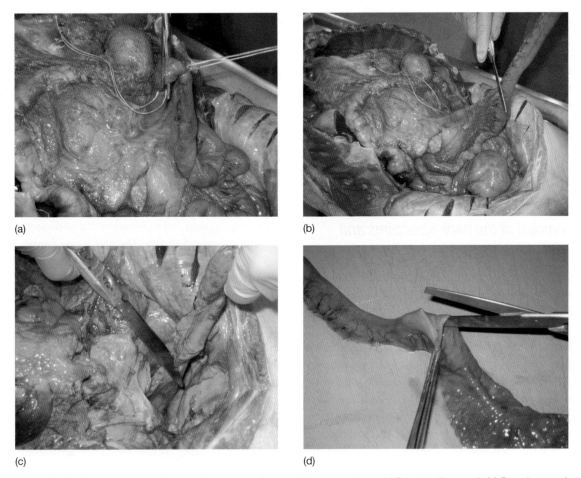

(a)　(b)　(c)　(d)

Figure 10.10 (a) Jejunum being ligated. (b) Intestine dissected from mesentery. (c) Rectum dissected. (d) Bowel opened.

knife down the whole length of the parietal pleura over the inner aspect of the ribs, and forcing a hand through the slit to form a cleavage plane between the parietal pleura and the chest wall (Knight, 1996).

Removal of the intestines

To remove the organs in one block, the eventual bulk of the block is first reduced by removing the majority of the intestines. They are examined *in situ* and if there are no contraindications may be removed. The origin of the jejunum is located immediately behind the transverse colon as it emerges from its retroperitoneal course and is tied off by making a hole in the mesentery, tying two ligatures using string and dividing the gut between them (Fig. 10.10a). The small and large intestines are dissected free of the mesentery in

continuity (Fig. 10.10b) down to the level of the rectum (Fig. 10.10c), which should be transected as distally as possible. If the pathologist intends to open the small intestine, it should be dissected from its mesentery as close to the intestinal wall as possible. This produces a straight length of intestine that can be easily opened with scissors. If the small intestine is not to be opened, it can be removed more rapidly by incising its mesentery along its root, which runs from top left to bottom right. The large intestine and rectum are freed from the posterior abdominal wall using blunt dissection. Care is needed to avoid tearing the capsules of the liver or spleen, and to avoid opening the stomach. In cases of intestinal infarction, the mesenteric vessels should be examined *in situ* prior to incision of the mesentery. The intestines can be

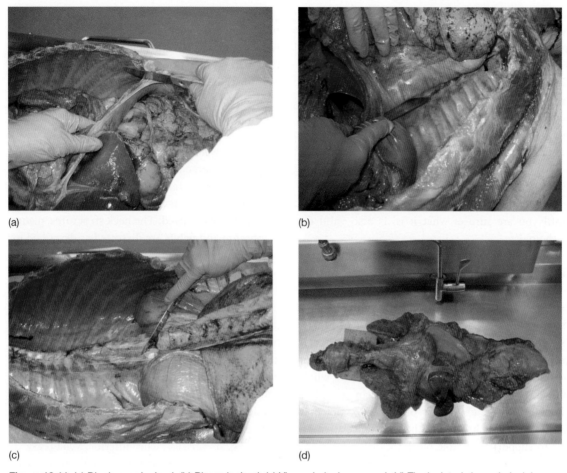

(a)

(b)

(c)

(d)

Figure 10.11 (a) Diaphragm incised. (b) Pleura incised. (c) Visceral pluck removed. (d) The isolated visceral pluck is examined for gross abnormalities.

opened along the anti-mesenteric border using bowel scissors (Fig. 10.10d), and this is made easier if the mesentery has been incised as close to the bowel as possible. If the contents of the gut do not need to be sampled for toxicology or microbiology, the bowel is opened and washed in cold water, taking care not to produce aerosols, and the luminal surface is examined. All abnormalities should be recorded, described, measured and related to some measured fixed anatomical site such as the ileoceacal valve. The specimen can also be photographed if desired before histological sampling.

Removal of the testes

No autopsy on a male is complete without an examination of the testes. The external genitalia are examined *in situ* before removing the testes. This is best done once the abdomen has been opened. The testes can then be removed from the scrotum via the inguinal canal using blunt dissection.

Removal of the abdominal and pelvic viscera (one-block technique)

Once the bulk of the intestines have been removed it is relatively simple to free the abdominal and pelvic viscera from the abdominal wall. The diaphragm is first incised as close to the abdominal wall as possible (Fig. 10.11a) and the retroperitoneal tissues are freed posteriorly with a combination of blunt and sharp dissection. The block of tissues containing the rectum, bladder and prostate (or the uterus and adnexa in the female) is freed by blunt dissection working anteroposteriorly. This block can then be separated from the pelvic walls by severing the tissues as close to the organ outlets as is possible without puncturing the skin or disrupting the perineum. Freeing the retroperitoneum and the pelvic blocks is the most difficult part of the evisceration to perform under direct vision. The temptation to free tissues by sense of touch alone and a knife wielded blindly should be strongly resisted. Such a technique is both dangerous and a bad dissection. The surgeon's dictum that 'you should never cut anything until you are sure of what it is' is also valid for pathologists.

When these blocks are cleared laterally and at the pelvic outlet, the dissection of the aorta from the anterior surfaces of the lumbar vertebrae and sacrum can be continued from the thoracic block downwards. Once again, this is made easier by incising the prevertebral fascia. The kidneys in their perinephric fat can be freed from the posterior abdominal wall using blunt dissection. The whole 'visceral pluck' can now be removed in one piece (Fig. 10.11b and c). This is often heavy and may require a helping hand from the APT, since attempting to support the whole block by lifting from the neck alone often breaks the hyoid bone or cartilages associated with the larynx.

The empty cavity should be dried with a sponge and the various surfaces examined for abnormalities. The intercostal muscles are incised, to facilitate the examination for posterolateral rib fractures. While the interior is dry, thus preventing aerosol formation, a broad-bladed chisel and a rubber-headed mallet can be used to strip off sections of the anterior aspects of several adjacent vertebral bodies looking for osteoporosis, fractures, tumours, infection, disease and amounts of marrow. Alternatively, 'vertebral strips' can be obtained using an oscillating saw with a fan-tailed blade.

Removal of the viscera in two blocks

The method described above for removing the organs in one block has the advantage that the organs can be subsequently dissected in anatomical continuity. Many pathologists, however, find that the organ block produced is heavy and unwieldy and prefer to eviscerate the thoracic organs separately from the abdominal and pelvic block. Such a dissection method may also be of particular value in the examination of patients who have had intra-abdominal surgery, sepsis or neoplasia with resultant multiple adhesions between the loops of small and large intestine. In such cases, it is often preferable to leave the bowel attached to the abdominal block and remove the thoracic organs separately.

To remove the organs in two blocks, the body cavities are opened as before and, if desired, the intestines are removed. The neck structures, pleura, diaphragm and pelvis are dissected as described for the single-block technique above, and the thoracic organs are freed from the vertebral bodies with blunt and sharp dissection. The thoracic aorta can now be divided at the level of the descending aortic arch and dissected off the back of the thoracic block. The oesophagus is similarly divided below the pharynx and dissected free, so that it remains in continuity with the stomach. Some pathologists prefer to ligate and divide the stomach at the level of the diaphragm. While it produces a more manageable block, this technique prevents a subsequent assessment for oesophageal varices. The inferior vena cava is divided and the thoracic organs can now be freed and removed. The abdominal and pelvic organs are then removed as before.

Whether removed in one or two blocks, the freed pluck can now be examined for gross abnormalities before proceeding to the systematic dissection (Fig. 10.11d).

Examination of the genital tract

On occasion it may be necessary to examine the male or female genital tract in association with the lower genital and gastrointestinal tracts. The procedures for each gender are outlined below.

Female genital tract

Removal of the intact female genital tract encompasses a block dissection and examination of the bladder, external and internal genital tract, rectum and anus. The procedure should be considered when

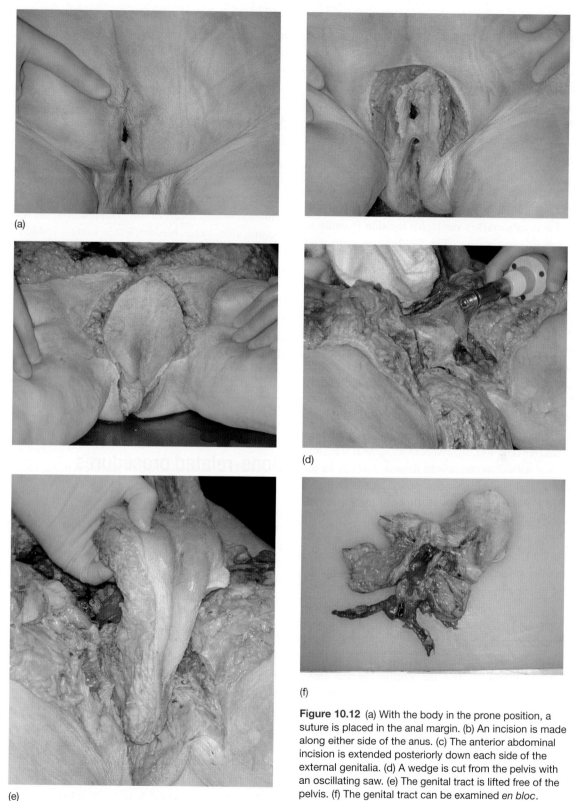

(a)

(d)

(e)

(f)

Figure 10.12 (a) With the body in the prone position, a suture is placed in the anal margin. (b) An incision is made along either side of the anus. (c) The anterior abdominal incision is extended posteriorly down each side of the external genitalia. (d) A wedge is cut from the pelvis with an oscillating saw. (e) The genital tract is lifted free of the pelvis. (f) The genital tract can be examined *en bloc*.

the deceased has any form of natural pathology that may involve two or more of the above structures, for example invasive tumours or fistulae, as well as the assessment of medical or surgical procedures to this area. The technique is also used in the assessment of genital tract and anal/rectal injuries in cases of suspected sexual assault.

To start the procedure, the body is placed in the prone position to enable examination of the anus. A suture is then placed at the posterior margin – the base of the natal cleft at the 6 o'clock position (Fig. 10.12a). This assists in the removal of the specimen and acts as a marker stitch. An incision is made to either side of the anus (Fig. 10.12b) and continued forwards on either side of the external genitalia. The anus and rectum are dissected free before returning the body to the supine position.

With the legs separated, the standard midline abdominal incision is continued downwards on either side of the external genitalia to join the posterior incisions (Fig. 10.12c). The skin and subcutaneous structures are then dissected free of the pubic rami and brought forwards. Using either an oscillating saw with a fan-tailed blade or a hand saw, two incisions are made to the front of the pelvis and the bone wedge lifted free (Fig. 10.12d). The bladder, genital tract and rectum with anus can now be dissected free from the lateral and posterior aspects of the pelvic wall and lifted forwards and upwards through the gap in the pelvic ring (Fig. 10.12e).

The genital tract can now be examined *en bloc* (Fig. 10.12f). With the specimen positioned with the anterior aspect uppermost, the urethra is identified and opened along its anterior aspect to the bladder. The bladder is similarly opened. The specimen is then rolled over and the marker stitch to the anus identified. At this point the anus is incised working posteriorly to examine the entire rectum. Finally the vulva is examined and the vagina opened along either lateral wall. The uterus is then cut in half to expose the os, cervical canal and endometrial cavity. Each fallopian tube and ovary is then examined. Using this technique all three structures can be examined independently and yet any pathology involving two or more structures can be identified and recorded.

To reconstruct the pelvis, the bone wedge is replaced in the pelvic ring. The skin incision is closed using a series of deep strong sutures, working anteriorly from the posterior aspect (Chapter 21). An excellent cosmetic result can be achieved.

Male genital tract

Examination of the male genital tract can be undertaken in the same way as that of the female. The only difference is that one has to decide whether to remove the entire penis, as with the female external genitalia, or not. It can be undertaken such that the rectum, anus, penis, bladder, testes, ureters and kidneys can all be removed *en bloc* or in an appropriate combination.

If the decision is made to leave a cosmetic penis intact, the skin of the penis must be dissected away from the internal structures from the base towards the glans, by inverting the skin as one proceeds. In this way the internal structures of the penis can remain attached to the bladder and prostate via the urethra and a good cosmetic reconstruction can occur by packing the skin of the penis afterwards with a suitable packing agent.

Bone-related procedures

The pathologist may be required to undertake a number of bone-related procedures at the evisceration stage. These relate to the assessment of the presence of osteoporosis, the consideration for specialist examination of the rib-cage and thoracic spine, and the removal of a whole long bone as typified by the removal of a femur.

Assessment of osteoporosis

The assessment of osteoporosis (or more accurately osteopenia) is of considerable importance, since death following fracture of the femur may be attributed to natural causes if severe osteoporosis is present, or may be viewed as a trauma case (therefore attracting the interest of the coroner) if no osteoporosis can be demonstrated.

The traditional method of assessing bone fracturability in the mortuary is to take the cut end of a rib

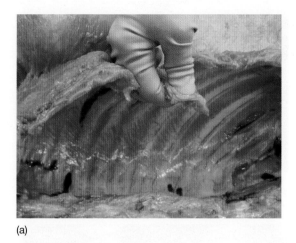

(a)

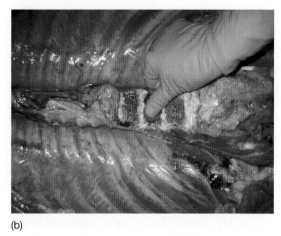

(b)

Figure 10.13 (a) The rib is squeezed, assessing for osteoporosis. (b) Assessing the vertebral medullary bone for osteoporosis.

between finger and thumb and deform it until it fractures (Fig. 10.13a). A range of subjective assessments (up to six) can be established with a little experience and this has been demonstrated to show good interobserver reproducibility (Harris *et al.*, 1991).

The second method is to assess the strength of the trabeculae of the medullary bone of the vertebral bodies by direct pressure after removing the anterior aspects (Fig. 10.13b). This has been shown to be less sensitive and reproducible than rib fracture at estimating bone fraturability, even though the ribs are mainly cortical bone, which is thought to be less significant than medullary bone in osteoporotic fracture.

Formal comparison of the mechanical strength of isolated femurs with these crude indices of bone strength in a small series has shown them to be better predictors of osteopenia than bone histomorphometry. More recent studies showed that DEXA scanning of isolated bones was an ever better indicator and correlated well with rib fracturability and direct quantitative femoral mechanical fracturability. Indices such as the Singh index, even when automated in a computerised morphometry system, showed very poor correlation with direct mechanical testing.

Removal of an infant's rib-cage for the examination of fractures

Prior to an autopsy of an infant a radiological survey should have been undertaken of the bony skeleton. If this reveals old or new rib fractures, or if a squeezing injury to the chest is suspected, then the entire rib-cage should be removed for further radiological and histological examination. Often the pathognomonic injuries of squeezing can be identified only on microscopic examination of the site of insertion of the rib head with the vertebrae.

The standard autopsy is first undertaken on the infant. The thoracic cavity will have been opened with the sternum removed by careful cutting through the cartilaginous insertions of the ribs. The thoracic pluck is removed. If the spinal cord is to be removed this should be undertaken from a posterior approach in this procedure so as not to cause any damage to the rib head insertion to the thoracic spine.

The thoracic skin, soft tissues and muscles are further dissected from the rib-cage, starting at the front and proceeding all the way to the back. A cut is made through an intervertebral disc above the level of the first thoracic vertebrae. This releases the upper end of the dissection block. A cut is then made through an intervertebral disc below the 12th thoracic vertebrae. This frees the lower margin of the dissection and the entire rib-cage and attached thoracic spine will lift free from the cadaver.

The dissection block should be fixed in formalin. It should then be x-rayed. The removal of the skin and soft tissue attachments will yield a higher quality x-ray examination of the rib-cage. Following this the entire specimen should be decalcified.

Following decalcification, the specimen is prepared for microscopic examination. The thoracic spine can be left intact or the specimen can be cut in half. Each rib insertion onto the thoracic spine should be identified and sectioned. Depending on whether the spine is cut in half, this will either yield 12 blocks composed of the vertebrae with both attached rib heads or 24 hemi-vertebrae with attached rib heads. The authors prefer the latter approach so that there is no possibility of mix up between the left and right sides. The anterior costal–cartilage junctions are then all sampled. Finally, any abnormality identified on x-ray or palpation of the ribs is sampled.

Removal of the femur

Removal of the femur starts with a medial incision to the superior aspect of the upper leg, just below the groin. The incision proceeds inferiorly along the medial aspect of the upper leg to the level of the knee where it sweeps below the patella to go to the lateral aspect of the knee. A shorter incision to the medial thigh, starting just above the medial femoral condyle, can also be used but this provides a more limited view of the femoral shaft. The cutting then proceeds superiorly along the lateral aspect of the upper leg to the level of the hip. Starting at the knee, the skin flap – including with it the patella – is reflected upwards to the hip, thus exposing the femur. The knee is then flexed and the lateral, medial and cruciate ligaments are divided (Fig 10.14a). The muscle is divided down to the bone and cleared from the periosteum with a PM40 blade. This starts at the knee and proceeds upwards until the hip is reached (Fig. 10.14b). Using this amount of clearance, division of the hip capsule and the ligaments and tendons is conducted under direct vision (Fig. 10.14c). Rotating the femur to enable complete freeing of the attachments at the hip, the femur is lifted free. Reconstruction can be performed as described in Chapter 21.

Dissection of the face

Examination of the face should not be undertaken by anyone who is not already proficient with standard autopsy techniques as there is a potential risk of

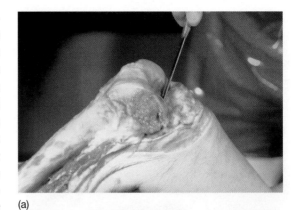

(a)

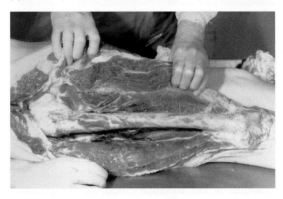

(b)

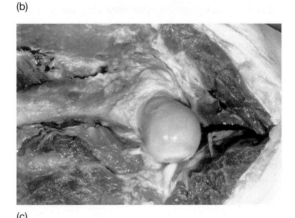

(c)

Figure 10.14 (a) The ligaments of the knee are divided. (b) The muscle is divided down to the periosteum. (c) The hip joint is exposed.

causing incisions to the skin of the face that may result in a poor cosmetic result. It is, however, an important technique for the assessment of facial pathology, including natural disease (e.g. tumours), maxillofacial surgery and blunt trauma to this area.

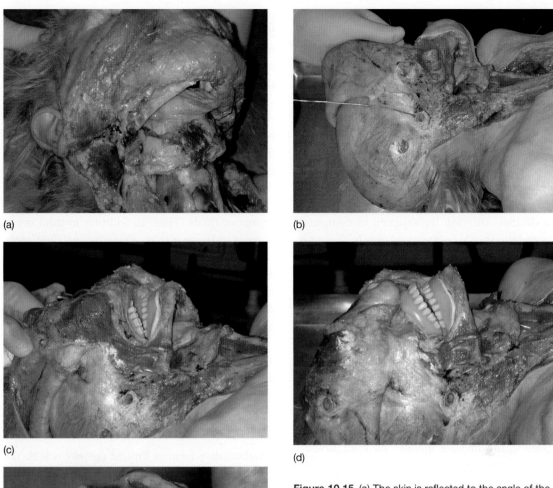

(a)

(b)

(c)

(d)

(e)

Figure 10.15 (a) The skin is reflected to the angle of the jaw; the tongue has already been released in this case. (b) The external auditory meatus has been divided, and the skin of the face reflected, working towards the nose. (c) The oral cavity has been opened and the gum margin incised. (d) Dissection stops at the bridge of the nose. (e) The dissection has been continued, to expose the bony orbit and stops at the bridge of the nose.

The standard Y incision is continued rostrally such that it joins the incision used for examination of the scalp. The skin of the neck is reflected to the level of the jaw (Fig. 10.15a). Starting laterally, the external auditory meatus is cut and the skin reflected forwards towards the nose (Fig. 10.15b). This is dissected off the musculature of the face. As one approaches the midline of the jaw extra care is required as the skin is thin at this site and punctures must be avoided. As one reaches the lateral part of the mouth the incision runs along the connection of the oral cavity to the bone and enters the oral cavity (Fig. 10.15c). The dissection stops on reaching the nasal structures (Fig. 10.15d). The same procedure is performed to the other side. This will result in the skin being attached only to the nose and around the eye sockets. The dissection can be continued by carefully advancing the PM40 blade between the outer aspect of the eye socket and the periorbital fat. By making a sweeping motion around the orbit the eye may be brought forward in continuity with the skin of the face. The muscles and optic nerve are cut and the orbital contents will come out of the eye socket. The dissection can continue towards the bridge of the nose, where most would stop. If repeated on the other side, the skin of the face now remains attached only along the ridge of the nose (Fig. 10.15e). Although the skin can be completely removed this should be attempted only by those performing this procedure regularly. The muscular and bony structures of the face, mouth and nasal cavity may now be examined through layered dissection.

Minimally invasive autopsies

To end this chapter we consider alternatives to full invasive autopsies. These are known as 'minimally invasive' procedures. With the exception of so-called 'view and grant' systems or radiological autopsies (see Chapter 19) all other published alternatives to the invasive autopsy have an invasive component, even if it is the insertion of a needle into the body (Rutty, 2007). The two principal groups of minimally invasive approaches are presented here.

The needle autopsy

Three types of needle autopsy are described in the literature (Underwood *et al.*, 1983; Dorsey, 1984; Walker and Going, 1994; Foroudi *et al.*, 1995; Suvarna and Start, 1995; Huston *et al.*, 1996; Dada and Ansari, 1997; Aranda *et al.*, 1998; El-Reshaid *et al.*, 2005; Hando *et al.*, 2005).

The first type uses a device such as a Tru-Cut needle. The advantage of doing this operation post-

mortem is that enough passes can be made through the same incision to quite adequately sample most organs. The cores of tissue can be processed in the normal way and the process can be undertaken on the ward if necessary, thus providing fresh tissue specimens. Generally the incisions can be covered with adhesive plasters or closed with adhesive glue. No suturing is required. Tru-Cut biopsy can be incorporated into so-called radiological autopsies (see Chapter 19).

The second type uses fine-needle aspiration. Cytological specimens can be retrieved from body organs or fluids. Thus, in addition to solid organ samples and bone marrow, cerebrospinal fluid, pleural effusions, ascites, urine and joint fluid can be obtained, processed and examined. It is considered a cheap, quick and reliable technique which assists but does not replace either a standard autopsy or limited histological examination.

A third type of 'needle autopsy' is in fact a variant of fine-needle aspiration: needle aspiration and microbiological culture. Samples are sent for culturing rather than histology.

The laparoscopic autopsy

An alternative form of limited autopsy is with the use of a laparoscope. This can be used only by a person skilled in the operation of such a device, and can be used only to sample areas of the body that will allow the passage of a laparoscope – for example the thorax or abdomen. Avrahami and colleagues draw our attention to examination of the abdominal cavity by laparoscope, claiming it to be a simple, clean and easy-to-perform procedure with results comparable to the conventional autopsy. It should, however, not be used as an alternative to a standard full autopsy but rather another form of a limited autopsy (Avrahami *et al.*, 1995; Catheline *et al.*, 1999; Damore *et al.*, 2000; Cacchione *et al.*, 2001).

References

Adams VI (1990). Autopsy technique for neck examination. I. Anterior and lateral compartments and tongue. *Pathol Annu* 25(2):331–49.

Adams VI (1991). Autopsy technique for neck examination. II. Vertebral column and posterior compartment. *Pathol Annu* 26(1):211–26.

Aranda M, Marti C, Bernet M, Gudiol F, Pujol R (1998). Diagnostic utility of post-mortem fine-needle aspiration cultures. *Arch Pathol Lab Med* **122**:1112.

Avrahami R, Watemberg S, Hiss Y, Deutsch AA (1995). Laproscopic vs conventional autopsy: a promising perspective. *Arch Surg* **130**:407–9.

Box CR (1919). *Post-mortem Manual: A Handbook of Morbid Anatomy and Post-mortem Technique*, 2nd edn. London: J&A Churchill.

Burton JL (2003). Health and safety at autopsy. *J Clin Pathol* **56**:254–60.

Cacchione RN, Sayad P, Pecoraro AM, Ferzli GS (2001). Laparoscopic autopsies. *Surg Endosc* **15**:619–22.

Catheline JM, Turner R, Guettier C, Chamault G (1999). Autopsy can be performed laparoscopically. *Surg Endosc* **13**:1163–4.

Dada MA, Ansari NA (1997). Post-mortem cytology: a reappraisal of a little used technique. *Cytopathology* **8**:417–20.

Damore LJ, Barth RF, Morrison CD, Frankel WL, Melvin WS (2000). Laparoscopic post-mortem examination: a minimally invasive approach to the autopsy. *Ann Diagn Pathol* **4**:95–8.

Dorsey DB (1984). Limited autopsies. *Arch Pathol Lab Med* **108**:469–72.

El-Reshaid W, El-Rashaid K, Madda J (2005). Postmortem biopsies: the experience in Kuwait. *Med Princ Pract* **14**:173–6.

Foroudi F, Cheung K, Duflou J (1995). A comparison of the needle biopsy post mortem with the conventional autopsy. *Pathology* **27**:79–82.

Gresham GA, Turner AF (1979). *Post-mortem Techniques (An Illustrated Handbook)*. London: Wolfe Medical.

Hando K, Maeada S, Hosone M *et al.* (2005). Usefulness of rapid cytological diagnosis at autopsy. *Rinsho Byori* **53**:284–9.

Harris SC, Cotton DWK, Stephenson TJ, Howat AJ (1991). Assessment of osteopenia at autopsy. *Med Sci Law* **31**:15–18.

Huston BM, Malouf NN, Azar HA (1996). Percutaneous needle autopsy sampling. *Mod Pathol* **9**:1101–7.

Knight B (1996). *Forensic Pathology*, 2nd edn. London: Arnold.

Maxeiner H (1998). 'Hidden' laryngeal injuries in homicidal strangulation: how to detect and interpret these findings. *J Forensic Sci* **43**:784–91.

Prinsloo I, Gordon I (1951). Post-mortem dissection artifacts of the neck: their differentiation from ante-mortem bruises. *S Afr Med J* **25**(21):358–61.

Rutty GN (2007). Are autopsies necessary? The role of computed tomography as a possible alternative to invasive autopsies. *Rechtsmedizin* **17**:21–8.

Rutty GN, Squier WMV, Padfield CJH (2005). Epidural haemorrhage of the cervical spinal cord: a post-mortem artefact? *Neuropathol Appl Neurobiol* **31**:247–57.

Start RD, Cross SS (1999). ACP Best Practice No. 155: Pathological investigation of deaths following surgery, anaesthesia and medical intervention. *J Clin Pathol* **52**:640–52.

Suvarna SK, Start RD (1995). Cytodiagnosis and the necroscopy. *J Clin Pathol* **48**:443–6.

Underwood JCE, Slater DN, Parsons MA (1983). The needle necropsy. *Br Med J* **286**:1632–4.

Vanezis P (1989). Techniques of dissection. In: Vanezis (ed.) *Pathology of Neck Injury*, pp. 22–4. London: Butterworth.

Walker E, Going JJ (1994). Cytopathology in the post mortem room. *J Clin Pathol* **47**:14–17.

Walker JEC, Rutty GN, Rodgers B, Woodford NWF (2002). How should the chest wall be opened at necropsy? *J Clin Pathol* **55**:72–5.

Weston J, Locker G (1992). Frequency of glove puncture in the post mortem room. *J Clin Pathol* **45**:177–8.

Wilson RR (1972). *Methods in Morbid Anatomy*. London: Butterworth.

Chapter 11

DISSECTION OF THE INTERNAL ORGANS

Julian L Burton and Guy N Rutty

Introduction

Irrespective of the suspected cause of death, dissection of the internal organs should be undertaken in a systematic and thorough manner. The temptation to begin with the organ system containing the suspected cause of death is best avoided. There are perhaps as many methods of dissecting the internal organs as there are pathologists performing autopsies. What is important, therefore, is not for every pathologist to undertake the dissection in an identical manner, but rather that each pathologist discovers the approach which works best and sticks to it. While on occasion the pathologist's normal routine will need to be modified because of the diseases present, dissection of the internal organs can generally proceed in the same order in every case. With the adoption of a systematic approach, the pathologist can be confident that the same level of vigilance will be maintained throughout the autopsy.

Some pathologists choose to begin their dissection with the heart, as this is the most common site of the cause of death. This may have the advantage of soothing the pathologist's nerves once a cause has been found, but there is a risk that, having found one possible cause of death, the true cause of death will be overlooked. The authors' approach is to begin with the retroperitoneal structures, before examining the pelvic organs and then the spleen, pancreas, upper gastrointestinal tract and liver. The lungs, neck structures and heart are then dissected before finally examining the brain. This approach is described here.

The collection of swabs for culture is described in detail in Chapter 16 and toxicology is described in Chapter 15. It is worth noting that consideration should be given to the collection of such samples at an early stage if they have not already been collected prior to evisceration, and before water is allowed to redistribute organisms. This is important when considering sampling for diatoms, algae or bacteria in relation to drowning cases as these samples must be taken prior to organ evisceration and must not come in contact with other water sources (Lucci and Cirnelli, 2007; Kakizaki *et al.*, 2008). Outside specific causes of death at all stages of the dissection, cold running water should be played on the tissues and these should be dabbed dry with a sponge to allow clear visualisation. In the past, there have been concerns that allowing the tissues to come into contact with water would impair subsequent histological assessment, but it has been established that this is not the case (Cotton and Stephenson, 1988). Further, it can be argued that the value of the macroscopic autopsy examination is severely limited if tissues are obscured by blood and other body fluids (Knight, 1996).

The retroperitoneum

The retroperitoneum is a common and convenient starting point for the systematic dissection of the organ pluck. The entire pluck (or the abdominal and

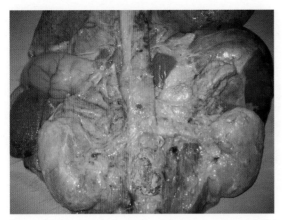

Figure 11.1 Adrenal glands dissected from perinephric fat.

pelvic pluck if the organs have been removed in two blocks) is placed on a well-lit dissection board, at a comfortable height, with the dorsal surface uppermost. The subsequent dissection is facilitated if the diaphragm is dissected free bilaterally at this point. This can then be laid out in a tray for demonstration if abnormal, or discarded for later return to the body.

The adrenal glands are exposed and examined (Fig. 11.1). In obese individuals, the adrenals are often difficult to locate and the best approach is to attempt to remove the surrounding fat with blunt dissection, either with fingers or by opening blunt-ended scissors within the fat using the outside edges of the blades rather than cutting with them. Although Shimuzi *et al.* (1997) described a method to assist with their location, the present authors find that blunt dissection to the anatomical area where the glands should be located will reveal their location. The adrenals are then trimmed of fat, weighed and sliced. Representative slices of the glands may be laid out for subsequent demonstration and retained for histopathological examination. The cut surfaces of the adrenal glands should be examined for the presence of haemorrhage, cortical atrophy, cortical hyperplasia, cortical tumours and medullary tumours. Incidental tumours of the adrenal cortex (mostly inactive cortical adenomas) are found in approximately 2–3 per cent of autopsies (Barzon *et al.*, 2003). Because malignant neoplasms (typically lung cancers) metastasise to the adrenal glands, any tumours identified should be sampled for histology.

A small transverse incision is made into the posterior aspect of the aorta (Fig. 11.2a), which can then be opened along its length with a pair of blunt-ended scissors. In this way, the aorta can be opened down to the cut ends of the common iliac arteries and up as far as the third part of the arch before it curves deeply towards the anterior of the chest (Fig. 11.2b). The patency of the ostia of the main branches, such as the coeliac axis, superior and inferior mesenteric arteries and renal arteries, can then be assessed using a probe (Fig. 11.2c) before opening the renal arteries out to the renal pelves. At this stage it is possible to dissect the aorta off the pluck, sacrificing the mesenteric branches but leaving it in continuity with the aortic arch and kidneys. The presence or absence of para-aortic lymphadenopathy is noted. Indeed, if there is no specific reason to keep these structures attached, it is acceptable to sever the aorta at the level of the third part of the arch, divide the renal arteries and place the aorta in a tray for later demonstration. Alternatively, the pathologist may choose to leave the aorta *in situ* at this stage, allowing the subsequent removal and demonstration of the retroperitoneal tissues *en bloc*.

The inferior vena cava is a thin-walled structure that ascends the retroperitoneum to the right of the aorta. It can be opened along its posterior aspect, taking care not to damage the right renal artery, and followed up to the liver and down to the leg branches (Fig. 11.2d). The renal veins should be opened. This is of special importance where renal tumours are suspected. Indeed, the kidneys should not be dissected off until the inferior vena cava has been opened, since the tumour may extend directly into it.

The remaining perinephric fat can be cleared with blunt dissection, exposing the kidneys. The ureters are best located with the fingers; fortunately the ureters tend to be the toughest structure in this region and blunt dissection usually leaves them intact. They can be freed down to the bladder and left in continuity with it. Manual compression of the bladder at this point may demonstrate outflow obstruction, particularly in the male, and sometimes reflux can be observed in either sex. The bladder (and prostate in males) can be dissected free of the pelvic block and opened. If they appear dilated or

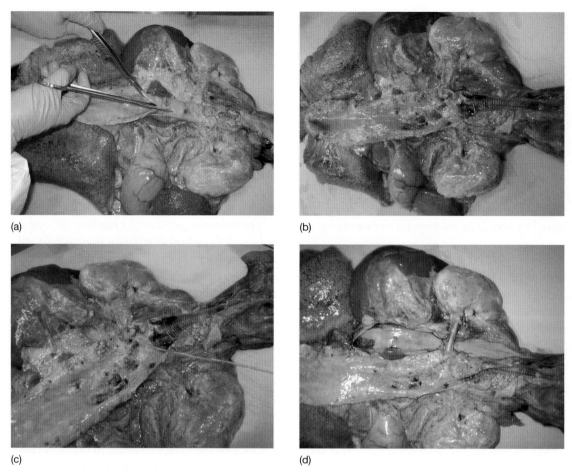

(a)

(b)

(c)

(d)

Figure 11.2 (a) Opening the posterior aspect of the aorta. (b) The aorta opened along its length. (c) Testing the patency of the ostia with a probe. (d) The vena cava opened.

otherwise abnormal, the ureters can be opened down to the bladder at one end and into the renal pelvis at the other by inserting scissors into the renal pelvis and cutting downwards towards the bladder.

The kidneys are usually opened by one clean cut extending along the long axis of the kidney, starting at the anti-ureteric surface and leaving the two halves connected by a small rim of tissue on the renal pelvic aspect (Fig. 11.3a). Regardless of whether it is first separated from the vascular and ureteric attachments, or left *in situ* for later demonstration of the intact retroperitoneal block, the safest way to open a kidney is to lay it on the dissection board and hold it in place with a large sponge. The kidney can then be cut using a long thin-bladed knife. The number of cut sponges in the average busy autopsy

room is mute testimony to the wisdom of this method. The cut renal capsule can be peeled back, noting the ease with which this can be done, allowing the external aspect of the kidney to be examined (Fig. 11.3b). The kidneys can then be removed from the ureters, weighed and laid out for subsequent demonstration. Traditionally, the ureter on the left is cut longer than on the right, facilitating differentiation between the two kidneys later. Alternatively, the kidneys may be left *in situ* to allow demonstration of the intact retroperitoneal block (see below). They should be removed from the ureters and weighed at the end of the demonstration.

The bladder can be opened from trigone to fundus using a pair of blunt-ended scissors inserted into the urethral channel. The tip of the scissors is

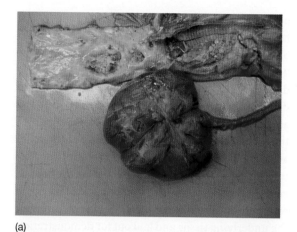

(a)

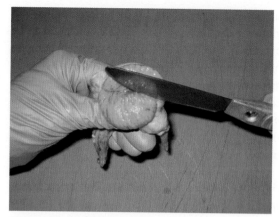

Figure 11.4 Testis being sliced.

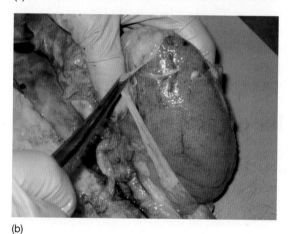

(b)

Figure 11.3 (a) Sliced kidney. (b) Capsule being stripped from the kidney.

inserted into the urethra and angled anteriorly. A linear vertical cut is used to open the bladder. Alternatively, if pathology is suspected on the anterior wall, a curvilinear incision is made around the lateral and superior borders of the bladder. The bladder mucosa can be inspected for trabeculation and the presence of tumours. Erythema of the trigone is a common feature in the catheterised bladder. The patency of the ureteric orifices can be assessed using a probe. It is often difficult to locate the ureteric orifice, particularly in tumorous and trabeculated bladders; in such cases it is much easier to insert the probe into the ureter and pass it into the bladder. In males, transverse slices should be made into the prostate. 'Ball valve' obstruction of the urethra by a hypertrophied median lobe is a common cause of

bladder outflow obstruction and commonly correlates with the degree of trabeculation. In cases of prostatic carcinoma there may be direct extension of the tumour into the bladder and/or seminal vesicles and this should be documented before the bladder is removed. As in the surgical pathology cut-up room, it is difficult at autopsy to detect the presence of carcinoma of the prostate with the naked eye, but the autopsy is a valuable tool for determining the extent of spread of the disease (Ono *et al.*, 2002).

In males, the testes should be removed and examined as described in Chapter 10. The testes can then be opened with a single clean cut extending along the long axis and aimed towards the epididymis using a PM40 blade (Fig. 11.4). Although frequently omitted from the autopsy examination, the testes may harbour significant pathology such as seminoma or teratoma and can be the site of bruising which may be overt in nature or due to, for example, squeezing of the testicles as a form of institutional bullying. The pathologist who does not examine the testes at autopsy but states in the report that they were normal will appear foolish if it later transpires that one or both of the testes were prosthetic!

The female reproductive organs are conveniently examined at this point. Dissection of the intact female and male genitourinary tracts is discussed in detail in Chapter 10. Anatomical anomalies can be demonstrated and documented. The presence of serosal fibroids (leiomyomas) and possible endometriosis can be sought. The condition of the ovaries is noted and the patency of the fallopian tubes can be assessed. The uterus should be opened with a longitudinal cut allowing the endometrium and myometrium to be examined. The cervix should be examined. Samples of any lesions noted can be taken for histopathological assessment. In women of child-bearing age, histological sampling can be useful to prove the absence of pregnancy. Measurements of uteri distorted by fibroids are difficult and, as in surgical pathology, the overall weight is the least misleading index.

Finally, while dealing with the pelvic structures, the rectum should be opened and its mucosa examined. Some pathologists (and anatomical pathology technologists) leave the rectum *in situ* when eviscerating the pelvis but this is not recommended. The rectum is the most common location of large intestinal malignancies. Examination of the rectal stump may also reveal the presence of colitis, solitary rectal ulcers, polyps or blood.

En-bloc retroperitoneal dissection

In cases of suspected genitourinary tract pathology, the pathologist may wish to demonstrate the retro-

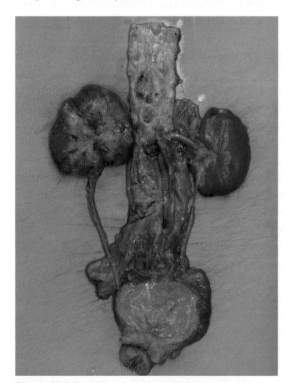

Figure 11.5 En-bloc retroperitoneal dissection demonstrated.

peritoneal structures in anatomical continuity. The technique takes some practice and care but is valuable when demonstrating findings in the genitourinary tract to interested parties An en-bloc dissection is achieved by undertaking the dissection described above but leaving the organs *in situ*. The aorta is then divided at the level of the third part of the arch and dissected free to the level of the renal arteries, sacrificing the mesenteric arteries. The inferior vena cava is divided at the level of the hepatic veins and dissected free of the liver bed. The entire retroperitoneal block can now be dissected free of the underlying tissue and laid out for demonstration (Fig. 11.5). The block includes the kidneys (attached to the opened aorta and inferior vena cava), ureters, bladder, and the prostate or female genital tract. The specimen should be trimmed of superfluous fat before demonstration.

The gastrointestinal tract

Once the retroperitoneal and pelvic tissues have been examined, attention can be turned to the gastrointestinal tract. Normal situs is confirmed and the various sites in which pus can accumulate and become walled off should be examined (subphrenic space, paracolic gutters). Adhesions of organs resulting from old or recent peritonitis, fistulae and perforations can be sought. The organ block is then positioned on the dissection bench with the posterior aspect uppermost.

If the organs were eviscerated in one block (Letulle technique), the oesophagus must first be dissected free. In cases where there is no suspicion of portal hypertension, the oesophagus is first opened along its posterior aspect down to the level of the diaphragm (Fig. 11.6a). It can then be divided from the pharynx and dissected from the posterior aspect of the trachea (Fig. 11.6b). If oesophageal varices are suspected, the oesophagus should not be opened, and is dissected free of the trachea intact and in continuity with the stomach prior to eversion.

The eversion technique is used to demonstrate the presence of oesophageal varices, since the thin-walled vessels tend to collapse if the oesophagus is opened without eversion and then become very dif-

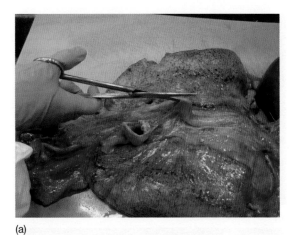 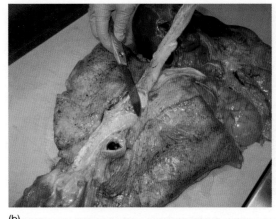

(a)   (b)

Figure 11.6 (a) Oesophagus opened. (b) Oesophagus dissected free.

ficult to identify. This procedure should be performed whenever there is a possibility of chronic liver disease and/or portal hypertension, and certainly when cirrhosis of the liver has been discovered during the preliminary evisceration.

The organs are removed so that the oesophagus and stomach remain in continuity. With the posterior surface of the organ block facing upwards, the oesophagus is first ligated and then dissected from the back of the trachea by dividing it below the larynx and holding the upper end with forceps. The diaphragmatic attachments are divided and the stomach mobilised. A transverse incision is made in the stomach about 10 cm below the gastro-oesophageal junction and the stomach contents are emptied. The upper end of the oesophagus is tied with string and a pair of clampable forceps (such as Spencer Wells) are passed up inside the oesophagus to grasp the tied end (Fig. 11.7a and b). The forceps are withdrawn and the oesophagus is everted (Fig. 11.7c) with the varices, if present, clearly visible on the mucosal surface (Fig. 11.7d).

Dissection of the remainder of the upper gastrointestinal tract is simplified if the omental fat is first dissected free from the greater curve of the stomach. The spleen and pancreas can then be examined, along with the portal venous system if needed.

Holding the spleen in one's non-dominant hand, the attachments between the spleen and the greater curve of the stomach are divided with scissors. The stomach falls away, exposing the anterior surface of the pancreas and the lesser sac. The portal venous

system can be opened at this point by first opening the splenic vein, which runs from the splenic hilum along the superior border of the pancreas into the portal vein, which is then opened. The spleen can be dissected free at this point having first identified and examined the splenic vessels. The presence of accessory spleens (splenunculi) can be ascertained. The spleen should be weighed and the condition of the splenic capsule noted before slicing the organ at no greater than 10 mm intervals (Fig. 11.8). If focal pathology is not identified, a single representative slice can be set aside for demonstration and a small sample is taken for histopathological assessment. In infective cases, the surface of the unopened spleen should be seared with a hot scalpel blade, palette knife or broad-bladed soldering iron to sterilise the capsule. Swabs can be plunged through this area to collect specimens for microbiological culture. Some pathologists prefer to examine the spleen by making a single slice through its longest axis. In our view, this is suboptimal and will miss small focal pathology (such as tumours or areas of infarction).

The oesophageal dissection can now be continued through the crura of the diaphragm and along the edge of the stomach. Before opening the stomach, consideration should be given to the collection of gastric contents for toxicological analysis (discussed in Chapter 15). There is little to choose between opening the stomach along the greater or the lesser curve, but the pathologist should have a routine preference, since it is easier to be certain of

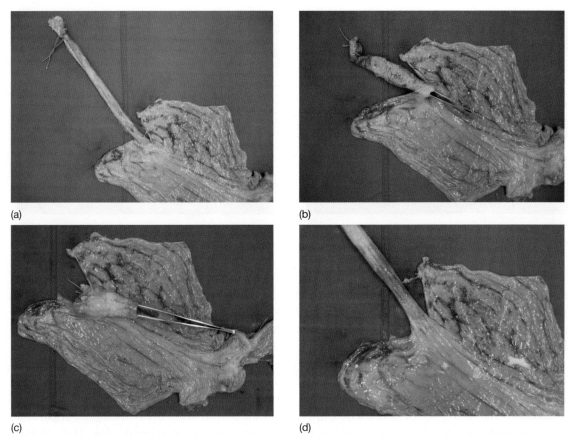

(a)

(b)

(c)

(d)

Figure 11.7 (a) The proximal oesophagus is tied with string. (b) Forceps are inserted into the oesophagus to grasp the string. (c) The forceps are withdrawn. (d) The oesophagus is everted.

the anatomy of the organ after the dissection if one always chooses the same approach. Even in cases where toxicological analysis is not required, the contents of the stomach should be collected and examined rather than allowing them to spill over the rest of the dissection or directly into the sink. Many people find this the most emetic part of the whole autopsy and, in their anxiety to get it over with, discard the stomach contents without looking at them. This is always a mistake. The volume and state of digestion of the food, the presence of tablet residues or blood and, in the elderly and demented, the presence of a wide variety of objects can prove informative. After removal of the contents, the mucosa of the stomach can be carefully washed and the presence of erosions, ulcers, perforations, gastritis and tumours can be ascertained (Fig. 11.9a).

An alternative method of examining gastric

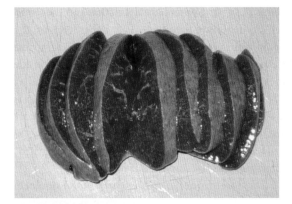

Figure 11.8 Sliced spleen.

mucosa is to invert the stomach. This has the advantage, when demonstrating the organs to clinicians, of leaving the stomach looking stomach-shaped. The oeseophagus is left unopened and is dissected free of

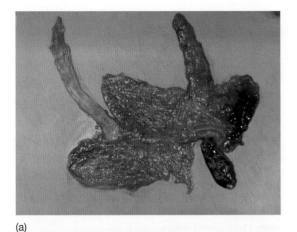

(a)

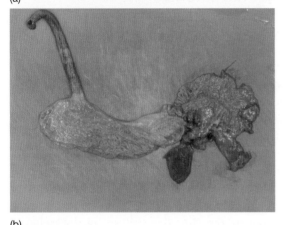

(b)

Figure 11.9 (a) Inspection of the gastric mucosa.
(b) Inspection of the everted gastric mucosa.

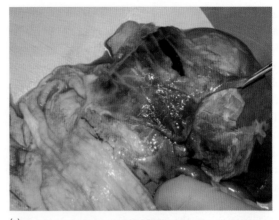

(a)

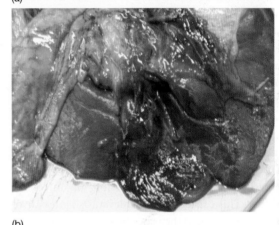

(b)

Figure 11.10 (a) Patency of the common bile duct.
(b) Gallbladder opened.

the trachea. The fat is removed from the greater and lesser curves of the stomach and an incision is then made into the greater curve at the gastric antrum using scissors. The gastric contents are collected with the help of a ladle and jug as described above. Long-toothed forceps are then inserted into the stomach via the antral incision and passed upwards into the proximal portion of the oesophagus. While gripping the inner portion of the proximal oesophagus, the forceps are then retracted, inverting both stomach and oesophagus. The mucosa can now be washed and inspected (Fig. 11.9b).

The incision used to open the stomach should now be continued through the pylorus and along the whole length of the residual duodenum, keeping the cut anterior so as to preserve the ampulla intact and to avoid damage to the pancreas. The patency of the

bile duct can be demonstrated by squeezing the gallbladder (Fig. 11.10a), and this also helps to locate the ampulla of Vater, which is not always obvious. The common bile duct can then be opened back to the liver (a probe inserted into the ampulla of Vater may be useful in guiding the dissection) using artery scissors and the cystic duct can be found from this end or by opening the gallbladder and following the duct out (Fig. 11.10b). Gallstones can be evaluated at this stage; the type can be noted and a few should be cut across to confirm this. The collection of bile for toxicology is discussed in Chapter 15.

The pancreatic duct can also be identified and opened along the length of the pancreas, and samples can be taken for histology. Alternatively, some pathologists prefer to slice the pancreas from tail to the head at intervals of no greater than 10 mm. As a minimum, the pancreas should be sliced longitudinally from the head to the tail using a PM40 blade. Large tumours of the pancreas, and pancreatitis, will be apparent if present. Neuro-endocrine tumours of the pancreas are typically small and wide histological sampling is generally required for their detection. The gallbladder and extrahepatic biliary tree are now dissected free from the liver, effectively separating the upper gastrointestinal tract from the liver and thoracic organs. These organs can be laid out in a tray for later demonstration.

At this point, consideration should be given to examination of the remainder of the intestines. Many pathologists do not routinely open these structures, finding the procedure unpleasant and unrewarding, and prefer to rely solely on an assessment of the serosal surfaces of these organs. This is not recommended, as mucosal lesions will be missed. In drug-related deaths, packages of drugs or failed wrappings may be found throughout the small and large intestine. The intestines should be opened in a sink under water (to minimise the risk of aerosol formation) along their anti-mesenteric border to prevent the aerosol transmission of infectious agents. This can be easily achieved using a pair of bowel scissors, and the procedure is facilitated if the mesenteries were divided as close to the bowel wall as possible during the evisceration. The mucosa is washed clean and inspected for the presence of inflammation, ulcers, diverticula and tumours. The presence or absence of the appendix is recorded.

The liver is examined *in situ* for 'cough grooves' (which can be correlated with the corresponding hypertrophic muscle bands in the diaphragm), tumour deposits, vascular lesions, and signs of trauma and developmental delay. If there are no specific contraindications, the liver can be freed of its 'ligamentous' and diaphragmatic attachments. The inferior vena cava is divided by sliding the blunt edge of a sharp long-bladed knife under the liver to the level of the diaphragm, and then rotating the knife to free the liver with the sharp edge. The liver should be weighed at this stage and then cut in serial slices at intervals of no greater than 10 mm as it lies on the dissection board with its posterior surface downwards (Fig. 11.11). Some pathologists prefer to

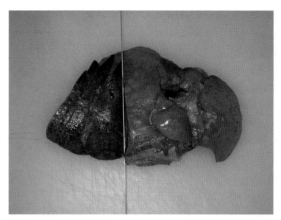

Figure 11.11 Sliced liver.

refrain from completing the cuts, thus leaving the organ with the structure of a book which allows the extent of large lesions such as tumours to be demonstrated. Alternatively, and especially where no lesions or only diffuse lesions are found, a single representative slice may be retained from each lobe for demonstration, samples taken for histopathological evaluation, and the rest discarded following careful assessment.

In some cases, such as bile duct problems or tumours of the head of the pancreas, it may be more helpful to the clinicians (and for photography) to keep the relevant organs in continuity while partially dissecting tissues to reveal the pathological and anatomical details.

In cases where the deceased underwent abdominal surgery, the dissection can be significantly hampered by the presence of recent or old adhesions and carcinomatosis peritonei. In addition, specific attention must be given to the presence of peritonitis, cutaneous perforations, enterostomies and colostomies. In such cases the organs should be eviscerated in one block (Letulle technique), leaving the large and small bowel mass attached. Ileostomies and colostomies are dissected free and clamps can be attached to facilitate identification during the dissection. Dissection of the retroperitoneal tissues and upper gastrointestinal tract can then be undertaken as described above. Removal of these organs leaves the matted bowel, which is first examined for signs of perforation. The extent of further examination of the bowel is dependent on the nature of the intra-abdominal pathology. The bowel may be opened under water or, in the case of dense fibrous adhesions, may be examined by making multiple slices in the coronal plane (Culora and Roche, 1996).

In cases where the deceased had undergone a liver transplant, the vascular and biliary anastamoses should be examined in detail for patency and leaks. The portal venous system is opened as described above, and the hepatic artery traced back from the porta hepatis. The presence or absence of a gallbladder is noted and the common bile duct is opened and traced to its insertion into the small intestine. The cut surface of the liver is examined carefully and widely sampled for the histological assessment of rejection. In patients dying after intraportal hepatocyte transplantation, the portal venous system should be opened to exclude portal vein thrombosis (Baccarani *et al.*, 2005).

The heart and major vessels

Demonstration of a cardiac air embolus

As with the demonstration of a pneumothorax, one must always consider a cardiac air embolus prior to opening the body, especially if there is a history of either trauma or a therapeutic procedure where air may have entered the venous or arterial system. Venous air embolism may occur with open systems of intravenous infusion, during parturition or abortion, during operations to the head and neck if the head is above the level of the heart, and during orogenital sex in a pregnant woman. A volume of 100–250 mL of air is estimated to be required to cause death from venous air embolus although greater or smaller amounts can occur. Again, as before, radiological imaging should be performed prior to the examination. Plain x-ray may reveal an over-distended heart and great vessels due to the abnormal presence of air (Fig. 11.12a and b). This examination has been superseded by the use of multi-slice computerised tomography, although caution must be expressed with the over-interpretation of air within the heart and great vessels when using this technique as this may be a pure post-mortem artefact owing to the rapid production of intravascular air due to decomposition.

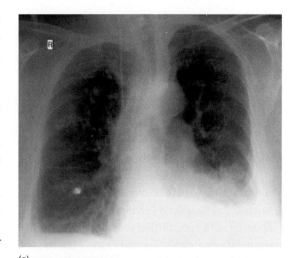
(a)

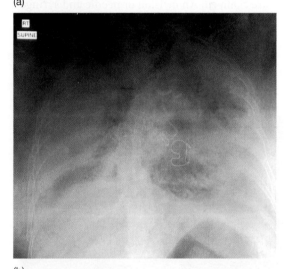
(b)

Figure 11.12 (a) Ante-mortem chest x-ray. (b) Post-mortem chest x-ray showing a cardiac air embolus.

Two methods have been described for the examination of the heart for the presence of an air embolus (Knight, 1983; Di Maio and Di Maio, 1989).

- *Method 1.* The chest cavity is opened as normal with great care being taken not to open the pericardial sac or cause any damage to the vessels entering and exiting the heart; this includes the vessels going to and from the arms and neck. To ensure that this happens, the heart can be examined via a window cut into the sternum. If the sternum is opened, the internal mammary vessels should be identified and clamped or ligated. The pericardial sac is opened and the epicardial veins examined for air bubbles. The coronary arteries are too thick to allow air bubbles to be observed at this stage. The pericardial sac is held open by an assistant and filled with water. As for a pneumothorax, a water-filled syringe and needle with the plunger removed can be advanced into the right ventricle, observing for air bubbles. Alternatively, an incision can be made, under water, into the right ventricle, again observing for bubbles.

- *Method 2*. The second method starts with the opening of the pericardial sac but then each of the great vessels entering and exiting the heart are clamped. An incision or needle and syringe procedure can be performed as before. When the right ventricle is opened, not only does one observe a stream of bubbles but also the ventricle is filled with frothy blood.

Pericardium

To examine the heart, the thoracic organ block is positioned on the dissection board with its anterior aspect uppermost. The pericardium is first incised by lifting it up free from the anterior cardiac wall and making a transverse cut near the base. This cut is then followed by a median inferior-to-superior cut forming an inverted T-shaped incision (Fig. 11.13a). Fluid in the pericardial sac can be sampled for microbiology or extracted and its volume measured in the case of effusions or haemopericardium. In subjects who have been actively resuscitated there may be a blood-stained effusion due to attempted pericardiocentesis or due to intracardiac injections which should be, but are not always, recorded in the notes. Active resuscitation can also rupture small epicardial vessels and these are often very difficult to demonstrate.

In some cases the heart is focally or diffusely adherent to the pericardium. Focal attachments are often

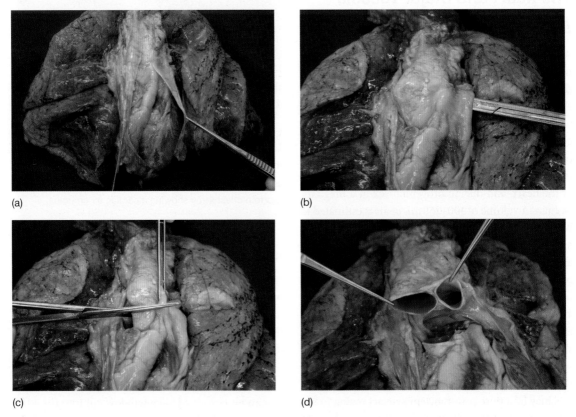

(a)

(b)

(c)

(d)

Figure 11.13 (a) The pericardial sac is opened. (b) The aortic and pulmonary arteries are identified. (c) While supported these structures are cut across using scissors. (d) The interior of the pulmonary artery is examined for thromboembolus.

due to infarction and are fibrinous in recent infarcts and fibrous in old ones. The extent and nature of the adhesions should be noted for subsequent correlation with the distribution of the infarct. Generalised adhesions can also be fibrinous in the early stages of pericarditis and fibrous in the late stages. The pericarditis can be due to primary inflammation or inflammation secondary to surgery or infarction. Dense fibrous pericardial adhesions are common in patients who have undergone a coronary artery bypass graft. Fibrous adhesion of the pericardium to the heart can be difficult or impossible to separate and one may have to dissect the heart with the pericardium attached. In any case, an attempt to remove the pericardium using blunt dissection should be employed and actual cutting is reserved for situations that have defeated the blunt approach. Post-surgical cases in which there has been coronary artery bypass surgery require special documentation and should be performed with the surgeons present wherever possible.

The heart may then be removed from the pericardial cavity. The aorta and pulmonary arterial trunk are identified and two fingers passed behind them; with the fingers slightly separated (to avoid cutting the glove rubber) the vessels can be cut (Fig. 11.13b and c). The lumen of the pulmonary arterial trunk should be checked for thromboembolus (Fig. 11.13d) since a large 'saddle embolus' lodged at the bifurcation of this trunk may be the cause of sudden death and is easily lost during later dissection. The temptation to probe the proximal pulmonary artery should be resisted; damage to the pulmonary valve may occur preventing subsequent assessment of pulmonary stenosis and regurgitation. Finally, the pulmonary veins and venae cavae are divided and the heart lifted clear of the pericardial cavity. In general it is desirable to remove the heart with a short cuff of the aorta, but a longer cuff of the superior vena cava should be removed to prevent damage to the sino-atrial node.

Coronary arteries

If coronary artery angiography is not to be performed then the dissection of the heart should follow the direction of blood flow around the heart in general terms. The main difference of opinion is whether or not the coronary arteries should be dissected first.

In favour of dissecting the coronary arteries first is the fact that they are not damaged by any other procedure. The limitation is that they are harder to locate in the unopened heart and more difficult to relate to areas of ischaemia. In either case, the location of the ostia of the coronary arteries is first confirmed. Normally, one orifice is present in each of the two forward-facing aortic sinuses (right and left). In cases where both ostia arise in one aortic sinus, the pulmonary artery should be dissected free of the aortic root to determine the path of the anomalous coronary artery. If the anomalous coronary artery passes between the pulmonary artery and aortic trunk there is a risk of sudden death on exercise (Davies, 1999). The proximal portions are probed to check their patency. Following this, they are traditionally examined by transverse cuts at 1–2 mm intervals (and certainly no greater than 5 mm) (Fig. 11.14a). Coronary artery atheroma is a focal or multi-focal disease. Overspacing of the cuts in the coronary arteries may miss a fatal stenosis or occlusion. Under no circumstances should the coronary arteries be opened longitudinally as this makes it impossible to determine the severity of atheromatous stenoses. The presence of thrombus and atheroma within the epicardial vessels is recorded. The point at which stenosis of the coronary arteries becomes clinically significant is contentious, but the finding of a 70–75 per cent stenosis (lumen diameter less than 1 mm) has a high probability of being the cause of death when no other cause is found macroscopically (Davies, 1999).

Heavily calcified coronary arteries are frequently encountered in elderly subjects. These may be very difficult to cut. The temptation to support the vessel from behind with a finger inserted through the valve may be strong but is extremely dangerous and should be resisted. Even when the heart is opened it is often impossible to cut heavily calcified vessels with a scalpel. Scissors may be used, but the value of this is in itself doubtful since the shearing action of the scissors inevitably causes compression and even obliteration of a tiny lumen. In such cases, consideration should be given to coronary artery angiography but this is generally unrealistic in routine practice in

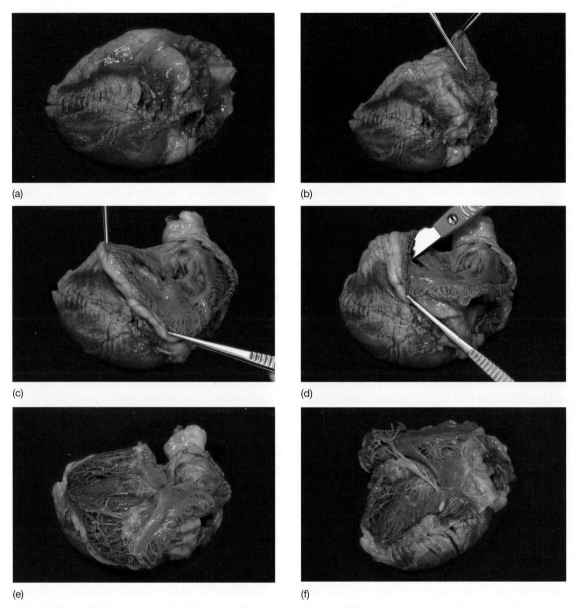

Figure 11.14 (a) The left anterior descending coronary artery is sliced at small intervals. (b) The right atrium is opened by a cut extending from the superior vena cava to the right atrial appendage. (c) The opened right atrium. (d) The right side of the heart is opened with a lateral incision made with a PM40 blade. (e) Tricuspid valve. (f) The opened right ventricular outflow tract.

most mortuaries. Alternatively, the intact coronary arteries can be dissected free of the heart, fixed, decalcified, and sliced when soft.

Cardiac chambers and valves

Whether the coronary supply is dissected before or after opening the heart, the actual opening of the heart can be achieved by a variety of techniques.

Prior to any incision of the heart it is possible to assess the valves semi-quantitatively. The integrity of the mitral and tricuspid valves can be determined by filling the heart with water via the atria, clamping the aorta and pulmonary valves, and gently squeezing the ventricles. Competent valves should prevent retrograde flow of water into the atria. Similarly, the aortic and pulmonary valves can be assessed by attempting to pour water into the heart via the aorta and pulmonary artery. Valvular stenoses can be assessed at this stage by inserting a graduated conical measure into the valves. This is also an important time to look at the valves for the presence of congenital abnormalities and vegetations, since the evidence for these may be lost when the valves are cut.

Zeien and Klatt (1990) provide a description of the examination of cardiac valve prostheses at autopsy. The following is adapted from this classic text; an x-ray examination to include the great vessels and the aorta should be considered in cases of sudden mechanical failure in an attempt to identify breakage and embolisation of valve components. If a radiological examination is not possible, then palpation of the vessels *in situ* should be undertaken. The heart is dissected carefully to allow for inspection of the prosthesis and annulus in the consideration of dehiscence and paravalvular leakage. A discontinuous ring of endothelialisation should lead to the consideration of a leak. Careful exploration with a probe should determine the site of leakage. The prosthesis is identified by its generic configuration and then, if possible, by its trade name. The integrity of the valve is checked. The component parts are determined to be present and functional. Abnormal motion due to the presence of thrombus is examined for. If present, the thrombus should be cultured and examined microscopically. Misalignment and disproportion are assessed by comparing the prosthesis with the ventricular chamber size and surrounding myocardium.

The general principle in dissection of the heart is to follow the route of blood flow. The heart is positioned with its posterior aspect uppermost and the apex of the heart away from the operator. The right atrium is first opened by a cut extending from the entry of the superior vena cava across to the right atrial appendage (Fig. 11.14b and c). Even in prolonged atrial fibrillation it is unusual to find thrombus in the right atrial appendage. The right atrium and ventricle can now be opened by inserting the tip of a PM40 blade through the tricuspid valve into the apex of the right ventricle and making a lateral incision from the apex to the atrium (Fig. 11.14d and e). Turning the heart over, the anterior wall of

the right ventricle is incised close to the anterior aspect of the septum, continuing up through the pulmonary valve into the pulmonary artery (Fig. 11.14e). The mirror image procedure is then followed with the left atrium, left atrial appendage, mitral valve, left ventricle close to the septum and up through the aortic valve and aorta (Fig. 11.15a–e).

It is often found that the left anterior descending coronary artery is not restricted to the anterior aspect of the septum and is consequently severed with the above technique. Some operators prefer to open the left ventricle along its left lateral margin and to open the aortic valve and aortic root directly, leaving the anterior wall of the left ventricle attached to the septum. Also, some operators find it easier to perform the whole cardiac dissection with scissors, while others prefer to make the ventricular incisions and cut through the valves with a large-bladed knife. There are variations on the method and it is possible to open the right side of the heart posteriorly, close to the septum, and the left side of the heart anteriorly, close to the septum, enabling the whole preparation to be laid flat and then viewed from either aspect.

The valve measurements can be confirmed at this stage, the circumference being measured along the valve ring. The nature of valvular lesions can also be confirmed and documented. It is also appropriate to weigh the heart, since it is empty of blood. The weight of the heart should be compared with tables of normal heart weights for height and body weight. Some pathologists choose to measure the thickness of the ventricles at the outflow tracts. This is a poor indicator of hypertrophy as the thickness of the myocardium will depend on whether the heart is affected by rigor mortis or not. A better method is that of Foulton *et al.* (1952), which involves dissecting the left ventricle off in continuity with the septum and comparing the weight with that of the right ventricle. If the ventricles are freed of epicardial fat and dissected along the valve rims, the normal ratio is between 2.3:1 and 3.3:1. Right ventricular hypertrophy is diagnosed if the right ventricle weighs more than 80 g and when right hypertrophy occurs alone the ratio is always less than 2:1. If biventricular hypertrophy occurs the ratio may be normal. If the left ventricle plus septum

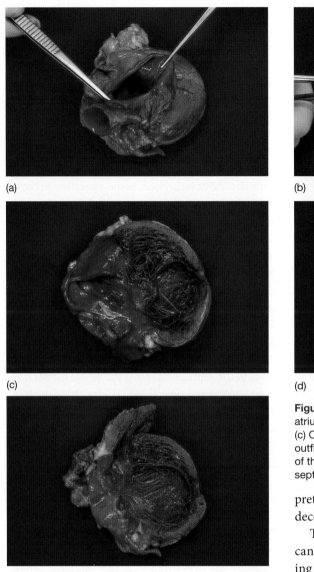

(a)

(c)

(e)

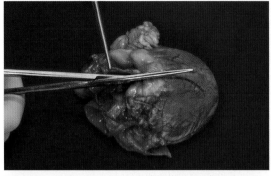

(b)

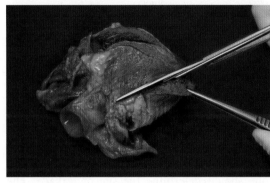

(d)

Figure 11.15 (a) Viewing the mitral valve from the left atrium. (b) The lateral border of the left ventricle is opened. (c) Opened left atrium and ventricle. (d) The left ventricle outflow tract is exposed by cutting up the anterior aspect of the left ventricular wall close to the interventricular septum. (e) Opened left ventricle outflow tract.

preted in the context of the weight and height of the deceased (Hangartner *et al.*, 1985).

The myocardium of the left and right ventricles can now be sliced across at 5–10 mm intervals, leaving thin connections to hold it together, and this allows the extent and distribution of ischaemic and fibrotic areas to be delineated (Fig. 11.16). Most pathologists will slice the myocardium transversely, parallel to the atrioventricular valve rings. Alternatively, and especially where myocarditis is suspected, the myocardium can be sliced longitudinally.

Some pathologists favour the removal of two or three slices from the apex of the heart, each 5–10 mm thick, before opening the remainder of the heart in the direction of blood flow. This has the advantage of presenting visiting clinicians (and examiners) with an echocardiographic view of the ventricles.

weighs more than 225 g, then left ventricular hypertrophy can be diagnosed. Ideally, Foulton's technique should be performed on the fixed heart as it is easier to remove all of the epicardial fat. Where consent cannot be obtained to retain the heart, the method can be successfully applied to the fresh heart. Other workers have found higher values for the isolated left ventricle (McPhie, 1957; Bove *et al.*, 1966), but Foulton's values are a reasonable approximation and the ratios remain useful. As with the whole heart, the left and right ventricular weights should be inter-

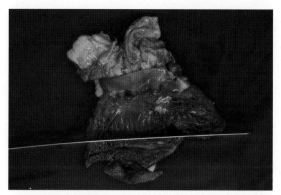

Figure 11.16 The left ventricular myocardium is sliced to look for abnormalities.

The most diseased sections of the coronary arteries can be placed around one of these slices in bottle caps, allowing coronary artery and myocardial disease to be easily related to each other (see below).

Examination of the conducting system of the heart

To examine the cardiac conducting system, the heart is fixed in a distended state after removing as much contained blood as possible and then packing with cotton wool. Care must be taken when removing the heart not to sever the superior vena cava too close to its cardiac insertion, or the sino-atrial node may be lost. The right atrium is then opened, allowing access to the interior. The superior vena cava (SVC) is left intact. The auricular appendage of the right atrium is identified and from this the crest extends to abut on the superior vena cava; the sino-atrial (SA) node is situated at this site (Fig. 11.17a) and the first block is taken from here. The interior of the right atrium has several landmarks (Fig. 11.17b); the key one is the coronary sinus. The atrio-ventricular (AV) node is just anterior to the coronary sinus and the bundle branches pass forwards at this point before dipping down into the septal myocardium. Two blocks are taken for the conducting system. The first is obtained by opening the SVC and continuing the cut into the right atrial muscle, taking the area where the auricular crest abuts onto the SVC (Fig. 11.17c). Longitudinal sections are then taken from this block, usually about five in number.

The AV node can be sampled by taking the area produced by a vertical cut anterior to the coronary sinus traversing the tricuspid valve ring and into ventricular muscle. A parallel cut is then made through the supraventricular crest and again down into ventricular muscle. The two incisions are joined above and below by two horizontal incisions (Fig. 11.17c). This block is divided into two halves horizontally, leaving the conducting system in the lower block, and horizontal slices can be taken through this. The upper block is sectioned vertically from anterior to posterior (Fig. 11.17d) and this contains the AV node and bundle branches.

Dissecting the heart after cardiac surgery

The post-mortem examination of the heart in patients dying after cardiac surgery has been discussed in detail by Lee and Gallagher (1998) and requires several modifications of the techniques described above. Briefly, it is of note that a detailed history, including the findings at operation and details of the operative procedure, should be obtained before commencing. The presence of cannulae, pacing wires, drains and intra-aortic balloon pumps are noted. On opening the thoracic cavity, the presence and volume of any intrathoracic haemorrhage is recorded. The pericardium should be examined, and the presence of surgical incisions into it recorded. All coronary artery bypass grafts, and the cannulation sites for cardiopulmonary bypass grafts, should be identified, checking that the suture lines are intact, before the heart is removed from the body. When the heart has been removed, any coronary artery bypass grafts should be examined, including a transverse cut across the distal anastamoses. The native coronary arteries, the cardiac chambers and valves are examined as described above. In cases of valve replacement, special attention should be paid to the presence or absence of thrombosis, vegetations, perforations, perivalvular leaks, abscesses, and structural deterioration. Sections of myocardium are taken for histopathological evaluation from any area of suspected myocardial infarction and the myocardium distal to any bypass graft anastamosis (Lee and Gallagher, 1998).

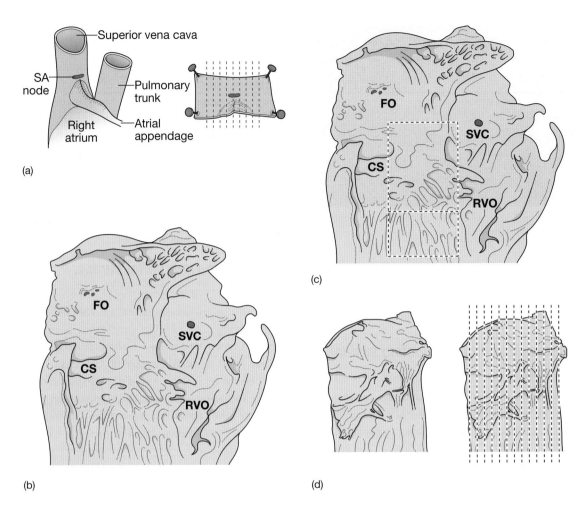

Figure 11.17 (a) Diagram showing the location and sampling of the sino-atrial (SA) node. (b) Internal anatomy of the right atrium with the foramen ovale (FO), the coronary sinus (CS), the supraventricular crest (SVC) and the right ventricular outflow tract (RVO). (c) Internal anatomy of the right atrium showing the conducting system with the area to be sampled (dashed lines). (d) The block indicated in (c) has been removed and is viewed in the same plane as in (c) and from the left. The vertical lines show the position of the blocks taken for histology.

Demonstrating the cardiac dissection

Having dissected the heart in the direction of blood flow and sliced the myocardium, many pathologists find it difficult to orientate the organ during the subsequent demonstration of pathological findings to students or colleagues. Abnormalities in the coronary arteries may be difficult to relocate once the heart has been opened. A suture placed under the affected portion of the artery is useful in this respect; alternatively, the section of interest can be dissected free of the heart and placed onto a tray for demonstration and later histopathological assessment.

Abnormalities in the cardiac chambers, myocardium and valves are demonstrated with the heart held with the posterior aspect uppermost (Fig. 11.18a). The upper flap of tissue is reflected, exposing the right atrium, tricuspid valve and right ventricle (Fig. 11.18b). Replacing this flap of tissue and opening the heart from the other side exposes the right ventricular outflow tract and pulmonary valve (Fig. 11.18c). Transferring the heart to the other hand so that the anterior surface is uppermost (Fig. 11.18d), and repeating the procedure, exposes first the left atrium, mitral valve and left ventricle , and then the left ventricular outflow tract and aortic valve (Fig. 11.18e and f).

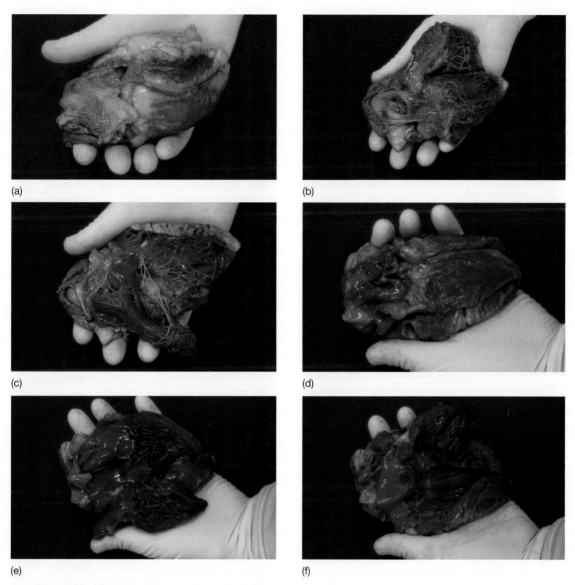

Figure 11.18 (a) Demonstrating the cardiac chambers and valves. The heart is held with the posterior surface uppermost. (b) The right atrium, tricuspid valve and right ventricle are exposed. (c) Right ventricular outflow tract and pulmonary valve. (d) The heart has been turned over into the other hand. (e) The left atrium, mitral valve and left ventricle are exposed. (f) Left ventricular outflow tract and aortic valve.

The respiratory tract

The upper respiratory tract

To examine the respiratory tract, the block of tissues containing the tongue, larynx, trachea and lungs is placed on the dissection board with the posterior surface uppermost. The tongue is first sliced transversely from base to tip, looking for abnormalities including tumours, fibrosis, bruising or the congestion that follows strangulation. The tongue may have been bitten in individuals dying during or after an epileptic seizure. Alternatively the tongue is cut longitudinally. This method is preferred by the authors as it demonstrates anterior and posterior, right- and left-sided pathology with the use of a single incision.

The epiglottis is visible at this stage and can be

examined to exclude epiglottitis. Lateral cuts are made along the hyoid bone and thyroid cartilage, and these are inspected before opening the larynx. The trachea can now be opened through the posterior membranous portion (Fig. 11.19) and the main bronchi pursued down to their entry into the lungs; this is the most common site for primary lung tumours, and foreign bodies have a predilection for the right main bronchus which slopes more rapidly downwards than the left.

At this stage, the pluck is turned over and the rest of the dissection proceeds from the anterior aspect.

The strap muscles of the neck may not be of interest in the routine autopsy, but have considerable forensic interest from the point of view of pressure applied to the neck. It is easy to confuse the bruising that can occur during intubation, epileptic seizures and cannulation of the central veins, but the history should help to clarify this. Dissection of the strap muscles is described in detail in Chapter 10. In the routine autopsy, the thyroid is best revealed by dissecting the strap muscles upwards from their inferior attachments *en bloc*. The thyroid has a relatively fixed site, but extreme variations can occur, including retrosternal. The parathyroids are more variable in position and commonly difficult to locate in the cadaver. The general principle supported by most pathologists is that if they are diseased you will be able to find them and if you cannot find them then they are most probably normal. Parathyroid glands can be distinguished from small lymph nodes by dissecting them free of any surrounding fat and placing

them in water; parathyroid glands will float (owing to their high fat content) whereas lymph nodes will sink. Often they may be found in a posterolateral position and should be sought while removing the oesophagus from the trachea; often they are missed and discarded still attached to the oesophagus.

The thyroid is freed from the anterolateral aspect of the trachea, weighed and sliced, noting the presence of any nodules. The extent of invasion of thyroid cancers is significant. In such cases consideration should be given to taking the neck block intact, fixing it whole, and treating it in a similar way to laryngectomy specimens.

The authors have seen at least one case in which a trainee mistook a heavily calcified colloid nodular goitre for a carcinoma of the thyroid. This error can be avoided by dissecting the gland free of the trachea (so demonstrating the absence of invasion) and by remembering that colloid nodular goitres not uncommonly undergo extensive calcification, especially in the elderly, whereas thyroid cancers do not.

The lungs

The lungs are best examined *in situ*, before their evisceration, to determine whether they have normal lobar isomerism and to see whether they overlap anteriorly (a finding seen in patients with status asthmaticus, chronic obstructive airways disease, mechanical hyperinflation, and drowning). The visceral and parietal surfaces of the pleura, including the diaphragm, are examined for the presence of plaques. The lungs can be removed from the mediastinum by cutting the bronchi and vascular attachments as far from their entry to the lungs as possible (Fig. 11.20a). This gives some lengths of bronchi that can be cannulated for inflation and fixation should that be necessary.

Lung inflation is a prerequisite for investigations of pneumoconiosis, for any diffuse lung disease, and for those conditions in which the preparation of Gough–Wentworth slices are needed (Gibbs and Attanoos, 2000). In cases of tuberculosis where permission cannot be obtained to retain a whole lung, inflation fixation of the lung should be avoided: the technique will not kill the organism, will hamper

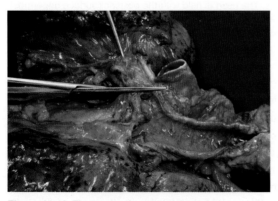

Figure 11.19 The trachea is opened posteriorly.

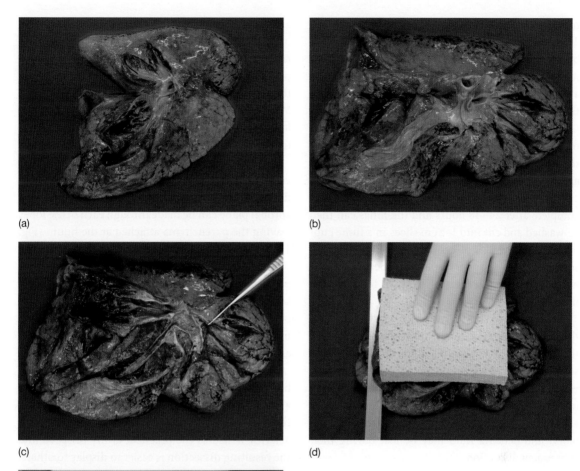

(a)

(b)

(c)

(d)

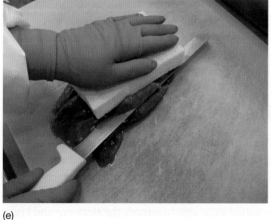

(e)

Figure 11.20 (a) The lungs are removed by cutting the bronchi and vessels as far from their entry to the lungs as possible. (b) The pulmonary arteries of the lower and middle lobe opened with blunt-ended scissors. (c) The pulmonary arteries to the upper lobe are opened from the hilum. (d) The bronchi are opened from the hilum. (e) The lung is held with a sponge and sliced.

microbiological investigation, and adds the hazard of formaldehyde inhalation to the dissection. In cases of suspected tuberculosis where the lung can be retained, microbiological samples should be taken prior to inflation and immersion fixation.

Attempts to inflate the lungs with fixative while still in the thoracic cavity leave the anterior portions of the lungs uninflated.

For inflation with formalin the lungs should be separated at the mediastinum with as long a length of bronchus as possible. It is, of course, feasible to retain the lungs in continuity with the trachea and to dissect this free of the rest of the chest structures. In either case a cannula should be inserted into the bronchus or trachea and fixed with a ligature. A tight seal and relatively intact pleura are required for inflation. It is not necessary to clamp the bronchus. The lung should then be placed in a container of buffered 10% formalin or formol-saline and the cannula connected to a reservoir via a manometer or to a container of fixative arranged above the lung so that a positive head (30 cm) of pressure is directed into the bronchi. With a pump system, the reservoir of fixative can be recycled into the lungs, reducing the total volume required, although no pressure is applied to the lungs by the pump. The procedure is carried out in a fume cupboard. Fixation should be complete after 24–48 hours and the lungs can then be washed and cut into 1–2 cm slices in a fume cupboard using metal L-pieces like those used for brain sectioning. In cases of suspected tuberculosis, the lung should be fixed for at least 72 hours before processing.

Care is taken not to dislodge any pulmonary thromboemboli. The lungs are next examined for the presence of congenital abnormalities, bullae, scars, areas of consolidation and visible emphysema, which should be recorded. Each lung is then weighed in turn prior to any further dissection. Lungs should always be weighed intact; a substantial volume of blood and oedema fluid may be lost during their subsequent dissection.

The lung is supported over a sponge, hilar side down, which exposes the interlobular fissure. If a knife is used to divide the visceral pleura directly opposite the hilum, the first structure encountered is the pulmonary artery. Care is needed to open the right lung in the oblique, and not the transverse fissure. This is opened and, without transecting the vessel, the arterial branches to the lower lobe can be opened with a pair of blunt-ended scissors. The branches to the middle lobe of the right lung and lingula of the left lung are opened in a similar fashion (Fig. 11.20b). The lung is now turned over, hilum upwards, and the arteries of the upper lobe, excluding the lingula on the left, are opened (Fig. 11.20c). Care is taken while dissecting the pulmonary arteries not to dislodge any pulmonary emboli. The risk of this is less than expected; post-mortem clot is not adherent, but pulmonary thromboemboli may be.

Having dissected the pulmonary arteries, the bronchi to the lower lobes, middle lobe and lingula are opened from the hilum. Finally, the upper lobe bronchi are opened with care. At this point there is a risk of transecting the vessels but it is possible to open the bronchi by going underneath the vessels if the scissors are advanced at an angle (Fig. 11.20d). With this technique, the airways and arteries of the lungs can be opened in a manner that keeps both intact (McCulloch and Rutty, 1998).

Having followed the various arteries and blood vessels out to the periphery, the lungs can be held down with a large sponge and a single cut in the coronal plane can be made through each of the lobes leaving the parenchyma attached at the hilum (Fig. 11.20e). This affords a good view of the extent and distribution of any pathology such as tumours, pneumonic consolidation, bronchiectasis, emphysema, pneumoconiosis, interstitial lung disease, the curious prominence of small bronchi in chronic obstructive airways disease, and mucus plugging in asthma.

Alternatively, the lungs may be examined, after being separated from their mediastinal attachments and weighed, by simply placing a single coronal slice through each, without opening the airways and arteries. This has the practical utility of speed and the resulting dissection is easier to display to others. If necessary it is still possible to revert to the more detailed examination described above.

Once the lungs have been opened and sliced, the parenchyma should be sampled for histology before squeezing it to detect the presence of oedema or pus.

The cranial contents

The procedure for removing the brain is discussed in Chapter 12 and does not differ between neurological and general cases. Candidates sitting the membership examination of the Royal College of Pathologists are expected to be able to remove the skull cap and brain once the scalp has been reflected and the skull incised by an anatomical pathology technologist. Where the brain is not thought to be the seat of problems requiring the specialised attentions of a neuropathologist it should be examined carefully externally, looking for the flattened gyri of oedema, or the depressions of infarcts or the grooves of bony projections in raised intracranial pressure, and the distribution of bleeding in various intracranial haemorrhages.

The superior sagittal sinus should be opened to exclude thrombus (Fig. 11.21a and b). The dura is stripped from the base of the skull and the inside of the skull should be stressed by pulling on the front and back to demonstrate basal fractures. The pituitary and its fossa should also be examined. The brain is then placed upside down on the dissecting board and the arteries at the base of the brain examined before removing the brainstem to examine the midbrain (Fig. 11.22a). The cerebellar hemispheres can be removed and examined with a series of radial slices. The cerebral hemispheres are sliced at 10–20 mm intervals looking for gross abnormalities. The first cut is usually placed at the level of the mamillary bodies (Fig. 11.22b), with further cuts placed anterior and posterior to this. Unexpected findings at this stage should be evaluated for referral to a neuropathologist. Removal and examination of the spinal cord, middle ears, eyes and vertebral arteries are described in Chapter 12.

Demonstration of the findings

At the end of the dissection the pathologist is left with a series of carefully dissected organs that can be displayed to students and colleagues. These will have been laid out as the dissection proceeds and will have a tendency to dry out with time. This can be prevented by keeping the dissected organs covered with a towel that has been dampened with water.

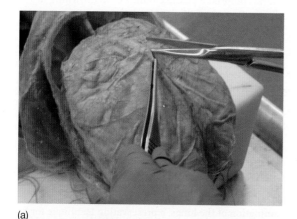

(a)

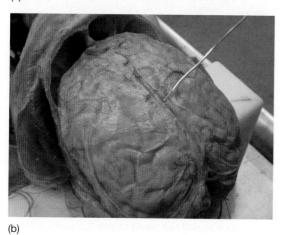

(b)

Figure 11.21 (a) The superior sagittal sinus is opened with scissors. (b) The superior sagittal sinus is examined to exclude thrombus.

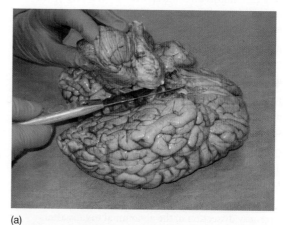

(a)

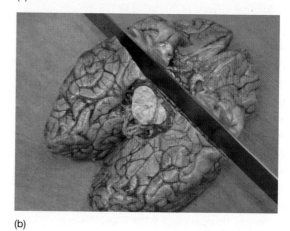

(b)

Figure 11.22 (a) The midbrain and cerebellum are removed. (b) Slicing of the cerebral hemispheres is started with a cut through the mamillary bodies.

Small tissue samples such as slices of the adrenal glands, parathyroid glands and slices of the coronary arteries are best placed into inverted bottle caps to prevent them sticking to the towel and being lost.

It is worth remembering that many of those who attend the post-mortem demonstration may have known the deceased in life, and may be less comfortable in the mortuary surroundings than the pathologist. The body should be washed down, and covered with a clean sheet or plastic apron. Similarly, the dissection area and instruments should be washed. The dirty apron, gauntlets and outer pair of gloves are removed. Thus the pathologist may demonstrate the findings to those in the viewing gallery while causing minimum distress to the onlookers.

Finally, small samples of tissue may be collected for subsequent histopathological assessment. Samples should be routinely collected from all organs and from any lesional tissue. Unless there is good reason, and express consent, whole organs should not be retained. All of the organs are then returned to the body in a strong watertight polythene bag, for subsequent reconstruction. This is the subject of Chapter 21.

References

Baccarani U, Adani GL, Sanna A *et al.* (2005). Portal vein thrombosis after intraportal hepatocytes transplantation in a liver transplant recipient. *Transplant Int* **18**:750–4.

Barzon L, Sonino N, Fallo F, Palu G, Boscaro M (2003). Prevalence and natural history of adrenal incidentalomas. *Eur J Endocrinol* **149**:273–85.

Bove KE, Rowlands DT, Scott RC (1966). Observations on the assessment of cardiac hypertrophy using a chamber partition technique. *Circulation* **33**:558–68.

Cotton DWK, Stephenson TJ (1988). Impairment of autopsy histology by organ washing: a myth. *Med Sci Law* **28**:319–23.

Culora GA, Roche WR (1996). Simple method for necropsy dissection of the abdominal organs after abdominal surgery. *J Clin Pathol* **49**:776–9.

Davies MJ (1999). The investigation of sudden cardiac death. *Histopathology* **34**:93–8.

Di Maio DJ, Di Maio VJ (1989). *Forensic Pathology*, pp. 405–10. New York: Elsevier.

Foulton RM, Hutchinson EC, Jones AM (1952). Ventricular weights in cardiac hypertrophy. *Br Heart J* **14**:413–20.

Gibbs AR, Attanoos RL (2000). Examination of lung specimens. *J Clin Pathol* **53**:507–12.

Hangartner JRW, Marley NJ, Whitehead A, Thomas AC, Davies MJ (1985). The assessment of cardiac hypertrophy at autopsy. *Histopathology* **9**:1295–306.

Kakizaki E, Takahama K, Seo Y *et al.* (2008). Marine bacteria comprise a possible indicator of drowning in seawater. *Forensic Sci Int* **176**(2/3):236–47.

Knight B (1983). *The Coroner's Autopsy*, pp. 116–17. Edinburgh: Churchill Livingstone.

Knight B (1996). *Forensic Pathology*, 2nd edn, pp. 1–47. London: Arnold.

Lee AHS, Gallagher PJ (1998). Post-mortem examination after cardiac surgery. *Histopathology* **33**:399–405.

Lucci A, Cirnelli A.(2007). A microbiological test for the diagnosis of death by drowning. *Forensic Sci Int* **168**(1):34–6.

McCulloch TA, Rutty GN (1998). Postmortem examination of the lungs: a preservation technique for opening the bronchi and pulmonary arteries individually without transection problems. *J Clin Pathol* **51**:163–6.

McPhie J (1957). Left ventricular hypertrophy; the determination of left ventricular weight. *Aust Ann Med* **6**:328–35.

Ono Y, Ozawa M, Suzuki K *et al.* (2002). Autopsy findings of patients with urological neoplasms. *Int J Clin Oncol* **7**:301–5.

Shimizu M, Sakurai T, Tadaoka Y (1997). A simple technique for identifying the adrenal glands at necropsy. *J Clin Pathol* **50**:263–4.

Zeien LB, Klatt EC (1990). Cardiac valve prostheses at autopsy. *Arch Pathol Lab Med* **114**:933–7.

Chapter 12

EXAMINATION OF THE NERVOUS SYSTEM

James Lowe

Introduction

Before commencing the autopsy it is essential to review the clinical history and, where relevant, any relevant imaging. This will indicate the broad planning and the consent that will be required to conduct a meaningful examination of the nervous system, relevant to clinical and medicolegal needs.

Clinical signs and symptoms involving the nervous system

Plan a full examination and sampling of the nervous system. In such cases, examination of the nervous system is expected to be essential to arriving at an accurate diagnosis of conditions contributing to the cause of death, including:

- cerebral hypoxia/anoxia;
- head injury;
- epilepsy;
- dementia;
- movement disorder;
- Creutzfeldt–Jakob disease;
- peripheral neuropathy.

Consent or authority should be sought for retention of the brain and/or spinal cord and peripheral nerve/muscle, depending on clinical indications.

No clinical indication of signs or symptoms directly referable to the nervous system

Plan an examination and sampling of the nervous system as part of a full general post-mortem. Findings in the nervous system are expected to give additional information. In such cases, a macroscopic examination of the fresh brain plus limited tissue sampling is typically adequate.

Limited post-mortem examination

In some circumstances it is appropriate to offer the choice of a post-mortem examination limited to the brain only or to the brain and spinal cord. Typically this is applied where there is a clinical history of a specific disease of the nervous system and the patient or family members seek further information on the diagnosis. This is also a common approach for patients and their families who seek to support research into diseases of the nervous system.

As with all limited post-mortems, it is possible that a full explanation for a disease may not be forthcoming. In the context of the central nervous system

(CNS), certain clinical situations would justify advising retention of the spinal cord in addition to the brain, detailed in later sections.

Consultation with a specialist neuropathologist is recommended before advising a family on the merits and potential drawbacks of a limited examination, as part of obtaining informed consent.

Retaining the brain and examination following fixation

The most reliable results are achieved if the brain and spinal cord are retained and examined following fixation. The benefits of retention of the brain and/or spinal cord should be explained to legal authorities or families considering a post-mortem. Pathologists should be familiar with the clinical context of neuropathological examination and be able to justify retention of brain and spinal cord, as appropriate.

In certain circumstances, retention of fresh material is desirable for possible genetic and microbiological investigations.

In some instances, authority or consent is restricted to the retention and examination of samples of the brain and spinal cord. It must be emphasised that in such circumstances strategic sampling is essential and that this has to depend on the clinical context. No diagnostic reliability can be placed on non-systematic histological sampling of the CNS.

If, in the course of a post-mortem to determine the cause of death, no apparent cause is found and the last hope is discovery of something in the brain, slicing in the fresh state is unlikely to be helpful and may in fact compromise a subsequent detailed examination.

Examination of the brain

Removal

Removal of the brain is indicated in all full post-mortems. In obtaining consent from a family or in providing information to a legal authority to justify the examination, it can be explained that secondary damage to the brain is common in a wide range of conditions. It is also not uncommon for an unex-

pected abnormality of the brain to be discovered, which then becomes of relevance to the immediate cause of death. There are no generally applicable studies that would inform quoting a precise probability that retention of the brain would give an answer to a clinical question.

The head should be supported by resting the occiput on a block such that the neck is slightly flexed. The operator should wear appropriate personal protective clothing including protection of eyes. The head and neck should be inspected for any operation scars, contusions or lacerations. Ventricular shunts for the treatment of hydrocephalus are best explored before the cranium is opened. The tube is exposed either in the subcutaneous tissues or, in the case of a ventriculoatrial shunt, in the internal jugular vein. After cutting the tube the patency of the proximal and distal parts can be tested with a syringe and water.

The scalp is incised using a scalpel. Start behind one ear, pass just behind the vertex, and finish behind the other ear. The scalp can be reflected from the skull using blunt dissection. Anteriorly, this should be as far as the supraorbital ridge. Posteriorly, the scalp should be reflected to the mid-occiput.

It is important to carefully examine the underside of the flaps for haemorrhage or bruising, which can be missed on external examination.

The temporalis muscles should be removed from the temporal regions of the skull using a scalpel as they can interfere with the cutting action of the saw. The skull is examined noting any fractures or operative procedures such as burr holes.

The skull-cap is normally sawn circumferentially using an oscillating saw, taking care not to penetrate the dura. Alternatively, a hand saw may be used. Anteriorly, the saw cut should lie 2.5 cm above the supraorbital ridge, and then be extended on each side to about 1 cm above the pinna of the ear. The cut is then angled across the back of the head to meet at the occiput. The purpose of the angled cut is to allow the calvarium to be fitted back without slipping, once the examination is finished. Notches placed in the incision will also help to prevent slippage following reconstruction (see Chapter 21).

The skull-cap is prised loose by twisting a T-shaped chisel in the saw cut. This movement separates the calvaria from the dura. However, in young people, the dura may be firmly adherent to the skull-cap and may need separating by means of a spatula. The dura is now exposed and can be inspected for extradural haematoma, which should be recorded by weighing as a means of estimating its volume. Careful correlation with any skull fracture is indicated.

The patency of the superior longitudinal sinus is next assessed by opening it with a scalpel and scissors. The dura is now incised on each side along the line of the saw cut, using small scissor cuts and thus avoiding damage to the underlying brain. Continue these cuts to – but not cutting through – the superior sagittal sinus. Reflect the dural flaps medially, taking care to cut through and not tear the bridging veins. Then free the anterior attachment of the falx and reflect the dura backwards.

The underlying brain, covered by the leptomeninges, can be seen. Any blood in the subdural space should be noted. The linear extent, location and thickness of a subdural haematoma plus its volume are measured. Histological sampling of subdural haematoma is indicated if there is any requirement to attempt to date the time of onset. This is done by looking for evidence of organisation. Purulent leptomeningitis will be evident on inspection, at which point samples of pus and/or cerebrospinal fluid (CSF) can be taken for microbiology.

The dural cap can be removed by careful blunt dissection and retraction, removing the falx from between the cerebral hemispheres.

To effect removal of the brain, the fingers of one hand are inserted beneath the frontal lobes to gently lift the frontal lobes from the floor of the anterior cranial fossa, so elevating the olfactory bulbs. The optic nerves, internal carotid arteries, pituitary stalk and oculomotor nerves now come into view and can be cut with a pair of long-bladed scissors or a scalpel close to the base of the skull. The temporal lobes are then gently retracted in turn to expose the tentorium cerebelli, which is incised along its attachment to the petrous temporal bone on each side, taking care to extend the incision as far poste-

riorly as possible. The brain can start to be delivered from the skull. At this stage it is important to support the occipital lobes with one hand to avoid excess traction on the midbrain. As the brain comes backwards, the midbrain, pons and medulla come into view and the remainder of the cranial nerves are cut as they pierce the dura. Finally each of the vertebral arteries is cut at its point of entry into the skull. The lower brainstem and upper cervical cord then rise into view and can be transected transversely with a scalpel. Avoid making a wedge-shaped cut as this prevents adequate examination of the cervical medullary junction. These final steps may have to be accomplished without direct vision, but a satisfactory specimen will soon be achieved with practice. The brain is then gently eased from the cranial cavity, elevating the cerebellar hemispheres with the fingers if necessary and leaving the flap of dura attached to the skull.

The approach of the pathologist should necessarily be flexible, and the procedure described above varied according to the needs of an individual case.

If one is particularly interested in the cervical–medullary junction, or if a section of the medulla is rendered difficult to visualise by cerebellar tonsillar herniation, it is preferable to remove the upper segments of the cervical cord attached to the brain. To achieve this a wedge of occipital bone and the arches of the upper few cervical vertebrae are first removed and the dura opened. The brain can then be delivered with the attached upper cervical segments of the cord.

In cases of suspected meningitis or encephalitis, it is desirable to take samples of the CSF which is uncontaminated by blood. This may be done either by needle aspiration from the anterior or posterior horn of the lateral ventricle, or from the fourth ventricle by gentle compression of the brain. Spinal CSF is obtained by tilting the patient's head down after removal of the brain.

Preliminary inspection and handling of the brain

The fresh brain and spinal cord are very soft. While it is possible to make an examination in the fresh state, only relatively obvious and gross pathology can be detected. If a more reliable examination is required, the whole organ should be retained and fixed before dissection. This is especially true in the more complex neurological cases that may prove difficult to elucidate and which may require referral to a specialist centre.

External examination of the brain will often reveal a considerable amount of information. The distribution and possible source of any haemorrhage in the subarachnoid space should be looked for in the fresh state, aided by gently washing blood away before fixation of the brain. Once fixed, blood becomes a hard craggy mass, making adequate dissection of (in particular) aneurysms a virtually impossible task.

The presence of any opacification in the subarachnoid space should prompt the use of swabs and collection of specimens for bacteriological examination. Less frank infiltration of the subarachnoid space may denote subacute, chronic or neoplastic meningitis. Smear preparations, fixed and stained, may be used to provide a rapid diagnosis.

Careful inspection of the surface features should be undertaken, noting any abnormalities – contusions, haemorrhagic infarction, areas of softening (gentle palpation may localise infarction), cystic areas, surface tumours, and atrophy, whether global or focal.

Features associated with brain swelling should be looked for including flattening of the cerebral gyri, uncal herniation with grooving of the parahippocampal gyri and foraminal herniation with impaction and moulding of the medulla and cerebellar tonsils.

The arterial supply to the brain is best identified and traced in the fresh state, when the possibility of seeing structural abnormalities such as a small aneurysm is greatest. To do this it is necessary to incise the arachnoid to gain access to the sylvian fissures and interhemispheric fissure.

At this stage any special procedures that may be required before fixing the brain should be performed. In cases of suspected encephalitis, representative samples of the fresh brain and CSF should be taken for rapid transport to the virology laboratory.

If there is a possibility of a neurometabolic disease (e.g. a neuronal storage disorder), portions of the brain should be deep-frozen for subsequent biochemical and genetic investigation.

The brain should be weighed. It is useful at this stage to also consider the benefit of photographic recording of any macroscopic pathology, particularly if there is no consent to retain the whole brain.

In certain cases, where there may be an active research interest, it may be appropriate to freeze representative samples of brain. If it is required to freeze a half brain, it is sagittally bisected using a long-bladed sharp knife. One half is fixed medial side

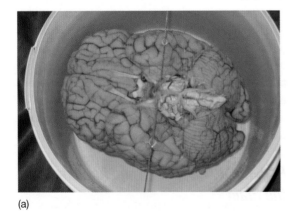

(a)

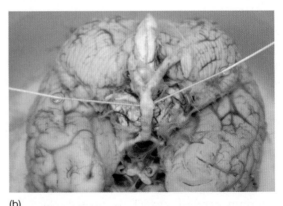

(b)

Figure 12.1 (a) Brain suspended by the basilar artery in a polythene bucket filled with neutral buffered formalin. (b) detail of point of suspension.

down in a bucket of formalin to be available for histological correlation with biochemical analysis obtained from the frozen hemisphere. Fresh frozen material may also be utilised in genetic analysis, an area that is becoming increasingly relevant in the neurodegenerative disorders.

Fixation of the whole brain is carried out with the brain suspended in a large bucket of 10 L capacity which is three-quarters filled with 10% neutral buffered formalin. A loop of string is passed between the pons and basilar artery, which is usually strong enough to support the brain in water. Alternatively, a plastic hook may be used, but either way suspension is from string attached to the ends of the handle of the bucket (Fig. 12.1). Great care must be exercised to prevent contact of the brain with the sides and the bottom of the bucket, as this may cause distortion and prevent adequate fixation. It is also important to ensure that the brainstem is covered with fixative. Diffusion of formalin entering normal brain tissue is usually sufficiently rapid to provide adequate fixation throughout the brain. Fixation may be impaired when there is cerebral oedema, however, and under these circumstances it can be improved by splitting the corpus callosum and making a small incision between the mamillary bodies, thus allowing the fixative access to the interior of the hemispheres. The fixative should be changed after 3 days, and then at weekly intervals. Brains should be fixed for approximately 4 weeks before further examination. Oedema and brain swelling are known to slow fixation.

Strategies for more rapid fixation of the brain have been proposed, including microwave-enhanced fixation. A recent audit and review of practice has suggested that a mixture of immersion and vascular perfusion using 10% formalin can achieve good results (Sharma and Grieve, 2006).

If authority to retain the brain for fixation is not available, it may be possible to obtain permission to fix the brain for 1–2 days. This allows some degree of hardening which can facilitate better slicing and allow more detailed macroscopic examination than in the fresh state. It must be emphasised that this is not best practice and should be subject to advice that it may not allow determination of all factors that may bear on a cause of death.

Slicing the brain in the fresh state and routine histological sampling

In many cases where there are no clinical signs or symptoms related to the CNS, it is appropriate to make an examination of the brain in the fresh state. Following external examination, as described in the previous subsection, the brain may be sliced and examined.

A single cut should be made to remove the brainstem and cerebellum from the cerebral hemispheres. This should be made with a scalpel, in the horizontal plane, through the midbrain at the level of the superior colliculi and above the origin of the third cranial nerves. This will allow inspection of the midbrain, an assessment of pigmentation of the substantia nigra, and an assessment of patency of the cerebral aqueduct.

The pons can be removed from the cerebellum by cutting through the cerebellar peduncles on both sides. The brainstem can then be sectioned at 3 mm intervals from the midbrain, through the pons to the medulla. The cerebellum can be sectioned radially to show the cortex, white matter and cerebellar dentate nuclei.

The cerebral hemispheres are sliced in the coronal plane using a long-bladed knife. A useful strategy is to place the cerebral hemispheres with the superior surface on the bench, and start making cuts from the frontal pole backwards at 1 cm intervals. In cases where the brain has undergone softening it may not be possible to make cuts this thin, and a thicker section may be necessary. An attempt should be made to place cuts at strategic levels, to become familiar with anatomy in a systematic manner. Sections can be made at the level of the tip of the temporal lobe, through the mamillary bodies, and through the mid-point along the length of the cerebral peduncle (to obtain a section of the hippocampus at the level of the lateral geniculate body).

In a case where it is appropriate to take routine samples from the brain, six blocks can encompass areas that have diagnostic utility for a range of pathological processes. The blocks are:

- midbrain including substantia nigra: detects a range of movement disorders and Lewy body diseases;

- cerebellum including dentate nucleus: hypoxic/ischaemic changes as well as neurodegenerative cerebellar disorders;
- hippocampus at the level of the lateral geniculate body: hypoxic/ischaemic changes and several dementing disorders;
- frontal cortex from the arterial boundary zone: hypoxic/ischaemic changes and several degenerative conditions;
- basal ganglia (caudate and putamen): several movement disorders and vascular disorders;
- occipital cortex: hypoxic/ischaemic changes, several degenerative conditions and amyloid angiopathy.

In addition to these screening blocks, any macroscopic focal lesions should be sampled. In cases of dysphagia or aspiration pneumonia, a block of the medulla at the level of the open IVth ventricle is useful. (Fig. 12.2)

Examination of the spinal cord

Examination of the spinal cord should be based on consideration of the clinical context of the case. Examination is likely to be essential to give a full explanation of clinical features in cases of paraparesis, paraplegia, clinically diagnosed motor neuron disease, multiple sclerosis, unexplained motor weakness, frontotemporal dementia, autonomic failure, cerebellar ataxia, and suspected Guillain–Barré syndrome. In trauma cases, examination of the spinal cord may reveal evidence of an unsuspected spinal injury.

There are basically three methods for removing the spinal cord. In the post-mortem room this can be

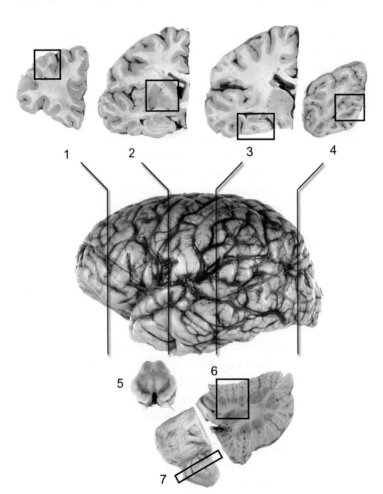

Figure 12.2 Routine histological sampling of the brain. 1, frontal cortex; 2, basal ganglia and internal capsule; 3, hippocampus; 4, occipital cortex; 5, midbrain; 6, cerebellar cortex and dentate nucleus; 7, medulla.

done by either the anterior or posterior approach. The third method involves removal of the entire vertebral column, the spinal cord being extracted following fixation. This last method avoids distortion artefacts of the cord and permits leisurely examination at a later date, but does require some skilled reconstruction by the mortuary technician; consequently, this approach is usually limited to specialist centres or cases of particular interest. The removal of short sections of the vertebral column, as for example at the site of a spinal injury, is, however, easily undertaken by saw cuts above and below the segment to be examined.

Whether the posterior or anterior approach is chosen tends to be a matter of personal preference. In general, mastering the anterior approach has wide applicability. Not only is there less risk of damaging the cord, but sampling of the dorsal root ganglia, nerve roots and the adjacent plexuses is definitely easier. The necessity for a further long skin incision is also avoided. Mastering the posterior approach is required when limited post-mortems are being performed.

An essential preliminary step in removing the spinal cord – whichever is the preferred method – is to free the dura around the foramen magnum from the cranial cavity. This is a difficult manoeuvre to perform from below. To do this, the dura around the upper end of the cord is held by toothed forceps, and a scalpel blade is inserted between the dura and the surrounding bone around the entire circumference of the cord. It is usually possible to do this to a depth of approximately 2 cm.

The anterior approach

The basic principle in the anterior approach to the spinal cord is to cut through the pedicles of the vertebra, so permitting removal of the vertebral bodies. Access to the spinal column is facilitated by using an initial Y incision when opening the body, followed by wide removal of the ribs, usually 10 cm lower than would normally be done in a routine examination of the thoracic organs. The lumbar and cervical paravertebral muscles are dissected free of the vertebra, thus exposing the emerging peripheral nerves of the lumbar and cervical plexuses. Sawing with a fan-tailed blade commences in the lumbar region with the blade placed immediately in front of the emerging nerve roots, and continues up the thoracic region in a line immediately lateral to the rib tubercles, then rostrally to the base of the skull. The angle of the saw blade varies in the different regions of the spinal column (Fig. 12.3), being horizontal in the lumbar region, becoming increasingly oblique in the thoracic region, and being almost vertical in the cervical region.

When sawing, care must be taken not to let the blade plunge too deeply once it has been felt to 'give' as it enters the spinal canal, particularly in the cervical region where one is cutting directly down onto the cervical nerve roots.

Finally, an oblique cut is made in the sacrum on each side, allowing the vertebral bodies to be pulled forwards. Adhesions with the underlying dura are freed with a scalpel and the process is continued rostrally until all the vertebral bodies are removed and the entire length of the spinal cord exposed.

The cord is now removed by dividing the nerve roots of the cauda equina and attaching a pair of Spencer Wells forceps to the dura. Only the dura should be handled, avoiding any trauma to the cord. The cord is now gently lifted from the spinal canal, freeing any adhesions and cutting through the spinal nerve roots. Representative dorsal root ganglia lying within the intervertebral foramina are easily included with the specimen. In the cervical region, however, further dissection is required to expose the ganglia as here they are more laterally situated. Great care must be taken not to angulate or pull on the cord as this will cause post-mortem artefactual damage.

Once removed, the spinal cord is then fixed before further dissection. Ideally, it should be suspended in a large tank or drainpipe so that no distortion occurs. A weight may be attached to the dura of the lower end to prevent shrinkage of the dura, which may cause buckling of the cord. If no suitable container is available it is acceptable to divide the cord into two or three sections for fixation by immersion. The cord is transected after opening the dura to avoid compression damage.

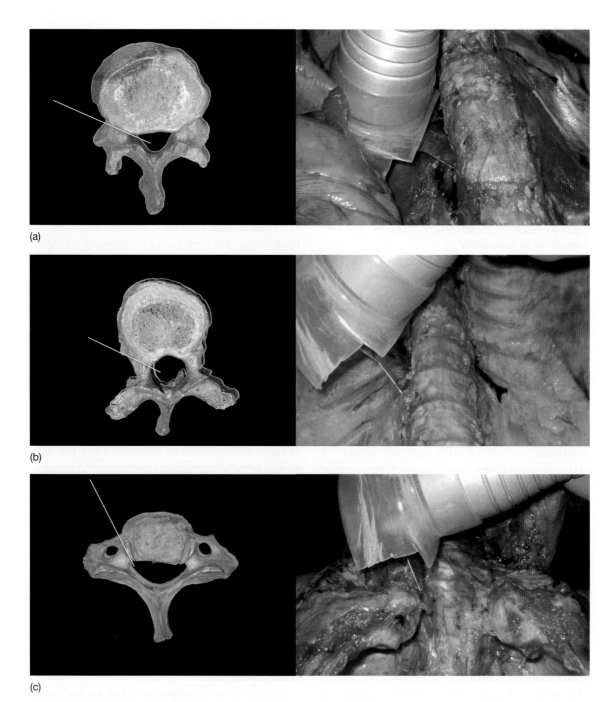

Figure 12.3 Anterior approach for the removal of the spinal cord, showing the angle of saw cut required for: (a) the lumbar vertebrae; (b) the thoracic vertebrae; and (c) the cervical vertebrae.

The posterior approach

The skin is incised from the occiput to the sacrum, and the paraspinal muscle mass is cleared to reveal the vertebral laminae; these are then sawn through on each side. The fan-tailed saw blade is directed forwards and slightly inwards, the line of the cut being approximately 2 cm from the midline (Fig. 12.4). The vertebral spines can then be elevated in a single

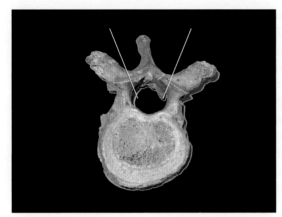

Figure 12.4 Posterior approach for removal of the spinal cord, showing the angle of saw cut required.

block, exposing the underlying cord. Using this approach further dissection with a knife and bony nibbler will be required to expose the dorsal root ganglia in the intervertebral foramina. The cord is now removed in a similar manner to that of the anterior approach.

Combined approach

A combination of the posterior approach in the cervical region and the removal of a wedge-shaped piece of occipital bone can be used in those subjects where the pathological lesion is thought to lie in the caudal brainstem or upper cervical cord. The spinal cord is transected below the level of the lesion and the upper end is delivered in continuity with the brain. The remainder of the spinal cord can then be removed separately.

Examination of the skull

Following removal of the brain, the dural lining and the base of the cranial cavity are checked for any abnormalities and the principal venous sinuses (petrosal, transverse, sigmoid, straight and the confluence) are examined for patency by opening using a scalpel and scissors.

In cases of known or suspected head injury, the dura should be removed to allow examination of the inside of the skull to detect possible fractures of the skull base. This is achieved by gripping the dura

with toothed forceps and forcibly stripping it from the bone surface. The internal surface of the skull should be wiped clean to remove blood and to reveal fractures.

Examination of the pituitary gland

Usually the pituitary gland is removed by first incising the posterior margin of the diaphragma sellae. The incision is necessary to avoid damage to the posterior lobe of the pituitary gland as the posterior part of the pituitary fossa is removed by means of a small-bladed chisel. The pituitary gland is then dissected out from the sella turcica using a scalpel, directing the blade away from the gland and grasping the diaphragm with a pair of fine forceps.

In patients with a tumour in the pituitary region, the central segment of the base of the skull can be removed using a Deseuter saw with a fan-shaped blade. This block is also to be recommended when a lesion of the cavernous sinus is present, and in addition to portions of the second to the sixth cranial nerves the trigeminal ganglia are also included. After fixation the block may be dissected or decalcified and sectioned in any suitable plane.

Removal of the eyes

It depends on one's practice as to whether removal of the eyes is a 'routine' or 'special' procedure (Parsons, 2006). Eyes may also be removed, in part or *in toto*, for the purposes of transplantation, usually by an eye surgeon, a trained transplant retrieval officer or an accredited anatomical pathology technologist.

There are five approaches to removal of the eye. The choice of which method to apply will depend on the purpose for the removal and the prosector's experience and preference with any particular technique that can be used alone or in combination: either the external or the internal approach (referred to by some as the anterior and posterior approaches, respectively). The internal (posterior) approach is easier to perform but requires the head to be opened and the brain to have been removed.

The external (anterior) approach

The approach is greatly facilitated by the use of lid retractors of the type employed by ophthalmic surgeons (e.g. a Weeks' lid speculum). These hold the lids firmly out of the way as the dissection proceeds and help reduce accidental damage to the lids, which can result in a poor cosmetic result. With the lids fully retracted, the conjunctival attachments of the globe can be cut using blunt-nosed curved scissors, the free edges attached to the globe giving purchase to forceps (preferably Spencer Wells) (Fig. 12.5). This allows continued dissection of the muscle attachments of the globe. The optic nerve is identified and cut under direct vision and the globe is brought forward to come free of the socket.

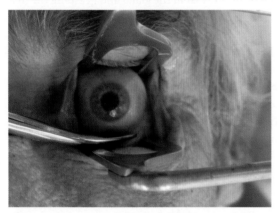

Figure 12.5 The conjunctiva is divided using curved scissors.

The internal (posterior) approach

The approach requires the brain to be removed and the dura to be stripped from the cranial bones. To remove the eye, one must remove the orbital part of the frontal bone. Using either an oscillating saw with a fan-tailed blade or a mallet and chisel, a cut is made to the bone running parallel to the cribriform plate of the ethmoid. A second cut is made to the bone running parallel to the lesser wing of the sphenoid. Finally both cuts are joined by a third cut through the orbital part of the frontal bone (Fig. 12.6). The bone is removed to expose the periorbital fat. Using a scalpel or blunt-nosed scissors, the fat and muscles are removed to visualise the globe. The optic nerve is cut and the globe lifted to release the inferior muscle attachments (Fig. 12.7). These can be left long for subsequent orientation of the globe. Care must be taken when incising the conjunctiva not to damage the eyelids or eyelashes, so many pathologists prefer to undertake this portion of the procedure under direct vision from the anterior approach. Once the last attachment is cut, the globe will lift out of the socket. A dot inked on the superior aspect of the globe with a marker pen at this point will aid subsequent orientation of the specimen, although other techniques such as leaving the superior rectus muscle longer than the others or the placement of a piece of card under the superior oblique muscle tendon are alternative methods.

The globe should be initially placed in formalin but later transferred into alcohol to stop it from collapsing prior to examination. The globe is then cut, photographed and processed using local protocols. Finally the orbit is reconstructed as outlined in Chapter 21.

Partial removal of the eye: the internal (posterior) approach

Occasionally permission is given for removal of the posterior part of the eye only, although wherever possible the entire globe should be removed. The technique is difficult and can result in retinal disruption and cosmetic defects. Therefore, approximately 30 minutes prior to the procedure 0.5 mL of 3% glutaraldehyde should be injected into the vitreous using the technique for vitreous fluid sampling (see Chapter 15). The eye is approached as described earlier for the posterior approach. The fat and orbital muscles are dissected as before and the optic nerve transected as posteriorly as possible. The eye is now cut along the equator superiorly with a knife and then with scissors to separate the posterior part of the eye from the anterior aspect. To enable orientation, a small nick is made in the superior aspect. Once the inferior rectus muscle is divided the eye will come free.

Removal of the intact eye, orbital contents and bony wall of the orbit

This technique is employed when orbital pathology extends to involve the orbital bony wall. To under-

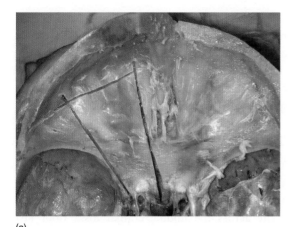

(a)

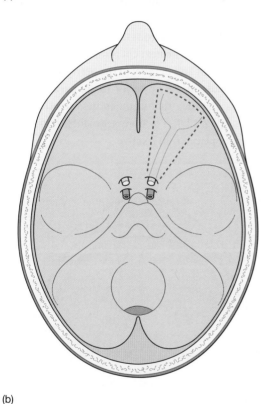

(b)

Figure 12.6 (a and b) Three cuts are made in the orbital plate.

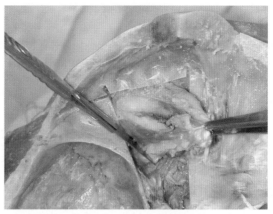

Figure 12.7 The globe is lifted and the inferior attachments released.

that the turcica is connected with the lateral border of the skull, the incision originating at the sella turcica and going to the squamous temporal bone. Now the ends of the cuts are continued anteriorly such that the medial one extends down through the frontal bone, along the medial border of the orbit and lateral border of the nose. It passes through the maxilla to end at a point close to the upper molar tooth. The lateral cut goes downwards through the greater wing of sphenoid, transects the zygomatic arch and joins the other cut at the upper molar area. The entire block of bone with the orbital contents can now be removed and processed.

Removal of the orbit, nasal passages and sinuses

On rare occasions it may be necessary to remove the orbits in continuity with the midline structures including the upper jaw and palate. Specific consent may be required for this procedure. Examples of when this may be required are granulomatous diseases involving the orbit, nasal passages and pharyngeal structures or malignancy.

The procedure commences as for the removal of the orbital contents and bony wall of the orbit. The facial bones are exposed and the cranial cavity emptied. The incisions are similar to those described above, except that the lateral internal incision goes more posteriorly through the squamous temporal bone, ending with a more posterior cut through the

take this procedure the facial bones and orbit must first be exposed. To do this, follow the procedure described for examination of the facial bones below. The bone incision then proceeds from inside the cranial cavity. A wedge of bone is cut interiorly such zygomatic arch. Anteriorly the incision passes vertically through the frontal bone, along the medial border of the orbit, along the lateral border of the nose, and ends at approximately the level of the upper canine. The entire block can now be removed and processed.

Reconstruction requires a skilled practitioner to rebuild the absent facial structures with a material such as plaster of Paris.

Examination of the middle ear

For most purposes, the middle ear, the eardrum and the intraosseous portion of the internal carotid artery can be satisfactorily examined by splitting the petrous part of the temporal bone with a chisel applied to the floor of the middle cranial fossa. The respiratory sinuses can be similarly opened for examination. This approach is appropriate for obtaining microbiological samples in cases of suspected otitis media.

The only really satisfactory way to examine the structures of the middle ear and inner ear is to remove a large wedge of temporal bone (as described below). The block is then decalcified and large serial sections are taken. This is usually undertaken only in selected cases where preservation of anatomic relations and histological correlation is required.

Removal of the temporal bone

There are three basic techniques for removal of the temporal bone (Nadol, 1980; Nadol *et al.*, 1996). The choice, as for removal of the eyes, depends on whether the head has been opened. It is of note that the removal of both temporal bones may render the skull unstable and complicate reconstruction.

The bone plug method

This uses an intracranial approach and is performed with the brain and dura removed. Using a specialist piece of equipment (a bone plug cutter), the entire inner ear and internal auditory canal, the medial part of the external auditory canal, the mastoid air system, a part of the venous sinus and the lateral half of the Eustachian tube are removed. The mastoid area is examined and the bony landmarks identified.

The bone plug cutter is centred on the arcuate eminence and advanced through the floor of the middle cranial fossa until it breaches the skull. The cutter is then removed. The bone plug is removed using forceps and scalpel and placed into fixative for subsequent examination.

The en-bloc method

This too uses an intracranial approach and produces a larger specimen. Using an oscillating saw, four cuts are made to the skull bones. The first cut is made laterally across the middle cranial fossa floor just medial to the squamous portion of the temporal bone. The second cut is made parallel to this one, being medial to the petrous tip into the basisphenoid and basiocciput. The next cut is made approximately 3.5 cm anterior and parallel to the petrous ridge with the last made in the posterior fossa, parallel to the petrous ridge such that it undercuts the other bony incisions (Fig. 12.8). The bony segment is removed as before and placed into fixative.

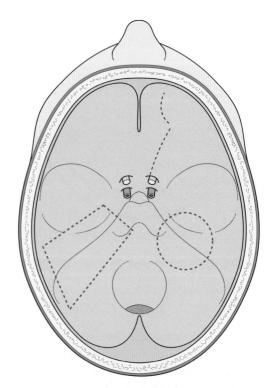

Figure 12.8 Methods of removing the temporal bones via an internal approach.

The extracranial approach

The temporal bone can be removed using an extracranial approach, avoiding the need to remove the calvarium. First, an incision is made behind the auricle and the external auditory canal transected. The soft tissue is removed and a long temporal bone plug cutter centred on the external auditory canal. The cutter is directed towards the opposite canal and advanced for its full length. The bony plug is freed and removed as before using a scalpel and forceps.

Dissection of the neck and examination of the extracranial vessels

Detailed dissection of the neck is an important procedure in a large number of neuropathological autopsies. Any subject with a history suggestive of cerebrovascular disease requires careful examination of the extracranial cerebral arteries. Cases of suspected peripheral nerve disease should undergo examination of the lower cranial nerves and possibly the autonomic nervous system.

The precise detail of the dissection and tissue samples will be dictated by knowledge of the patient's clinical history.

The first muscle encountered is the sternomastoid. This, supplied by its spinal accessory nerve, is divided at the mid-point. Samples may be taken and the cut ends then reflected upwards and downwards, thus exposing the carotid sheath. At this point, if required, the two bellies of the digastric muscle can be dissected out and sampled. The anterior belly is innervated by the trigeminal nerve and the posterior belly by the facial nerve. The carotid sheath containing the common and internal carotid arteries, internal jugular vein and the vagus nerve can now be explored. The internal carotid artery and vagus nerve are dissected upwards up to their point of entry into the skull. The swelling of the vagus nerve below the skull denotes the position of its inferior ganglion. The hypoglossal and accessory nerves emerge close to the vagus at this point. The glosso-

pharyngeal nerve is to be found between the internal carotid artery and the internal jugular vein running towards the pharynx.

Deeper dissection of the neck will reveal the cervical sympathetic chain lying in the loose connective tissue on the prevertebral muscles (Fig. 12.9). Of the three cervical sympathetic ganglia, the superior is the largest and lies behind the internal carotid artery opposite the second and third cervical vertebra. Following the chain downwards one encounters first the smallest, then the middle cervical ganglion, and finally, just below the level at which the vertebral artery enters the spinal column, the inferior cervical ganglion. The last is sometimes fused with the stellate ganglion. Sampling of the cervical sympathetic chain and the vagus nerve should be performed in any case with a history of autonomic failure.

Once the appropriate dissection of the neck nerves and musculature has been undertaken, attention can be directed towards the vessels. Although the usual method of dissection removes the vessels 'en bloc' with the rest of the neck structures, their separate dissection can be undertaken for more detailed study or demonstration purposes. Having already exposed the carotid arteries and transected them as rostrally as possible, the dissection is continued downwards, exposing the innominate artery and the origins of the subclavian and vertebral arteries on each side. The vertebral arteries are transected as they enter the foramina in the transverse processes of the sixth cervical vertebra. The subclavian vessels are cut and the transected vessels reflected downwards to the arch of the aorta. The final step involves cutting a wedge from the arch of the aorta incorporating the origins of the major neck arteries.

Examination of the vertebral arteries

Examination of the vertebral arteries is an often neglected aspect of the autopsy, in part due to their relative inaccessibility and the fiddly, time-consuming procedures required for their exposure. Their

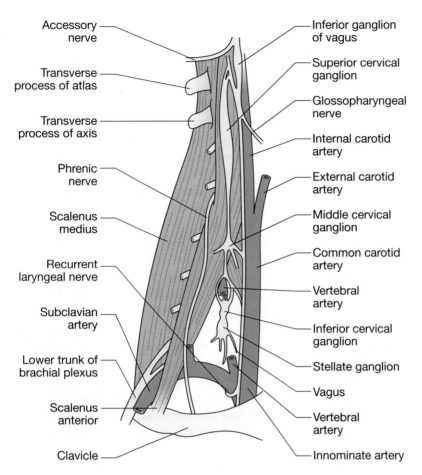

Accessory nerve

Transverse process of atlas

Transverse process of axis

Phrenic nerve

Scalenus medius

Recurrent laryngeal nerve

Subclavian artery

Lower trunk of brachial plexus

Scalenus anterior

Clavicle

Inferior ganglion of vagus

Superior cervical ganglion

Glossopharyngeal nerve

Internal carotid artery

External carotid artery

Middle cervical ganglion

Common carotid artery

Vertebral artery

Inferior cervical ganglion

Stellate ganglion

Vagus

Vertebral artery

Innominate artery

Figure 12.9 Deep dissection of the neck, showing the positions of the major vessels, nerves and ganglia.

examination can be considered from two perspectives: their cervical path and their intracranial path (Fig. 12.10) (Bromilow and Burns, 1985).

The en-bloc method

There are two described methods for examining the cervical path of the vertebral arteries. The first requires the removal of the entire cervical portion of the vertebral column (Vanezis, 1979). A Y-shaped incision is made to the neck and the anterior neck structures are removed along with the thoracic contents as described in Chapter 10. Next, the inner third of each clavicle is removed to ease access to the origins of the vertebral arteries. The head is then opened in the normal manner and the cranial contents removed, taking care to incise the medulla oblongata as close to the foramen magnum as possi-

ble. The ligaments and muscles attached to the cervical vertebrae are released taking care to leave the posterior skin and muscles attached to the back of the skull, thus avoiding decapitation. The neck is now removed *en bloc*. This should preferably include the base of the skull including the foramen magnum, which is removed with the use of an oscillating saw and a fan-tailed blade. The entire specimen is placed in formalin for fixation and then decalcified. This may take up to 8 weeks. The specimen may then be sectioned with a bacon slicer or the vertebral arteries dissected out with a scalpel.

The in-situ method

The second method examines the vertebral arteries *in situ* and is favoured by many in view of the fact that a large specimen of human tissue does not have

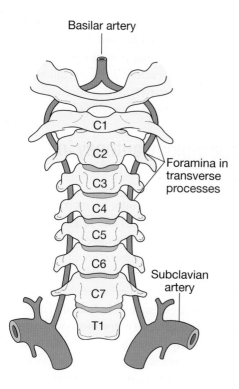

Basilar artery

C1
C2
C3
C4
C5
C6
C7
T1

Foramina in transverse processes

Subclavian artery

Figure 12.10 The path of the vertebral arteries.

blade as far as the axis. The sharp lateral turn of each vessel is identified before removing the bony boundary of the axis and atlas. The artery then goes posteriorly and turns into its cephalic portion. Further dissection requires the removal of the foramen magnum as before.

Autopsy imaging and injection technique

Further examination of the vertebral arteries can be facilitated by two methods. In the case of vertebral artery trauma, post-mortem angiography should be considered (Karhunen *et al.*, 1990). Alternatively, if an intracranial tear is suspected, a simple method to examine for leaks is as follows. The cranium is opened and, after careful examination of the vasculature, the cerebral hemispheres are removed by an incision through the pons. Cannulae are inserted into the proximal cervical parts of both vertebral arteries. With the aid of an assistant, water is simultaneously injected into both vessels while observing the cranial portions. Any tear should be demonstrated by the leakage of water.

Sampling of muscles and peripheral nerves

In cases where the clinical history and findings are those of a neuromuscular disorder, sampling of peripheral nerves and muscles will be required. This is in addition to removal of the spinal cord, with attached anterior and posterior nerve roots, and representative dorsal root ganglia. The precise pattern of sampling required will be largely determined by a detailed study of the clinical findings. Peripheral nerve involvement can be selective as in, for example, cases of multifocal mononeuropathy.

Many of the specialised techniques, such as enzyme histochemistry, which are routinely used in specialist neuropathology laboratories, can still be applied to post-mortem muscle up to 24–36 hours after death. Samples from areas regularly used in clinical diagnostic work (vastus lateralis, deltoid, gastrocnemius) should be orientated in the transverse plane and fresh-frozen for preservation at −80°C. Before sampling, the muscle should be widely

to be retained after the autopsy. A Y-incision is made to the neck with the neck well extended and the skin reflected to the edge of the mandible. The neck structures and chest cavity contents are removed as usual but the subclavian arteries are severed proximal to the origins of the vertebral arteries. The calvarium and its contents are removed as usual. The longus colli and longus capitus muscles are dissected off the anterior aspect of the cervical spine and the inner third of each clavicle is removed as before. The proximal parts of both vertebral arteries are dissected free as far as the foramen transversarium of the sixth cervical vertebra. Using a pair of small bone clippers or wire cutters, the anterior bony boundary of the foramina is removed from the sixth to the third cervical vertebrae. This is done by making two incisions to each bone – one to the anterior border as close to the body as possible and the other to the anterior tubercle of each transverse process. The vertebral arteries are then mobilised using a scalpel with a no. 11

exposed and the actual removal carried out as atraumatically as possible in order to avoid the production of artefacts. Samples of muscle should be excised as far as possible along the line of the fibres, thus facilitating the preparation of accurate cross-sectional and longitudinal sections. Ideally, a strip approximately 1 × 3 cm should be removed.

If it is not possible to preserve muscle for enzyme histochemistry, much information can still be gained from correctly handled samples of nerve and muscle fixed in 10% buffered formalin. To avoid distortion during fixation, the specimens of muscle can be laid on labelled card to which it becomes adherent and remains orientated in the fixative.

Peripheral nerve sampling is dictated by the distribution of clinical signs. Samples can be taken proximally from the main plexus regions (brachial and lumbar) and also peripherally as different disease processes affect different parts of the peripheral nervous system. In general, one should avoid superficial segments of nerve, such as the sciatic at the buttock, the median at the wrist and the ulnar at the elbow, which tend to be traumatised during life. The median, ulnar and radial nerves are easily accessible in the upper arms. With regard to the lower limbs, the femoral nerve is readily identified as it emerges from the lower border of the psoas muscle in the abdominal cavity. The sciatic nerve and the median and lateral popliteal nerve are accessed by dissection in the popliteal fossa. The sural nerve (a purely sensory nerve) is the most frequently biopsied nerve in clinical practice and is therefore usually included in any examination of the peripheral nervous system. It lies superficially posterior to the lateral malleolus. Finally, a U-shaped incision on the palm of the hand will expose the distal nerves and musculature of the upper limb. These small hand muscles are a rich source of motor end-plates and muscle spindles with which they are abundantly supplied.

Samples benefit from atraumatic handling and rapid fixation. There is a benefit in having material fixed in glutaraldehyde for resin processing, as applies to nerve biopsy samples in the living.

Dissection of the lower cranial nerves and muscle innervated from the brainstem has already been mentioned. The pattern of lower cranial nerve involvement in any disorder can be assessed by examining the anterior and posterior bellies of the digastric muscle (innervated by the trigeminal and facial nerves, respectively), the sternomastoid (accessory) and the tongue (hypoglossal).

Neuropathology autopsy in stroke

Stroke can be classified into haemorrhagic and ischaemic patterns (Boxes 12.1 and 12.2).

In haemorrhagic stroke, bleeding may be intracerebral, intraventricular, subarachnoid or have a mixed pattern. In post-mortems of the brain, a careful examination of the cerebral arteries attached to the brain in the fresh state is indicated. This will allow the detection of small berry aneurysms, which will otherwise escape detection if the brain is fixed and the blood becomes hardened. Large haematomas can be evacuated to facilitate later fixation when the whole brain is being retained for detailed examination.

Ischaemic stroke may be caused by thrombosis in a large cerebral vessel, small vessel disease, or be due to embolic phenomena. A small proportion of cases are due to rare and unusual conditions or remain unexplained despite post-mortem examination. In all cases of ischaemic stroke a full examination of the heart, great vessels and cerebral circulation is required, including the vertebral arteries. Clinically new approaches to stroke subtyping are being developed and post-mortem examination may be required to audit performance of such clinically applied schemes. The 'ASCO' scheme assigns a numeric probability to patients against criteria for Atherosclerosis, Small vessel disease, Cardiac source and Other cause (Amarenco et al., 2009).

Neuropathology autopsy in head injury

Head injury is a common cause of death in a range of ages, but especially in young adult males. Deaths from head injury constitute 1–2 per cent of all deaths

Box 12.1 Haemorrhagic stroke

No identifiable lesion

- *Associated with impaired coagulation.* Check bone marrow for leukemia as well as clinical notes for therapeutic anticoagulation. May be a complication of a procedure such as cardiac surgery.
- *Associated with recreational drug abuse.* Perform toxicology.
- *Idiopathic.* No cause identified despite macroscopic examination, toxicology and histology of brain.

Identifiable lesion

- *Aneurysm.* Ascertained in the fresh state by careful removal of blood and examination of cerebral arteries. Common 'missed' aneurysms are at the tip of the basilar artery and those that become embedded in the brain parenchyma leading to intracerebral or intraventricular bleeds.
- *Arteriovenous malformation.* Usually ascertained in the fresh state, supplemented by histological examination
- *Hypertensive vascular damage.* Suspected from location of bleed (deep hemispheric, pontine or cerebellar), and confirmed by histology of deep cerebral vessels together with supplementary information from the general post-mortem.
- *Amyloid angiopathy.* Suspected by the context of the bleed – a common cause of lobar haemorrhage in older patients. Confirmed by histology of vessels from the region of the bleed.
- *Venous sinus or cortical vein thrombosis.* Haemorrhagic infacts may mimic primary haemorrhage. Ascertained in the fresh state by examination of venous sinuses and noting thrombosis in cortical veins.
- *Trauma.* Usually evident from the context of the case.
- *Tumour.* May be difficult to delineate from damaged brain at the periphery of a bleed. Ascertain by histology from the margins of the bleed.
- *Iatrogenic.* Interventional procedures may give rise to bleeding. It is advisable to have the practitioner present to describe the procedure and highlight relevant imaging features so that a true explanation of the complication may be ascertained.

Box 12.2 Ischaemic stroke

- *Atherosclerosis.* Ascertained in the fresh state by noting atheromatous vascular disease. Inspection and histology of the carotid bifurcations may reveal complicated atheroma. Thrombosis of cerebral vessels may be seen, and must include examination of the vertebral arteries in the neck.
- *Small vessel disease.* Linked to previous hypertension and diabetes mellitus. Clinically linked to syndrome of lacunar infarction and imaging feature described as leucoaraiosis and microbleeds. May be suspected by noting lacunar infarcts in the fresh state and should be confirmed by histological examination of the brain
- *Cardiac.* Suspected at the time of post-mortem by examination of the heart, noting a potential site for embolism or primary cardiac disease. In young patients a patent foramen ovale may allow paradoxical embolism.
- *Other.* A range of rare causes can be established. Unusual causes of ischaemic stroke may be identified only with histology of cerebral vessels and brain such as cerebral vasculitis, arterial dissection and fibromuscular dysplasia (particularly affects vertebral arteries). Consider taking blood for serology to look for SLE or thrombophilia syndrome. Check bone marrow for haematological causation. A small proportion of patients with stroke have an inherited cause for disease, the risk being highest for young-onset disease – retain brain if possible, take histology plus consider preserving fresh material for genetic studies.

The identification of the type and amount of pathology that is responsible for death or disability is especially important in medicolegal cases in which consideration needs to be given to the various types of pathology and their causation.

The aim is to document injuries, provide an interpretation as to primary and secondary causes of damage, and to ascertain whether natural disease in the brain may have contributed to the causation of the original trauma or contributed to death. In patients who have been admitted to hospital and who have had imaging, careful review of imaging results usually assists in macroscopic interpretation of post-mortem findings.

from all causes. Between 1 and 5 per cent patients with a head injury remain vegetative and 5–18 per cent are severely disabled 6 months after their injury.

Careful documentation of soft tissue injuries to the scalp is important, supplemented by photographs when appropriate. The dura should be stripped from the skull to allow for the examination of skull fractures and photography. Histological sampling of the dura is appropriate when there has been a haematoma in relation to the dura (subdural or extradural) so that the tissue response to the haematoma can be assessed and hence an estimate of timing of injury be made. The dura can be sampled by taking the section of dura adjacent to and including the haematoma margin, and rolling it up like a swiss-roll. A thin 0.5 cm cross slice is then taken and placed directly into a processing cassette for fixation and histology – a so-called dural roll.

In many cases of head injury it is possible to achieve the three main aims of post-mortem brain examination by careful macroscopic examination of the brain supplemented by photography when appropriate. Examination of the brain in the fresh state may not allow macroscopic detection of subtle and important lesions related to the mode of death following trauma. It is often possible to obtain authority to fix the brain for 24–48 hours in formalin, followed by slicing, photography and histological sampling. This allows early return of the brain to the body and even the short fixation allows for better macroscopic assessment. It is appropriate to recommend to the legal authority authorizing the examination that the most reliable assessment can be obtained following retention of the brain for detailed examination. This recommendation is most important where criminal involvement is suspected or, in non-criminal cases, when death has occurred following head injury in the absence of obvious focal brain injury (for example with brain swelling alone) such that diffuse brain injury is likely. If authorization is not given for retention of the whole brain then it should be recommended that there is retention of a single coronal slice of brain together with additional samples of the corpus callosum, cerebellum and brain stem (Fig. 12.11). It is recommended that in such circumstances the pathologist documents limitations imposed on the examination in the post-mortem report, together with a statement as to how this may affect reliability of interpretation.

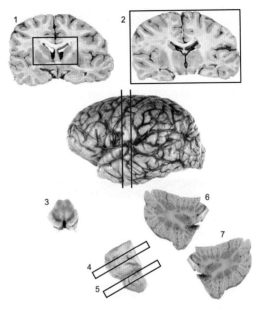

Figure 12.11 Head injury tissue retention when retaining the whole brain is not permitted. 1, block of both sides of anterior corpus callosum and internal capsule; 2, whole slice 1 cm thick taken from a level 1 cm caudal to the mamillary bodies (this is blocked for histology *in toto* as six large blocks); 3, midbrain; 4, pons; 5, medulla; 6 and 7, cerebellar hemisphere from both sides.

Macroscopic description of the site and size of contusions and subarachnoid bleeding can be related to the severity of head injury. Careful documentation of the extent of brain swelling and any consequential damage secondary to brain herniation is an important part of the examination.

Histological sampling may not be necessary in many cases, particularly where there is clear macroscopic evidence of focal brain injury, provided that a careful macroscopic examination has been performed and documented. If there is a question in relation to the timing of a head injury then histology of focal lesions can be helpful. Where the immediacy or adequacy of care following the injury is in question then it can be helpful to use histological sampling to detect secondary brain damage. It is especially important to perform wide histological sampling when diffuse traumatic axonal injury or diffuse ischaemic brain injury is suspected. This should be considered when a patient has been

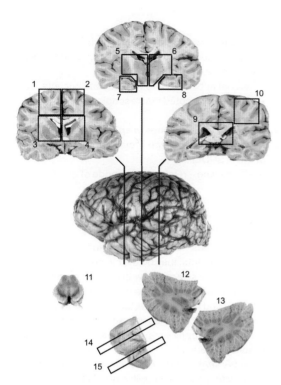

Figure 12.12 Head injury histological sampling to detect diffuse brain injury. 1 and 2, frontal cortex with parasaggital white matter; 3 and 4, corpus cellosum, anterior limb of internal capsule and basal ganglia; 5 and 6, basal ganglia and thalamus with internal capsule; 7 and 8, hippocampi at level of lateral geniculat body; 9, splenium of corpus callosum; 10, centrum semiovale in parietal lobe; 11, midbrain; 12 and 13, bilateral samples of cerebellum; 14, pons; 15, medulla.

unconscious but the brain examination has not revealed a focal mass lesion. A full sample set in the assessment of a head injury should include the following areas taken from both sides, as shown in Fig. 12.12: frontal cortex at the level of the head of the caudate to include parasagittal white matter, anterior corpus callosum at the level of the basal ganglia, anterior limbs of the internal capsule with basal ganglia, basal ganglia and thalamus including posterior internal capsule, parietal lobe with white matter from centrum semiovale, splenium of the corpus callosum, both hippocampi, midbrain, pons, medulla, cerebellum including the dentate nucleus. Any focal lesions should also be sampled histologically. In paediatric head injury, and especially if non-accidental injury is suspected, extensive histo-

logical sampling of the cervico-medullary region to look for axonal injury is important. The detection of traumatic axonal injury is facilitated by immunostaining for beta amyloid precursor protein (β-APP). In patients who die with a period of survival histological assessment with CD68 allows detection of the microglial responses to axonal injury.

In many cases the post-mortem does not discover anything beyond what had been established clinically and using imaging in life. In other instances detailed assessment is required, especially where evidence of the existence or absence of secondary patterns of damage is required to link to suggestions of inappropriate clinical management. In such cases examination in the fresh state with limited histology may not be adequate to give a full explanation of the cause of death. As has been noted, particular difficulty may be encountered in the ascertainment of diffuse brain injury and traumatic axonal damage, where macroscopic evaluation is unreliable and limited histological examination is inadequate (Smith *et al.*, 2003)

Neuropathology autopsy in epilepsy

As with many diseases, there is an increasing realisation that genetic causes underlie some of the epilepsy syndromes, contributing to the pathogenesis of the idiopathic epilepsies. Other forms of epilepsy may be classed as secondary. Recent review of the expectations of families, faced with the unexpected death of a person with epilepsy, has led to recommendations being made for appropriate post-mortem investigations. The majority of post-mortems on patients who die associated with epilepsy are conducted under a legal authority with the aim of ascertaining the cause of death. In planning such an examination, there is a differential diagnosis with syndromes that produce paroxysmal loss of consciousness, particularly syndromes which lead to cardiac arrhythmias.

The post-mortem plays an important part in assigning the cause of death into three major categories as follows.

Box 12.3 Epilepsy: investigations and findings

- *External examination.* Look for evidence of tongue biting and petechial haemorrhages in the skin and eyes that may indicate asphyxia.
- *Full post-mortem with histology.* Exclude other causes of death. It is recommended to take multiple samples from the heart and lung as well as sampling macroscopic abnormalities in other organs.
- *Toxicology.* Exclude death due to alcohol or abuse of drugs. Best practice recommendations are to preserve blood, urine and gastric contents for estimation of a range of potential investigations, including levels of therapeutic drugs.
- *Neuropathological examination.* The pathologist should always recommend, to a legal authority and family, retention of the brain for detailed examination . It has been stated that pathological findings will be seen in about 60 per cent of cases (Black and Graham, 2002). If it is not possible to retain the whole brain, it is recommended to retain two full coronal sections, 1.5 cm thick: one just in front of the midbrain, and one just behind the midbrain. These will allow histological sampling of the following regions (see Fig. 12.13):
  - cingulate gyrus;
  - hippocampus and parahippocampal gyrus from both sides;
  - superior and middle temporal gyri;
  - caudate nucleus, putamen and globus pallidus;
  - cerebellar vermis;
  - cerebellar hemisphere with dentate nucleus;
  - focal lesions noted macroscopically.

Neuropathological findings in epilepsy
- *Agonal hypoxic damage* – related to the mode of death in SUDEP.
- *Brain swelling* – related to the mode of death in SUDEP.
- *Head injury* – recent injury sufficient to cause death may be classed as epilepsy-related death rather than SUDEP.
- *Old contusions* – evidence of previous head injury (in some patients, may be the cause of epilepsy).
- *Hippocampal sclerosis* – with loss of neurons in this structure, may be seen in patients with chronic epilepsy and it is still uncertain whether this is a cause or effect of epilepsy in some patients.
- *Cerebellar atrophy* – may be related to medication in some patients.
- *Previous surgical lesions* – patient may have had surgery for epilepsy, or epilepsy may be a complication of surgery for an unrelated condition.
- *Vascular malformation, cortical malformation or tumour* – recognised as causes of epilepsy.

- *Non-epilepsy related.* People with epilepsy can die of any unrelated cause, for example myocardial infarction. A family should be offered the opportunity to have the brain examined in relation to the epilepsy even if another cause is ascertained.
- *Epilepsy-related.* This category includes drowning or accidents that could be attributed to an epileptic seizure, precipitating the event. A full post-mortem will reveal the cause of epilepsy-related death. A family should be offered the opportunity to have the brain examined in relation to the epilepsy. Blood levels of anti-epileptic medication may reveal non-compliance with medication that may have a bearing on the circumstances leading to death.
- *Sudden unexplained death in epilepsy* (SUDEP). This is a diagnosis of exclusion, supported by a full post-mortem with histological and toxicological investigations. SUDEP is defined as the sudden, unexpected, witnessed or unwitnessed, non-traumatic, and non-drowning death of patients with epilepsy with or without evidence of a seizure, excluding documented status epilepticus, and in whom the post-mortem does not reveal a structural or toxicological cause for death (Nashef, 1997). Studies have identified the risks of SUDEP with chronic uncontrolled epilepsy and have also suggested that SUDEP is likely to be a seizure-related event. The mechanism of death is still debated (cardiac or respiratory). An important risk factor is non-compliance with anti-epileptic medication, but detecting suboptimal levels (rather than absence) is difficult because of reliability issues with post-mortem drug testing (Tomson *et al.*, 2008). The Royal College of Pathologists (UK) has approved a protocol in suspected SUDEP (Box 12.3; Thom, 2005).

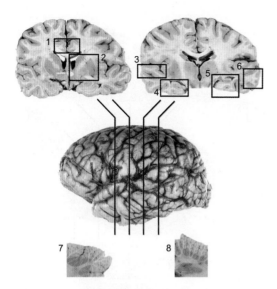

Figure 12.13 Tissue retention and sampling in epilepsy. Two slices of the cerebral hemisphere are retained, anterior and posterior to the midbrain, together with samples from vermis and cortex of cerebellum. Histological sampling from 1, cingulate gyrus; 2, caudate, putamen and globus pallidus; 3, superior temporal gyrus; 4 and 5 hippocampus and parahippocampal gyri; 6, middle temporal gyrus; 7, vermis of cerebellum; 8, cerebellar cortex and dentate nucleus.

Neuropathology in neurodegenerative diseases

The neurodegenerative diseases can be grouped into three main types: dementia syndromes, movement disorders and prion diseases. Several general concepts underpin the approach to post-mortem examinations.

- The immediate cause of death may be related to a complication or specific manifestation of the disease. Simply stating that a patient has died of a pneumonia without characterising a clinically recognised neurodegenerative disease may not be reliably ascertaining the true cause of death.
- Families increasingly recognise that some diseases are associated with a genetic cause and seek to characterise disease as a basis for future advice.
- Clinical features cannot predict the pathological cause of disease with certainty, so the post-mortem continues to provide important information. New entities continue to be described.
- There are overlap syndromes, and clinicopathological correlation continues to help refine approaches to diagnosis, disease classification and patient management. Several diseases previously felt to cause only a movement disorder are now recognised to also cause an associated dementia syndrome.
- New therapies are being developed and a post-mortem confirmation will increasingly be used as part of the evaluation of novel therapies for neurodegenerative diseases.
- Families wish to ascertain a diagnosis by post-mortem examination and subsequently seek to have retained tissues used for medical education, training or research.
- There are important public health implications for maintaining surveillance for transmissible diseases such as the prion diseases.

Dementia

Dementia syndromes are common and there is a benefit in full neuropathological ascertainment of the diagnosis (Box 12.4). In addition to providing a full explanation for the cause of death and signs seen in life, there is increasing awareness of genetic causes of dementia and families seek a diagnosis on which to base later advice. In some causes of dementia a specific complication may have a direct bearing on the cause of death. Consent advice should recommend retention of the whole brain plus the spinal cord in cases of frontotemporal dementia. There is a benefit in preserving fresh-frozen brain tissue for possible genetic investigation, with consent. If consent cannot be obtained for retention of the whole brain, limited sampling may be undertaken with the caveat that this may not give a full explanation of the disease or relationships to a cause of death (Fig. 12.14).

In most cases, referral to a specialist neuropathology service is required for diagnosis. A scheme for the staged examination of the brain in cases of dementia has been proposed (Dickson, 2005).

Box 12.4 Dementia syndromes

- *Alzheimer's disease.* This is the most common cause of dementia. It is most prevalent with increasing age, but may affect younger patients especially when there is an underlying genetic cause.
- *Dementia with Lewy bodies.* This has emerged as a common form of dementia. The regional neuropathology may link to and explain certain causes of death. Some patients with this syndrome die as a result of neuroleptic sensitivity to administered drugs. Pneumonia may be linked to dysphagia, associated with degenerative changes in the medulla (dorsal vagal nucleus).
- *Frontotemporal dementia syndromes.* These may be linked to degeneration of motor systems and link with the pathology of motor neuron disease, thereby explaining dysphagia and aspiration pneumonia (hypoglossal nucleus) or respiratory failure (deneravation of respiratory muscles).
- *Vascular dementia syndromes.* These are common, both in a pure form as well as contributing to neurodegenerative diseases as 'mixed dementia'. A small proportion of vascular dementia cases are caused by defined genetic causes.
- *Prion disease.* Rarely a prion disease may be the cause of a dementia syndrome.
- *Rare causes of dementia.* A very wide range of uncommon pathological causes of dementia have been described.

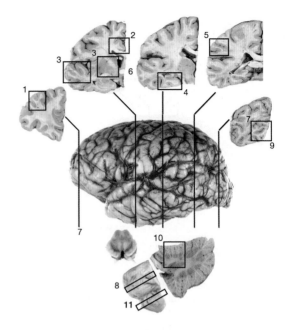

Figure 12.14 The minimum set of small blocks of brain sufficient to establish the diagnosis in most cases of neurodegenerative disorders. 1, middle frontal gyrus; 2, cingulate gyrus; 3, superior and middle temporal gyri; 4, hippocampus and parahippocampal gyrus; 5, inferior parietal lobule; 6, putamen and globus pallidus; 7, midbrain; 8, pons; 9, occipital cortex; 10, cerebellar hemisphere (including the dentate nucleus); 11, medulla. The blocks should be supplemented with samples of any macroscopically visible lesions. (Modified with permission from Love, 2004). The spinal cord should be retained in suspected cases of motor neuron disease.

Movement disorders

Movement disorders represent common forms of neurodegenerative diseases. They can be divided into several main categories according to the dominant clinical features. In all cases advice should be to retain the brain and spinal cord for detailed neuropathological examination.

Prion diseases

Prion diseases (transmissible spongiform encephalopathies) are rare fatal degenerative diseases with an incidence of about one per million population per year. The agent responsible for prion disease is believed to be a protein-only infective particle and is classified in hazard group 3 according to the advisory committee on dangerous pathogens. These diseases are not contagious but can be transmitted by inoculation, by ingestion and by iatrogenic routes. The agents are resistant to normal disinfection procedures and infectivity persists in formalin-fixed tissue.

Guidance on clinical risks and laboratory handling of potentially infected material has been published by the ACDP TSE Working Group (2003a,b), and regular updates are available online.

The cases covered include possible Creutzfeldt–Jakob disease (CJD), variant CJD, those in receipt of a blood transfusion from someone subsequently diagnosed with CJD or vCJD, those in receipt of pituitary-derived human growth hormone, gonadotrophins or dural grafts, the Gerstmann–Straussler–Scheinker syndrome, and fatal familial insomnia.

These last conditions are inherited forms of prion disease associated with mutation in the prion gene. Patients who have had genetic testing and those with a family history of disease should also be considered in the risk group. In terms of risk, any person who had undergone an intradural neurosurgical procedure or operation on the spinal cord prior to August 1992 is now classed as at risk of CJD.

In the evaluation of case notes prior to postmortem examination in patients with a neurological disease, it is usual for a clinical team to have already suspected the diagnosis of a prion disease. However, this is not always the case and pathologists need to be aware of the key features that would suggest the possibility of CJD. These are a rapidly progressive dementia, with a duration of less than 2 years, associated with two of the following features: myoclonus; visual or cerebellar signs; pyramidal or extrapyramidal movement disorder; akinetic mutism. In the UK the National CJD Surveillance Unit is available to provide advice, and in most other countries a similar national surveillance group can be contacted.

Autopsies for possible CJD and vCJD have assumed increasing importance following the bovine spongiform encephalopathy (BSE) epidemic, since it is an essential component of diagnosis and a vital way of confirming the diagnosis. Autopsies on cases of suspected spongiform encephalopathy may be safely undertaken in a hospital mortuary if published guidelines are followed (Box 12.5; Ironside and Bell, 1996; ADCP, 2003a,b).

Neuropathology autopsy in autonomic failure

There are many causes of autonomic failure, which may be divided into primary and secondary types. Some conditions are caused by pathology in the central nervous system, most commonly related to a neurodegenerative disease, while others are caused by disease in the peripheral nervous system. Central causes of autonomic failure associated with parkinsonism has been termed 'Shy–Drager syndrome'. The term 'Bradbury–Eggleston syndrome' is used to describe patients with isolated autonomic failure.

Box 12.5 Special procedures for suspected prion disease

In addition to the pathologist carrying out the autopsy with a trained skilled anatomic pathology technologist, a third 'clean' attendant should be present. Disposable personal protective equipment should be worn and disposable mortuary instruments used where possible. The minimum examination required is removal of the brain.

To prevent spillage, the body is retained within the body bag with appropriately placed absorbent wadding. The head is encased in a large, clear, polythene bag with an opening through which instruments can be introduced to prevent droplet and aerosol contamination. The skull can be opened either with a hand saw or with an autoclavable electric saw. The latter affords less risk for the operator as the increased local contamination can be contained by the plastic bag. If examination of abdominal or thoracic organs is undertaken it should be performed *in situ*. The greatest risk for infection during the autopsy is the accidental inoculation of either lymphoid or neural tissue. This may be minimised by wearing chain mail gloves layered between two pairs of rubber gloves.

Before fixation of the brain, $5\,cm^3$ samples of frontal lobe and cerebellum (as a minimum) should be frozen and stored at −70°C. In cases of vCJD, where peripheral lymphoid tissues are recognised to contain the transmissible abnormal prion protein, fresh samples of appendix, tonsil, gut and lymph node should be preserved.

The brain is then fixed as usual in 15% buffered formalin for further dissection later. This may be carried out in a class 1 microbiology safety cabinet, but after fixation in formalin it can be carried out on a ventilated bench provided that care is taken not to contaminate the area. Once again, disposable instruments should be used wherever possible, and the dissection carried out in a shallow tray lined with a disposable layer of material such as Benchcoat. Before wax processing, the blocks are placed in 96% formic acid for 1 hour (which substantially reduces infectivity) before being returned to formalin. Tissue-processing fluids do not need to be treated as potentially contaminated and can be disposed of using routine precautions (ACDP TSE Working Group, 2009)

Clinical information usually offers important clues as to the cause of autonomic failure, particularly disease of the peripheral nervous system associated with diabetes mellitus, alcoholism, amyloidosis, renal failure and connective tissue disease. Even in the presence of a known clinical association, thorough investigation of central and peripheral autonomic pathways is always indicated. Post-mortem consent should require retention of the brain, spinal cord and samples of the peripheral nervous system.

Initial histological investigation of a central cause for autonomic failure usually reveals the inclusions of multiple system atrophy in spinal cord and brain, or less commonly Lewy body pathology. Peripheral causes should initially concentrate on excluding the presence of a diabetic neuropathy, inflammatory disease or amyloid.

Further reading

Dawson TP, Neal JW, Llewwellyn L, Thomas C (2003). *Neuropathology Techniques*. London: Arnold Hodder Headline.

Ellison D, Love S, Chimeli L *et al.* 2003). *Neuropathology: A Reference Text of CNS Pathology*. New York: Mosby.

References

ACDP TSE Working Group (2003a). *Transmissible Spongiform Encephalopathy Agents: Safe Working and the Prevention of Infection in Clinical Laboratories*. London: HMSO. Available at www.advisorybodies.doh.gov.uk/acdp/tseguidance/tseguidancepart3.pdf

ACDP TSE Working Group (2003b). *Transmissible Spongiform Encephalopathy Agents: Safe Working and the Prevention of Infection. Annex H. After death*. London: HMSO. Available at www.advisorybodies.doh.gov.uk/acdp/tseguidance/tseguidance_annexh.pdf.

ACDP TSE Working Group (2009). *Transmissible Spongiform Encephalopathy Agents: Safe Working and the Prevention of Infection. Annex K. Guidelines for pathologists and pathology laboratories for the handling of tissues from patients with, or at risk of, CJD or vCJD*. London: HMSO. Available at www.advisorybodies.doh.gov.uk/acdp/tseguidance/tseguidance_annexk.pdf

Amarenco P, Bogousslavsky J, Caplan LR, Donnan GA, Hennerici MG (2009). New approach to stroke subtyping: the A-S-C-O (phenotypic) classification of stroke. *Cerebrovasc Dis* **27**:502–8.

Black M, Graham DI (2002). Mini-Symposium. Autopsy pathology: sudden death in epilepsy. *Curr Diagn Pathol* **8**:365–72.

Bromilow A, Burns J (1985). Technique for the removal of the vertebral arteries. *J Clin Pathol* **38**:1400–2.

Campbell J (1979). Examination of eyes and their adenexa. In: Ludwig J (ed.) *Current Methods of Autopsy Practice*, pp. 120–1. London: WB Saunders.

Dickson DW (2005). Required techniques and useful molecular markers in the neuropathologic diagnosis of neurodegenerative diseases. *Acta Neuropathol* **109**:14–24.

Ironside JW, Bell JE (1996). 'High risk' neuropathological autopsy in aids and Creutzfeldt–Jacob disease: principals and practice. *Neuropathol Appl Neurobiol* **22**:388–93.

Karhunen PJ, Kaupplia R, Penttila A, Erkinjuntti T (1990). Vertebral artery rupture in traumatic subarachnoid haemorrhage detected by postmortem angiography. *Forensic Sci Int* **44**:107–15.

Love S (2001). Sampling of brains at autopsy. In: Love S (ed.) *Neuropathology: A Guide for Practicing Pathologists*. Current Topics in Pathology, vol. 95. Berlin: Springer-Verlag.

Nadol JB (1980). Extracranial technique for temporal bone removal. *Ann Otol Rhinol Laryngol* **89**:251–2.

Nadol JB *et al.* (1996). Techniques for human temporal bone removal: information for the scientific community. *Otolaryngol Head Neck Surg* **115**:298–305.

Nashef L (1997). Sudden unexpected death in epilepsy: terminology and definitions. *Epilepsia* **38**(Suppl. 11):S6.

Parsons MA (2006). A histopathologist's guide to ocular pathology. In: Rutty GN (ed.) *Essentials of Autopsy Practice: Current Methods and Trends*, pp. 87–129. London: Springer.

Sharma M, Grieve JHK (2006). Rapid fixation of brains: a viable alternative? *J Clin Pathol* **59**:393–5.

Smith DH, Meaney DF, Shull WH (2003). Diffuse axonal injury in head trauma. *J Head Trauma Rehabil* **18**:307–16.

Thom M, on behalf of the RCPath Working Party on the Autopsy (2005). *Guidelines on Autopsy Practice. Scenario 6: Deaths associated with epilepsy.* London: Royal College of Pathologists, UK. Available at www.rcpath. org/resources/pdf/AutopsyScenario6Jan05.pdf.

Tomson T, Nashef L, Ryvlin P (2008). Sudden unexpected death in epilepsy: current knowledge and future directions. *Lancet Neurol* **7**:1021–31.

Vanezis P (1979). Techniques used in the evaluation of vertebral artery trauma at post-mortem. *Forensic Sci Int* **13**:159–65.

Chapter 13

FETAL, PERINATAL AND INFANT AUTOPSIES

Marta C Cohen

Introduction

Fetal, perinatal and paediatric autopsies differ considerably from those of adults. These autopsies should be undertaken only by those trained in these examinations, especially in medicolegal cases where a joint autopsy or double-doctored approach should be adopted unless the pathologist is an accredited forensic paediatric pathologist. The clinical questions raised are unique, requiring a different tactical and technical approach that necessitates specialised diagnostic skills to integrate the findings with the relevant obstetric and clinical history and with the results obtained from other disciplines such as cytogenetics, radiology or microbiology (Laing, 2004).

Fetal and perinatal autopsies

Objectives

The objectives of fetal and perinatal autopsies are:

- to determine, as far as possible, the gestational age;
- to determine, as far as possible, the time of death;
- to determine any underlying unsuspected abnormality or genetic metabolic disease;
- to evaluate the pregnancy and birth;
- to document growth and development;

- to establish the factors contributing to death and (if possible) the immediate cause of death;
- to evaluate the delivery of obstetric care;
- to evaluate the delivery of intensive care (if given);
- to assess the efficacy of new diagnostic or therapeutic procedures;
- to generate data for clinical audit;
- to generate data for confidential enquiry proceedings;
- to provide information that will aid in the counselling of parents as to the most likely outcome of future pregnancies

Historical information should be sought in connection with:

- the mother's general health;
- family history: consanguinity, malformations, genetic metabolic disease;
- previous pregnancies;
- maternal obstetric history;
- the current pregnancy: data should include the date of the last menstrual period, pregnancy complications such as hypertension, toxaemia, diabetes, infection, fetal growth restriction, bleeding, and exposure to chemicals or drugs (including tobacco and alcohol), results of ultrasonographic, in-utero magnetic resonance and amniocentesis or chorionic villi sampling examinations;

- labour and delivery: data should include time of onset of labour, the time of rupture of membranes, the amount and characteristics of the amniotic fluid, vaginal bleeding, length of labour, drugs administered, and mechanical intervention;
- the baby's postnatal course if liveborn: pharmacological and mechanical interventions, etc.

The standard protocol

(See RCPath, 2002; Siebert, 2007)

This protocol is applicable to all fetuses of more than 10 weeks gestation (or a body weight of 14 g):

1. Full skeletal x-ray.
2. Full body photographs (front and back).
3. Assessment of intrauterine growth. These measurements should be compared with standard charts. Standard physical measurements include (a) occipito-frontal circumference; (b) body weight; (c) crown-to-heel length; (d) crown-to-rump length; (e) foot length.
4. Maceration (if born dead).
5. Meconium staining.
6. Detailed external examination for anatomical deformity with photographic documentation, to include fontanelles, eyes, nose, ears, mouth and palate, digits, palmar creases, anus, umbilical cord, skin, etc.
7. Systematic inspection of internal organs and body cavities. Provide organ weights for all major organs using a digital balance (to 0.1 g). Examination of small fetuses is helped with the use of a dissecting microscope. Macerated and traumatised fetuses should not be disregarded as external malformations and major abnormalities can still be identified.
8. Additional investigations if clinically indicated: bacteriology, virology, karyotype, fibroblast culture, etc.
9. Removal and examination of the fetal brain. This is best performed under water. Two small paintbrushes help to manoeuvre the brain and thus facilitate examination of the surface (Figs 13.1 and 13.2). While still under water the brainstem and cerebellum are separated at the level of the midbrain. A coronal section of the

hemispheres is then performed at the level of the mammillary bodies with the help of a skin-graft blade or a double-edged razor blade and a spatula (Dean and Whitby, 2007). Using the latter, both sections are transferred to a sheet of dental wax where further slicing is performed. The low-friction surface of this wax minimises disruption of the brain when sections are taken.

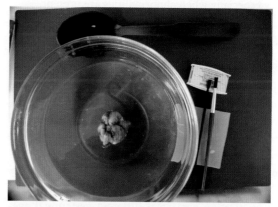

Figure 13.1 Toolkit used for underwater examination of the fetal brain.

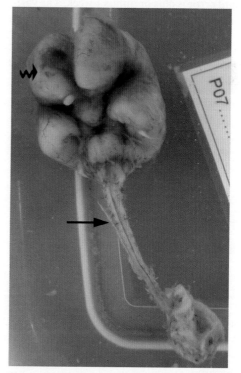

Figure 13.2 Inferior surface of the brain (wavy arrow indicates frontal lobe) with spinal cord (straight arrow) attached in an 18/40 fetus with myelomeningocele.

10. Sampling of tissues for histological studies. The extent of sampling in individual cases depends on the clinical situation. One block per organ is recommended, including the costochondral junction (this allows assessment of the growth plate and bone marrow). In the anatomically more complex organs, such as the brain, more extensive blocking is usually necessary, especially when abnormalities are present.

Pathological assessment of gestational age

This is best carried out by physical measurements such as crown-to-rump length, foot length and biparietal diameter and comparison made with normal reference data. A timetable of normal developmental milestones in fetuses is also helpful (Table 13.1) (Siebert, 2007).

Radiological assessment based on the appearance of ossification centres at different gestational ages may be used, but this is not a very reliable method as the standard error is plus or minus 1 week. The variability for the specific appearances of ossification

Table 13.1 Gestational milestones

Features	Body weight (g)	Gestational age (weeks)
Intestine in abdomen		
Fusion of palatal shelves		
Early fingernail development	14	10
Differentiated external genitalia	45	12
Early toenail development	320	18
Fingernails present		
Lanugo visible		
Skin red	460	20
Eyelids separate		
Eyelashes present	1000	26
Fingernails reach fingertips		
Toenails present	2100	32
Testes in scrotum		
Fingernails beyond fingertips	3400	38

centres increases with gestational age (Schumacher et al., 2004). The cerebral gyral pattern develops progressively in complexity with gestational age and is a useful alternative marker of maturity (Larroche et al., 1998).

In several organs (cerebellum, lung and kidney) the microscopic structure changes with developmental age and their histological appearances may be used in the assessment of gestational age.

Examination of the placenta and attachments

Examination of the placenta is an integral part of perinatal and fetal autopsies. The placenta should be submitted to the pathologist in the fresh state. Sampling of unfixed tissue may be needed for bacterial or viral cultures, cytogenetics, electron microscopy, vascular perfusion studies (monochorionic twins), and metabolic and molecular studies (Langston et al., 1997). Examination of the placenta should include naked eye inspection of the following.

- *Fetal membranes.* These must be checked for completeness, colour and the point of rupture.
- *Fetal and maternal surfaces of the placenta.* The maternal surface is examined for completion, adherent clot and surface depression which may indicate previous retroplacental haemorrhage. Evidence of subchorial haemorrhage, fibrin deposition or amnion nodosum should be sought on the fetal surface.
- *Umbilical cord.* Note the insertion (central, marginal, eccentric or velamentous) and number of vessels (assess this at least 3–5 cm above the chorionic plate, as the two arteries may fuse near the insertion). Focal abnormalities such as strictures, haematomas, thrombi, knots and varicosities should be sought. The presence of two vessels reflects a single umbilical artery (more frequent in diabetic mothers and when there are chromosomal abnormalities).
- *Villous tissue.* This is inspected through serially slicing the placental disc (at about 1 cm intervals). The cut surfaces are carefully inspected for infarction, pale areas,

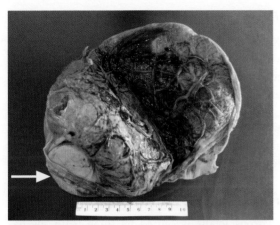

Figure 13.3 Trimmed placenta depicting a papyraceous fetus (arrow) at the edge of the chorionic surface.

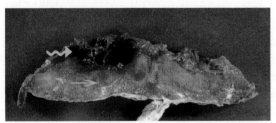

Figure 13.4 Cut surface of placenta showing a retroplacental haematoma (wavy arrow) with an underlying infarcted area (straight arrow).

haemorrhage, intervillous thrombus, etc. All significant lesions are described, measured and their locations noted.

Gross abnormalities of the placenta can be documented with a photograph (Figs 13.3 and 13.4)

The following measurements are important and should be compared with standard charts (Kraus *et al.*, 2004).

- *Placental weight* (after trimming the cord and membranes). Two placental diameters should also be measured as well as the maximum placental thickness.
- *Weight of any accompanying blood clot.*
- *Umbilical cord length.* Short cords predispose to rupture; long cords predispose to entanglement.
- *Feto-placental weight ratio* (FPR). The placental nutrient supply to the fetus (dependent on the size, morphology, transporters and blood supply of the placenta) is a determinant of fetal growth.

The FPR assesses placental efficiency and fetal growth. It increases from 4 at 25 weeks to 7 at term. Abnormal FPRs are related to abnormal fetal or placental weight (Langston *et al.*, 1997). FPR values should be compared with standardised charts (Kraus *et al.*, 2004).

Samples should be taken from the placenta for histology. A minimum of four blocks should be taken: two full-thickness blocks from the parenchyma (one including the chorionic plate and the other the maternal surface), one of the umbilical cord and one of the fetal membranes. The placental margin should be avoided. A sheet of fetal membrane should be rolled and a block taken from the roll.

The neonatal autopsy

(See RCPath, 2006)

A neonate is a newborn of up to 4 weeks of life. When examining the neonate, items 1, 2, 3 (assessment of post-natal growth), 8 and 9 of the protocol for fetal and perinatal deaths still apply.

External examination

In addition to the description of any dysmorphic features, the external examination should include an assessment of the nutritional status, muscle bulk, presence of oedema, pallor, jaundice and medical intervention (describing all puncture marks, catheters, drains, etc.).

Systematic inspection of internal organs and body cavities

Provide organ weights for all major organs. Include identification of pneumothorax, in-situ segmental examination of the heart and great vessels to confirm or exclude malformations, and removal of the organs in blocks.

Sampling of tissues for histology

Follow the recommendations provided for fetal and perinatal autopsies (see above). In addition, sampling of the brain should cover major areas: cortex, basal ganglia, thalamus, hippocampus, ventricles, midbrain, pons, medulla oblongata and cerebellum.

Clinical situations requiring additional investigation

Multiple pregnancies

Identification of the twins by the pathologist should match that assigned by the obstetrician. Twins or other multiple births must be compared for body size, sex, and external and internal features. Complications that are especially related to twinning include twin-to-twin transfusion syndrome (TTS), conjoined twinning and cord entanglement. These complications are more likely to occur, or can only occur, in association with monozygous twinning. Hence ascertainment of zygosity is important and can usually be assessed on the basis of:

- pattern of placentation (the usual method);
- blood group analysis;
- DNA 'finger printing';
- human leucocyte antigen (HLA) typing.

In the TTS, vascular communications may be demonstrated in the placenta by injecting a barium/gelatine mixture into the umbilical vessels of the donor twin. In chronic TTS there is discrepancy in the amount of amniotic fluid and body growth between the twins. Conjoined twinning requires more extensive dissection for accurate categorisation. The use of post-mortem MRI can assist in the dissection of conjoined twins (Roberts *et al.*, 2007).

Monochorionic placentation indicates that the twins are monozygotic; if placentation is dichorionic, the twins are either monozygotic or dizygotic. The assessment is made based on the pattern of chorionic vascularisation and on the gross and histological characteristics of the dividing membrane This is thick and opaque and shows a chorionic ridge along the base of the septal attachment in the dichorionic fused placentas. In contrast, the dividing membranes are thin and translucent with no chorionic ridge in mono chorionic twins. On histology, the dividing membranes contain fused chorion intervening between the amnions in the former but the chorion is lacking in the latter (Kraus *et al.*, 2004). The fused placentas of monochorionic twins depict vascular communication between the two fetal circulations.

Fetus or infant with skeletal dysplasia

X-rays are mandatory (anteroposterior and lateral views of the whole body). The diagnosis is made primarily on radiological features. Clinical photographs are essential.

Histology must include the epiphysis (growth plate) of a long bone and the trachea. Frozen tissues should be stored at $-70°C$ to allow for further genetic testing.

Fetus or infant with hydrops

Hydrops fetalis is caused by three main mechanisms: anaemia, hypoproteinaemia and cardiac failure. The number of known associated causes of hydrops is extensive. Investigations should be directed at the possible causes; these may be separated into those that are structural and those that are non-structural. In the former, a thorough routine examination should reveal an underlying mechanism. Examples of *structural causes* of hydrops are:

- twin-to-twin transfusion syndrome;
- chromosome abnormalities (e.g. Turner's syndrome, trisomy 21 and trisomy 18);
- developmental abnormalities related to heart, larynx, lung, kidney, blood vessels and lymphatics (including cystic hygroma);
- fetal tumours (e.g. sacrococcygeal teratoma, neuroblastoma);
- skeletal dysplasias (e.g. chondroplasia, osteogenesis imperfecta);
- placental haemangiomatosis.

Non-structural causes of hydrops include immune and non-immune types. Non-immune causes are:

- haematological disorders (mainly homozygous α−thalassaemia);
- feto-maternal haemorrhage;
- infection (usually viral, mainly parvovirus B19 and cytomegalovirus);
- genetic metabolic disease (GMD).

When feto-maternal haemorrhage is suspected, a Kleihauer test may provide useful information. A comprehensive list of causes of hydrops fetalis is provided by Machin (2007).

Investigation of the fetus or infant with suspected GMD

The examination must be carried out as soon as possible after death (where practicable, ideally within 6 hours) to avoid autolysis and to ensure that histological, histochemical, biochemical and molecular investigations are optimal (Ernst *et al.*, 2006).

Genetic metabolic disease may be suspected in pregnancies that have been terminated following a previously affected sibling, or subsequent to a positive antenatal diagnosis. The type of investigations will generally be determined by the precise genetic metabolic condition being considered. Sudden death can be produced by a metabolic disease in 5 per cent of cases (Ernst *et al.*, 2006). The majority of these cases belong to the category of fatty acid oxidation defects (medium-chain acyl-CoA dehydrogenase deficiency, very-long-chain acyl-CoA dehydrogenase deficiency, and short-chain 3-hydroxyacyl-CoA dehydrogenase deficiency) (Ernst *et al.*, 2006). The procedures to be followed will usually depend on the degree of suspicion. When the index of suspicion is high, the following protocol is recommended.

1. Skeletal survey.
2. Skin biopsy for fibroblast culture and enzyme analysis. Gonadal tissue or fascia lata are useful alternatives to skin. Amniotic membrane or chorionic plate are used in the presence of fetal autolysis. The sample should be placed in culture medium at 4°C.
3. Retain samples of urine, cerebrospinal fluid, bile and plasma (store at –70°C) for organic acids, amino acids, acylcarnitines.
4. Prepare a smear from peripheral blood to assess the presence of vacuolated lymphocytes.
5. Blood should be preserved in heparin and in fluoride. Plasma should be separated and stored at –20°C.
6. Sample the bone marrow to assess the presence of storage cells (e.g. Gaucher disease, mucopolysaccharidosis).
7. Sample cartilage and bone (e.g. mucopolysaccharidosis).
8. Fix tissue in glutaraldehyde for possible electron microscopy. Suitable tissues include liver, kidney, brain, muscle and placenta.
9. Snap-freeze portions of unfixed organs in liquid nitrogen and store at –70°C (placenta, muscle, brain, liver, spleen and kidney) for enzymatic studies.

When the level of suspicion of a genetic metabolic disease is low, steps 1, 2, 3 and 7 are probably sufficient.

The preterm infant

Prematurity is defined as an infant born at a gestational age of less than 37 weeks. Infants of less than 1500 g at delivery are referred to as 'very low birth weight' (VLBW) infants.

The autopsy should focus on recognising complications associated with prematurity. These may be roughly separated into those related to organ immaturity and those that are iatrogenic in nature (Table 13.2). The sites of drains, catheters or surgical incisions should be noted.

Intraventricular haemorrhage should be graded (Table 13.3) (Larroche *et al.*, 1998). This assessment is ideally carried out after the brain has been hardened in fixative. The recommended period of formalin fixation is 2–3 weeks. A method that reduces the fixation time and allows return of the brain to the body prior to the funeral consists in fixing the brain in 20% buffered formalin at 37°C for 4–6 days. The addition of a teaspoon of salt to the formalin will make the brain float. The formalin should be changed every day. Two hours prior to the examination the brain is placed in cold water in a refrigerator to maximise the stiffness of the tissue.

Table 13.2 Complications associated with prematurity

Related to organ immaturity	Iatrogenic
Hyaline membrane disease	Pneumothorax
Neonatal necrotising enterocolitis (NNEC)	Tubal injuries (especially trachea)
Intraventricular haemorrhage (IVH)	Necrotising tracheobronchitis
Periventricular leucomalacia	Bronchopulmonary dysplasia
Kernicterus	Neonatal necrotising enterocolitis
Infection (localised or generalised)	Retinal injury
	Hepatic injury

Table 13.3 Germinal matrix haemorrhage and intraventricular haemorrhage

Grade 0	No haemorrhage
Grade 1	Germinal matrix haemorrhage (GMH)
Grade 2	GMH or choroid plexus haemorrhage (CPH) with intraventricular haemorrhage (IVH) without ventricular dilatation
Grade 3	GMH or CPH with IVH and ventricular dilatation
Grade 4	GMH or CPH with IVH and parenchymal haemorrhage

This part of the examination is effectively carried out by serial transverse slicing of the brain. Naked eye evidence of periventricular leucomalacia is sought at the same time. An exception to the routine examination of the brain after formalin fixation is when kernicterus is suspected, as this is only effectively evaluated in the fresh specimen. Its presence may be confirmed in unstained frozen sections. Microbiological investigations in these infants should be rigorous and include culture of cerebro spinal fluid, blood, lung and the tips of catheters.

The infant with intrauterine growth restriction

This is defined as an infant whose birth weight is less than the 10th percentile of that expected for gestational age. This cause may be constitutional (symmetrical intrauterine growth restriction (IUGR)) or nutritional (asymmetrical IUGR). In the first category, brain and liver growth are proportionate whereas in the second category their growth is disproportionate (i.e. the ratio of brain weight to liver weight exceeds 2.8). The fetus appears small with a relatively large head. Causes of symmetrical IUGR include syndromes, genetic and chromosomal disease and viral infections.

The hypoxic term infant

These infants are usually born with low Apgar scores and require active resuscitation at birth, often followed by a period of endotracheal intubation and intermittent positive-pressure ventilation (IPPV). Death may result from cerebral hypoxic damage or

from the complications of resuscitation/ventilation. The site of drains, catheters or surgical incisions should be noted. Assessment for the presence of pneumothoraces is essential (Siebert, 2007); this is achieved by means of a post-mortem x-ray or by opening the thoracic cavity under water. An alternative method to check for pneumothoraces consists in the placement of a water-filled syringe into the unopened thoracic cavity and aspirating any gas present. If bubbles are formed these are indicative of pneumothorax (unless the lung has been punctured).

The dysmorphic fetus or infant

Precise documentation is imperative and, in this regard, radiological investigation, detailed photography and chromosome analysis are important. Tissue for cytogenetic culture should be taken using a sterile procedure. Skin, fascia, lung, chorionic villi from the placenta and cartilage are regarded as the best sources for culture (Siebert, 2007). It is prudent to retain a sample of tissue (e.g. spleen or muscle) for cryopreservation and potential molecular analysis in some cases.

The ultimate aim of precise categorisation is accurate prediction of the recurrence risk and appropriate counselling of the family. The pathologist must determine whether deformity is single or multiple; if multiple, consider categorisation into 'syndrome', 'association' or 'sequence'. The question of whether the malformation was lethal or simply an incidental finding should also be addressed. Dysmorphia may be produced by intrauterine infections (cytomegalovirus, rubella, toxoplasmosis); such cases will require appropriate microbiological studies.

The stillborn infant

This term applies to all infants born after the twenty-fourth week of gestation who do not breathe or show any other signs of life after complete separation from the mother. Stillborn fetuses may be macerated when death has occurred prior to delivery (decomposition begins immediately *in utero*) or they may be non-macerated. They may also be separated into those who die before labour (prepartum) and those

Table 13.4 Post-mortem changes after intrauterine death

Time	Feature
12 hours	Skin appears parboiled or little changed
12–48 hours	Blistering of skin and overriding of cranial bones
48 hours	Sloughing of skin, especially on hands and feet; increased joint mobility
72 hours	Massive sloughing; mobility of symphysis mentus and pubis

whose deaths occur during established labour (intrapartum). The presence of visceral petechiae, inhaled amniotic material and hypoxic–ischaemic injury of the brain may be present in this scenario (RCPath, 2006). There is no reliable method to accurately determine the interval between intrauterine death and delivery, although this could be attempted using some of the available data (Table 13.4; Singer and Macpherson, 1998). Precise timing of the period of intrauterine death is difficult.

The basic protocol should be applied, including the weighing of all organs. Organ weights are decreased by autolysis. The extent to which tissues are sampled for histology will depend on the degree of maceration. Viral inclusions may still be seen in autolysed tissues. A stain to assess the distribution of fat in the adrenal and connective tissue on sections from severely autolysed tissue may yield important information. The placental examination constitutes an important component of the stillborn autopsy and many variables should be considered when exploring the maternal–fetal–placental unit (Siebert, 2007).

The possibly infected fetus or infant

Whereas most situations would usually require some degree of microbiological study, fetuses or infants more strongly suspected of having infection should be more rigorously investigated and further sampling should be carried out. Clinical situations indicating a strong likelihood of infection (bacterial or viral) include:

- maternal vaginal discharge;
- discoloured or malodorous placenta and/or membranes;
- premature prolonged rupture of membranes;
- maternal pyrexia, before or after delivery;
- fetal skin lesions;
- intrauterine growth retardation;
- TORCH syndrome (toxoplasmosis, other infection, rubella, cytomegalovirus, herpes simplex);
- non-immune hydrops (usually viral aetiology);
- following a period of intensive care (especially preterm infants).

Blood cultures and tracheal/bronchial swabs are the minimum requirements when bacterial infection is suspected. When more rigorous investigation is indicated, cerebrospinal fluid, lung and splenic tissue, tubes and cannulae may be cultured, in addition to the minimal procedure. Blood for culture may be aspirated from the left side of the heart using a sterile needle and syringe. Portions of tissue (lung, heart and spleen) should be sent for viral culture, placed into sterile transport medium. The results of maternal blood cultures and a high vaginal swab may provide useful information when bacterial infection is suspected. Information on the rubella-immune status and from the Venereal Disease Research Laboratory (for syphilis) may be available in the maternal clinical notes.

The following viruses may be implicated in intra-uterine infections: cytomegalovirus, herpes simplex, rubella, parvovirus and HIV. Cytomegalovirus and rubella infection may be associated with dysmorphia. In presumed viral infection, a serum sample should be sent for viral antibodies. Frozen tissue may also be retained for study using in-situ hybridisation and/or PCR.

Indications for chromosome analysis

Indications include:

- possible specific chromosome syndromes;
- one or more malformations;
- fetuses of more than 13 weeks gestation with ambiguous genitalia or dysgenetic gonads;
- severely macerated fetus or stillborn with suspicious finding (best to use placental amnion or chorionic plate);

- fetus or stillborn with severe unexplained IUGR;
- non-immune hydrops;
- recurrent fetal loss;
- family history of genetic abnormality.

In the fresh specimen, a skin culture taken under sterile conditions is usually adequate. In the presence of fetal maceration, a sample should be obtained from the placental amnion. The specimen is placed and transported in culture medium. Fetal specimens sent over long distances may be received in the laboratory fixed in formalin; the referring clinician should be advised to sample skin or a sample of blood for culture prior to fixation.

Post-mortem magnetic resonance imaging

Magnetic resonance imaging constitutes a useful ancillary investigation in the fetal, perinatal and paediatric autopsy (Cohen *et al.*, 2008). MRI can determine structural normality or abnormality. Its main benefit is in the examination of the central nervous system owing to the high incidence of malformations (20 per cent of fatal congenital abnormalities), the difficulties in dissecting the high-water-content fetal brain, and the quick maceration that occurs after intrauterine fetal death or termination of pregnancy. In addition, central nervous system MRI can 'complete' the post-mortem when consent has been restricted to the chest and abdomen. MRI also provides a permanent comprehensive digital record of each case that is available for future reference and can be used in court. This has proved useful in cases of suspected infanticide as the lungs are fluid-filled in cases that were stillborn, or air-filled in cases that have died immediately after delivery (Cohen and Whitby, 2007).

Dissection techniques

A detailed autopsy technique is outlined by Siebert (2007). Embryos and fetuses of less than 10 weeks gestation or weighing less than 14 g may be examined by the free-hand sectioning method, in which the trunk of the embryo is cut into transverse slices of about 1 cm thickness. The small specimens are

examined in a Petri dish under a dissecting microscope fitted with a camera for photographic documentation. For fetuses above 10 weeks gestation the dissection starts with a Y-shaped or midline thoraco-abdominal incision. The organs are removed *en bloc* for inspection, leaving the kidneys, ureters and bladder *in situ*.

Blocking

Blocking of tissue should be standardised, so far as possible, for several reasons.

- It allows the pathologist to become familiar with the microanatomy of a particular area of the organ. This is especially important in more complex organs such as the brain.
- It permits effective comparisons to be made between cases of similar areas.
- Quantitative evaluation is only possible when the same anatomical areas are used for assessment.

Classification of perinatal deaths

In the UK this comprises stillbirths and early neonatal deaths. Several classifications have been proposed for the purpose of classifying perinatal deaths. One that is used in the UK is that of the extended Wigglesworth classification (1998), as shown in Box 13.1. It has the merit of simplicity and should be useful in general practice.

Box 13.1 Wigglesworth classification of perinatal deaths

- Congenital defect/malformation (lethal or severe)
- Unexplained antepartum fetal death
- Placental abrubtion before labour
- Death from intrapartum 'asphyxia', 'anoxia' or 'trauma'
- Immaturity (liveborn)
- Infection
- Other specific causes (includes twin-to-twin transfusion, tumours, inborn errors of metabolism, etc.)
- Accidental (non-intrapartum trauma)
- Sudden infant death, cause unknown
- Unclassifiable: to be used as a last resort

Box 13.2 Classification system according to relevant condition at death (ReCoDe) (Gardosi _et al._, 2005)

Group A: Fetus
1. Lethal congenital anomaly
2. Infection
   2.1 Chronic
   2.2 Acute
3. Non-immune hydrops
4. Isoimmunisation
5. Feto-maternal haemorrhage
6. Twin-to-twin transfusion
7. Fetal growth restriction

Group B: Umbilical cord
1. Prolapse
2. Constricting loop or knot
3. Velamentous insertion
4. Other

Group C: Placenta
1. Abruptio
2. Praevia
3. Vasa praevia
4. Other placental insufficiency
5. Other

Group D: Amniotic fluid
1. Chorioamnionitis
2. Oligohydramnios

3. Polyhydramnios
4. Other

Group E: Uterus
1. Rupture
2. Uterine anomalies
3. Other

Group F: Mother
1. Diabetes
2. Thyroid disease
3. Essential hypertension
4. Hypertensive disease in pregnancy
5. Lupus or antiphospholipid syndrome
6. Cholestasis
7. Drug misuse
8. Other

Group G: Intrapartum
1. Asphyxia
2. Birth trauma

Group H: Trauma
1. External
2. Iatrogenic

Group I: Unclassified
1. No relevant condition identified
2. No information available

Unfortunately, two-thirds of the fetal deaths end up in the unexplained or unclassifiable categories of any classification system available. In order to overcome this problem, Gardosi _et al._ (2005) developed the 'Classification of stillbirth by relevant condition at death (ReCoDe)'. The authors developed it by defining relevant clinical categories for stillbirth that were tested in a dataset of stillbirths in the West Midlands.

The system, shown in Box 13.2, is hierarchical and aims to identify what went wrong _in utero_, not necessarily why. The hierarchy starts from conditions affecting the fetus and moves outwards in simple anatomical groups, subdivided into physiopathological conditions. The system allows more than one category to be coded: the primary code is the more relevant condition applicable to the case while secondary coding can be used to increase descriptiveness. According to Gardosi _et al._ (2005), the ReCoDe classification system can identify relevant pathology in 85 per cent of cases.

Sudden unexpected death in infancy

The age covered by the category 'sudden unexpected death in infancy' (SUDI) is 1 week to 2 years. A detailed description is provided in an appendix to this chapter (see page 198).

Background

Infant deaths are unique in several aspects: most deaths occur at home and the majority are sudden and unexpected. Consequently, infant autopsies are different because baseline (control) data – morphological and non-morphological – are generally lacking and the cause of death is frequently elusive, despite extensive and in-depth investigation. Unexpected infant deaths at home form the most important group, and the approach outlined below is principally focused on this problem. The methodology can be

Table 13.5 Non-infectious recognisable causes of sudden death in infants

System	Cause of death
General	Genetic metabolic disease
Cardiovascular system	Congenital heart disease (including vascular and valve causes and anomalous coronary arteries) Endocardial fibroelastosis Cardiomyopathies Conduction system defects
Respiratory system	Asthma Upper airway obstruction Tension pneumothorax Massive pulmonary haemorrhage Primary pulmonary hypertension
Gastrointestinal system	Intestinal obstruction Gastrointestinal haemorrhage Pancreatitis Cystic fibrosis
Endocrine system	Congenital adrenal hyperplasia
Central nervous system	Trauma Cerebrovascular accidents (including arteriovenous malformation and haematological conditions) Epilepsy Tumours
Metabolic conditions	Acyl-coA dehydrogenase deficiencies Carnitine deficiency Glutaric aciduria type 2 Propionic acidaemia

Table 13.6 Infectious causes of sudden infant death

Condition	More frequent aetiology
Myocarditis	Coxsackie B, coxsackie A, echovirus, human immunodeficiency virus, cytomegalovirus, parvovirus
Bacterial pneumonia	*Streptococcus pneumoniae, Staphylococcus aureus, Haemophilus influenzae*
Bronchiolitis	Respiratory syncytial virus, adenovirus, parainfluenza virus, *Bordetella pertussis, Haemophilus influenzae*
Meningitis	*Neisseria meningitides, Streptococcus pneumoniae, Haemophilus influenzae*
Encephalitis	Herpes virus
Septicaemia	Group B *Streptococcus*
Acute laryngo-tracheo-bronchitis	Viruses, *Staphylococcus aureus*
Epiglottitis	*Haemophilus influenzae* type B
Gastroenteritis	Viruses
Haemolytic uraemic syndrome	*Escherichia coli* O157

modified to meet the precise situation so far as other deaths are concerned within this age category.

Recognisable causes of sudden infant death are shown in Tables 13.5 and 13.6 and the goal of the autopsy should aim at excluding such causes (Byard, 2004). Lethal diseases of this type are usually obvious at the macroscopic or microscopic level. Figure 13.5 shows possible lethal mechanisms that are not necessarily associated with overt pathological changes; some of these mechanisms are potentially diagnostically resolvable, others are not.

Traumatic deaths in this age group, and those due to other recognisable causes, are an important source of material against which to assess data obtained from SUDI. Thus, it is imperative that those involved in the investigation of unexplained

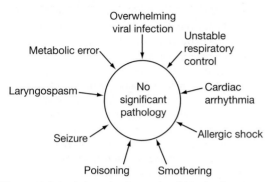

Figure 13.5 Lethal mechanisms of sudden death not necessarily associated with overt pathological changes.

infant deaths also be given access to such material. To facilitate comparison, the autopsy protocol for the two groups (i.e. unexplained and those likely to be explained) should be identical.

Protocol

In accordance with other post-mortem examinations, a detailed clinical history is very important. A significant proportion of these deaths in the UK come under the jurisdiction of the coroner. The Kennedy report, *Sudden Unexpected Death in Infancy* (2004), was the result of the working group convened by the Royal College of Pathologists and the Royal College of Paediatrics and Child Health. The multiagency protocol guides the investigation and care of families after the sudden and unexpected death of an infant or child. Key elements of the Kennedy protocol are as follows.

1. Staff involved should retain an open mind: natural death versus neglect or abuse (the minority of cases).
2. The coroner has jurisdiction over the body.
3. Babies found dead at home are always taken to the Accident and Emergency Department (not to the mortuary).
4. After the baby has been declared dead a paediatrician takes a clinical history from the parents. The baby is examined carefully. The presence of bruises, injuries, or retinal haemorrhages should raise suspicion. The police would lead those cases that will be done by the forensic pathologist (ideally as a joint post-mortem with the paediatric pathologist).

5. A standard set of samples are taken after death is confirmed (unless unnatural death is suspected). Consent from the appropriate medicolegal authority or the relatives must be obtained before these samples are collected and the Accident and Emergency Department must be licensed for these activities.
6. Ideally within 24 hours, a police officer trained in SUDI cases and the on-call SUDI paediatrician visit the home to talk with the parents and examine the place where the baby died.
7. The SUDI paediatrician inquires about the clinical history, including details of 'the last sleep', and prepares a report for the coroner and the pathologist. Parents must be informed that such a visit is routine but that the police have to thoroughly investigate the circumstances of all unexpected deaths of children (Box 13.3).
8. The paediatric pathologist performs the autopsy as soon as possible.
9. A multidisciplinary meeting chaired by the SUDI paediatrician takes place after the post-mortem report is issued (usually 8 weeks after the death). This meeting should be attended by all agencies involved: police, pathologist(s), social services, health visitor, the general practitioner of the baby and the coroner's officer.
10. The purpose of the meeting is to share information, agree the cause of death and plan future care for the family. Relevant information concerning the circumstances of the death, the infant's history, family history, risk factors for SUDI and subsequent investigations are reviewed. An explicit discussion of the possibility of abuse or neglect happens and, if no evidence is identified to suggest maltreatment, this should be documented as part of the report of the meeting. The death is classified according to the Avon classification of SUDI (Fleming *et al.*, 2004) (Table 13.7).
11. The SUDI paediatrician discusses the findings and future care with the parents.
12. The coroner holds the inquest and registers the cause of death.

Box 13.3 Information collected by the SUDI paediatrician at the home visit (Sheffield SUDI protocol)

1. Full name, date of birth and address of baby, mother and baby's father.
2. Detailed family medical history with special emphasis on any deaths in infancy or childhood of any offspring, siblings or other close relatives of any member of the current household.
3. Social and family history: social structure and composition, including information on alcohol, tobacco and other drug use and medications.
4. Detailed medical history of mother including obstetric history.
5. Medical and developmental history of the baby who has died: gestation, birth weight, perinatal or neonatal problems, type of feeding (and date and reason for changing type of feeding), growth, development and past assessments (e.g. health visitor or GP routine, well-baby checks), immunisations, any known contact with infection, medication (either prescribed or over-the-counter).
6. Account of the baby's feeding, sleeping, activity and health over the 2-week period prior to the death. Include information on: changes in feeding or sleeping patterns, changes in place of sleep, changes in individuals responsible for providing care to the baby, any social, family or health-related changes in routine practices over the past 2 weeks, any illness, accident or other major event affecting other family members in the past 2 weeks.
7. Account of events within the 48 hours prior to the

infant being found dead. Description of: precisely where the baby was placed for sleep, duration of sleeping period, position at the end of the sleeping periods, any changes in routine care or routine activity levels, any disruptions to normal patterns, information on the activity and location of all significant members of the household, information on alcohol intake and recreational drug use by members of the household during this period.
8. The final sleep: when and where the baby was placed to sleep, nature of the surface, clothing, bedding, arrangement of bedding, precise sleeping position, who was sharing the surface on which baby was sleeping (e.g. bed or sofa), how often the baby was checked, when he or she was seen or heard, the times at which the baby awoke for feeds, when and by whom the baby was found, the appearance of the baby when found, the position of the baby when found, where the bedding was, any covers over the baby (had the covers and the position of the covers moved?), whether the heating was on, the type of heating.
9. Action after baby was found: events that followed the discovery of the baby collapsed or apparently dead, to include details of: when, how and by whom the emergency services were called, who was with the baby at each stage, whether resuscitation was attempted and if so by whom, any responses obtained from the baby, how long it took for the emergency services to arrive.

Procedure

A whole body x-ray should be undertaken, with particular attention paid to signs of injury. Routine full-body photographs (front and back) are taken. Certain basic measurements are important to evaluate development; these include:

- body weight;
- crown-to-heel length;
- crown-to-rump length;
- occipito-frontal circumference;
- chest circumference;
- abdominal circumference.

Several of these measurements may be plotted against normal standard centile charts to evaluate premortem growth.

A careful search should be made on external examination for:

- marks of violence (when this suggests non-accidental injury this should be reported to the coroner, who will order a joint post-mortem with a forensic pathologist);
- distribution of post-mortem hypostasis (this may have forensic implications);
- evidence of malformation;
- evidence of medical intervention.

When there are positive findings in relation to the first two points, careful documentation and photography are essential.

External dissection

External incisions should be located to allow maximal exposure of the internal organs while at the same time permitting optimal cosmetic reconstruction after the autopsy has been completed. Y-shaped

Table 13.7 Avon classification chart, to be completed in cases of sudden unexpected death in infancy

Classification	0	IA	IB	IIA	IIB	III
Contributory or potential causal factors	Information not collected	Information collected but not factors identified	Factor present but not likely to have contributed to ill-health or possibly to death	Factor present and may have contributed to ill-health or possibly to death	Factor present and certainly contributed to ill-health and probably contributed to death	Factor present and provides a complete and sufficient cause of death
History[a]						
Death scene examination[b]						
Pathology[c]						
Other (specify)						
Other evidence of neglect or abuse?						
Overall classification[d]						

[a] Detailed history of events leading up to the death and including medical, social, family history plus to include any past evidence of neglect or abuse in this or other children in the family.

[b] Results of a detailed review of the scene of death by a paediatrician and police child protection officer in the light of the history given by parents or carers.

[c] Pathological investigations to a standardised protocol including gross and histological examinations, microbiology, toxicology, etc.

[d] This will generally equal the highest individual classification given above.

Reproduced with pernmission from Fleming et al. (2004)

incisions at the neck and groin can be joined by a central midline incision; after autopsy the sutured incisions will be hidden by clothing. (See also Chapter 21.)

Internal examination

Microscopic evaluation and the quality of specimen for special studies may be significantly influenced by the length of the post-mortem interval, the extent to which the body is handled after death, and the intervention of resuscitative measures. All the internal organs should be carefully inspected. A semi-quantitative assessment of the number (i.e. 0, +, ++, +++) and distribution of petechiae over the intrathoracic serosal surfaces is important. The larynx, trachea and its bifurcation should be assessed for structural abnormality; their lumina should be carefully inspected for foreign bodies, gastric contents and evidence of infection. The middle ears should be exposed and a record made of any abnormal content (e.g. pus, mucus). A swab should be taken if pus is present or suspected. One costochondral junction should be removed for microscopy. The brain and spinal cord should be removed *in toto* and fixed in formalin for a

period of 2–3 weeks or using the 'quick' method described above, prior to serial slicing and blocking. The posterior approach to the brain is preferred (see the appendix to this chapter). A detailed dissection technique is outlined by Siebert (2007). Recommended special investigations include those shown in Table 13.8.

Microscopic investigations

At least one histological section should be prepared from each major organ. More complex organs such as the brain and lung will require more extensive histological sampling. Blocks from these organs may be shaped differently so as to identify their origin at the time of microscopy.

Other considerations

Instances of unexplained sudden deaths that require further consideration include: a second unexpected death in the family, or an unexpected infant death in a family with a previous unexplained neonatal death. Such cases should be subject to toxicological screening, investigation of the cardiac conduction system, and immunological studies.

Table 13.8 Recommended special investigations

Sample	Send to	Handling	Test
Skin	Tissue culture	In transport culture medium	Fibroblast culture for inborn errors of metabolism
Blood (serum) 1–2 mL	Clinical chemistry	Spin, store serum at −20°C	Toxicology
Blood cultures: aerobic and anaerobic, 1 mL	Microbiology	If insufficient blood, aerobic only	Culture and sensitivity
Blood from Guthrie card	Clinical chemistry	Fill in card; do not put into plastic bag	Inherited metabolic diseases
Blood (whole)	Toxicology*	With and without fluoride	Toxicology screen
Cerebrospinal fluid (CSF) (a few drops)	Microbiology		Microscopy, culture and sensitivity
Nasopharyngeal swab	Virology		Viral cultures and DNA amplification techniques
Nasopharyngeal swab	Microbiology		Culture and sensitivity
Swabs from any identifiable lesions	Microbiology		Culture and sensitivity
Urine (if available)	Clinical chemistry	Spin, store supernatant at −20°C	Toxicology, metabolic diseases
Stomach contents	Toxicology*		Toxicology screen
Intestinal content	Virology		Viral cultures
Lung swab	Microbiology		Culture and sensitivity
Vitreous	Clinical chemistry		Urea/electrolytes/osmolality
0.5 cm² of heart, liver, kidney and muscle	Histopathology	Cryostat sections	Oil Red O stain or similar to search for excess fat deposition

*Chain of custody procedures should be followed.

Factors that should prompt consideration of genetic metabolic disease in cases of sudden death are parental consanguinity, maternal HELLP syndrome, previous Reye-like illness, or infant deaths in the family (from known genetic metabolic disease or unexplained), a previous acute life-threatening event (near-miss cot death), fasting or recurrent hypoglycaemia, neonatal hypotonia, dysmorphism, or enlargement of the liver and/or spleen. A pale (fatty) liver or hepatic fibrosis, cardiomegaly and severe brain oedema are important markers of metabolic disease at autopsy.

The most common metabolic disorders leading to sudden death in infancy are those associated with β-oxidation of fatty acids; the most frequently encountered defect is medium-chain acyl-CoA dehydrogenase (MCAD) deficiency (Ernst *et al.*, 2006). The sampling recommended in Table 13.8 should be sufficient for the post-mortem diagnosis of most defects of β-oxidation of fatty acids, but the predominant MCAD deficiency mutation can be detected by DNA analysis of the stored dried blood spot sample taken for mass neonatal screening of phenylketonuria.

Appendix: Protocol for paediatric post-mortem examination (1 week to 2 years)

The following measurements are carried out: crown-to-heel length, crown-to-rump length, head circumference, abdominal circumference (at the level of the umbilicus), and chest circumference (at the level of the nipples). The body is weighed.

A careful search is made for evidence of injury. The frenulum is assessed and the buccal cavity is examined for evidence of injury or other lesions. The presence of a vaccination scar is noted. Check the face for areas of pallor and, when present, note their distribution. Palpate for enlarged lymph nodes. The eyes are examined, looking for malformation, abnormal pupillary size or conjunctival petechiae. Probe the nasal passages to exclude choanal atresia or stenosis. Examine the external genitalia. A sample of vitreous humour is obtained for biochemistry (unless the death is suspicious and the eyes need to be removed to search for retinal haemorrhages). This is achieved by inserting a needle into the lateral aspect of the globe of the eye behind the cornea and applying gentle suction pressure on the plunger of the syringe.

The following incisions are made: a wide collar-shaped incision from shoulder to shoulder; a vertical Y-shaped midline incision extending from the centre of the collar down to the umbilicus; an inverted V-shaped incision from the umbilicus down to the groins. If necessary complete the incision through the abdominal wall using a pair of scissors.

An area of skin is swabbed with spirit and a small piece of skin (about 0.5 cm maximum dimension) is removed and placed in transport medium (TC-199).

The skin is reflected off the thoracic cage with the aid of a scalpel. The procedure is extended into the neck separating the skin from underlying muscle. The sternum and adjacent cartilages are removed by cutting through the cartilages near the costochondral junctions and dissecting the sternum off the mediastinum.

The superficial muscles of the neck are separated to expose the thyroid and the cervical component of the thymus. The thyroid is examined *in situ*. Examine the pleural cavities for fluid excess or other abnormality. The right lung is mobilised out of the thoracic cavity and a piece of right lower lobe removed for microbiologial study and/or imprints for viral study (use a sterile pack for this purpose). Check for the presence of petechiae over the visceral pleura. The capsule of the thymus is also examined for the presence of petechiae. The pericardium is opened using a 'no-touch' technique and a sample of blood is aspirated from the right atrium for culture; our practice is to take a large volume for other investigations if necessary. If sufficient blood is not obtained from the heart, further samples may be obtained from the inferior vena cava (facilitated by elevating the lower part of the body) or from the superior sagittal sinus (by inserting the needle

through the anterior fontanelle and directing it posteriorly). Samples for toxicology should be taken whenever possible from the femoral vein.

An assistant exposes the upper anterior neck by retracting the skin in the direction of the chin. A deep incision is made around the inner aspect of the mandible allowing the tongue to be freed. The neck structures are now dissected *en bloc* from the cervical spine; this dissection is continued into the thorax, allowing the thoracic contents to be separated from the dorsal spine. The heart is examined *in situ* to check for malformations and abnormal venous return. The pericardial sac, oesophagus and aorta are now divided just above the diaphragm and the entire thoracic and cervical structures are removed intact for dissection. The pathologist must be willing to adapt the technique when circumstances require it. A full in-situ neck and facial bone dissection may be required. In cases of suspected smothering the lips may have to be resected and blocked.

The peritoneal cavity is assessed and the abdominal organs are examined to check for situs. Also check the patency of the processes vaginalis using a probe. Ensure that both hypogastric arterial remnants are present. Remove three short segments of intestine from different levels and place in fixative. Varying lengths of segments are taken in order to aid identification of the original level at the time of blocking. This method also allows rapid fixation and so enhances the preservation of the mucosa for microscopy. Distal small bowel content is removed for microbiological examination. If stool is required for viral study, the content of a loop of small bowel can be 'milked' by gentle pressure. The remainder of the small and large bowel is removed. The liver, pancreas, stomach and spleen are removed intact by cutting around the attachment of the diaphragm and through the coeliac axis.

Check the bladder for any urine. Remove a sample if possible for refrigeration and potential biochemical investigation: 0.1 mL of urine is the minimal requirement and, even if the bladder seems empty, swabbing the bladder mucosa with a cotton ball provides a sufficient volume for analysis for a β-oxidation fatty acid defect. The kidneys and bladder are dissected off the posterior abdominal wall.

Further dissection of pelvic content is facilitated by cutting through the symphysis pubis. The symphysis is separated by abducting the legs. The penile shaft may be removed in continuity with the rest of the urinary tract if urethral pathology is suspected. This is achieved by separating the shaft from the inner aspect of the skin. This procedure is facilitated using a pair of long, thin scissors inserted from above the pubis. The penile shaft is retracted into the pelvic cavity and the inverted skin is cut away from the shaft near the glands. The skin is restored to a normal anatomical position. Further pelvic dissection allows the entire urinary tract to be removed *en bloc*. The testes may be removed by cutting into the scrotal sac from above.

A sample of muscle is taken, usually the middle of psoas on the left. For microscopy of bone marrow, remove a segment of right 5th rib close to the costochondral junction. Waldeyer's ring is inspected *in situ* and the entire ring is freed by stabilizing the uvula with forceps and cutting through the anterior part of the soft palate; then around and above the tonsils and adenoids.

The next stage is to remove the brain and spinal cord. The body is placed prone and a 'question mark'-shaped incision is made in the scalp over the back of the head, commencing in the midline at the base of neck and extending this upwards towards the left ear and across the scalp towards the other ear (Fig. 13.6). Keep the incision as posteriorly as possible to ensure good cosmetic reconstruction. Reflect the scalp off the posterior cranium to expose the arch of atlas. The arch is cut through on either side to expose the underlying dura (Fig. 13.7). The dura is incised with a sterile scalpel blade and a sample of CSF is aspirated into a sterile pipette for microbiological investigation. The approach allows the cerebellar tonsils to be viewed directly from below, assessing for the presence and degree of caudal dislocation. Cerebellar coning will be obvious when present. Cut through the upper cervical cord at the level of the foramen magnum. The upper cervical cord may be exposed and freed posteriorly to facilitate its subsequent removal.

The scalp over the upper and anterior part of the cranium is freed and folded forward. The parotid gland is exposed and separated. While the sutures

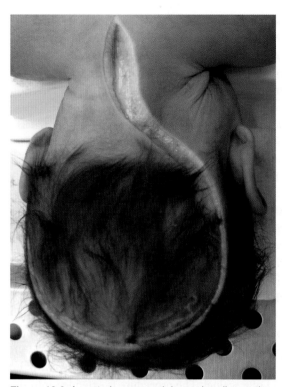

Figure 13.6 A posterior approach is used to dissect the brain in all cases of sudden unexpected death in infancy. A 'question mark'-shaped incision is made in the scalp commencing in the midline at the base of neck and extending this upwards towards the left ear and across the scalp towards the other ear.

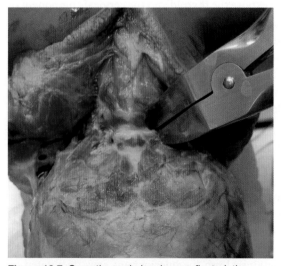

Figure 13.7 Once the scalp has been reflected, the atlas is cleared from the adjacent muscle and the lateral processes are cut with a pair of angled scissors.

are still unfused, the skull bones can be separated with a sharp scalpel blade. Great care should be exercised not to allow the blade to slip during the procedure. An electric plaster saw should be used to remove the skull bones in the older infant with fused sutures. The brain is finally freed by cutting through the falx, cranial nerves, vessels and finally a cut is made along the lateral attachments of the leaves of the tentorium cerebelli.

The pituitary is dissected out by making incisions into the cartilaginous part of the sella turcica. A permanent scalpel allows the pituitary to be elevated and freed intact within its bony/cartilaginous casing. Expose the middle ears; after cutting the dura over the petrous roof of the temporal bones with a scalpel remove the bone over the middle ears with a pair of heavy-duty bone cutters. A swab is taken if pus is found. The tympanic membranes are inspected for perforation. Repeat the procedure for the other side.

To remove the spinal cord, separate the psoas muscles at their proximal attachment, then cut through the costo-vertebral junctions on either side. The spinal canal itself is entered by cutting through the intervertebral disc just below L5. A pair of angled scissors allows the vertebral bodies to be removed from the vertebral arches to expose the spinal cord. The spinal cord is then separated and freed by cutting through the nerve roots with a pair of scissors or scalpel. All organs are now ready for dissection.

Acknowledgements

The author and editors are grateful to Dr. S Variend who contributed the chapter on this topic in previous editions of the book.

References

Byard RW (2004). *Sudden Death in Infancy, Childhood and Adolescence*. Cambridge: Cambridge University Press.

Cohen M, Whitby E (2007). The use of magnetic resonance in the hospital and coronial paediatric post mortem. *Forensic Sci Med Pathol* 3:289–96.

Cohen M, Paley P, Griffiths P, Whitby E (2008). Less invasive autopsy: benefits and limitations of the use of magnetic resonance imaging in the perinatal post-mortem. *Pediatr Dev Pathol* 11:1–9.

Dean AF, Whitby EH (2007). Contribution of antenatal magnetic resonance imaging to diagnostic neuropathology. *Curr Diagn Pathol* 13:171–9.

Ernst LM, Sondheimer N, Deardorff MA, Bennett MJ, Pawel BR (2006). The value of the metabolic autopsy in the pediatric hospital setting. *J Pediatr* 148:779–83.

Fleming PJ, Blair PS, Sidebotham DP, Hayler T (2004). Investigating sudden unexpected deaths in infancy and childhood and caring for bereaved families: an integrated multi-agency approach. *Br Med J* 328:331–4.

Gardosi J, Kady S, McGeown, Francis A, Tonks A (2005). Classification of stillbirth by relevant condition at death (ReCoDe): population-based cohort study. *Br Med J* 331:1113–17.

Kennedy H (2004). *Sudden Unexpected Death in Infancy*. London: RCPath and RCPCH. Available at www.rcpath.org/resources/pdf/SUDI%20report%20for%20web.pdf (accessed October 2009).

Kraus FT, Redline RW, Gersell DJ, Nelson DM, Dicke JM (2004). Placental pathology. In: King DW (ed.) *Atlas of Nontumor Pathology*, Fascicle 3. Washington, DC: American Registry of Pathology and Armed Forces Institute of Pathology.

Laing IA (2004). Clinical aspects of neonatal death and autopsy. *Semin Neonatol* 9:247–54.

Langston C, Kaplan C, Macpherson T *et al.* [Task Force of the College of American Pathologists] (1997). Practice guideline for examination of the placenta. *Arch Pathol Lab Med* 121:449–76.

Larroche JC, Encha-Razavi F, Wigglesworth JS (1998). The central nervous system. In: Wigglesworth JS, Singer DB (eds) *Textbook of Fetal and Perinatal Pathology*. Oxford: Blackwell Science.

Machin GA (2007). Hydrops: cystic hygroma, hydrothorax, pericardial effusions and fetal ascites. In: Gilbert-Barness E (ed.) *Potter's Pathology of the Fetus, Infant and Child*, Vol. 1, pp. 333–54. London: Mosby Elsevier.

RCPath (2002). *Guidelines for Autopsy Investigation of Fetal and Perinatal Death*. Available at www.rcpath.org/resources/pdf/appendix_6.pdf (accessed October 2009).

RCPath (2006). *Guidelines on Autopsy Practice: Best Practice Scenarios*. Available at www.rcpath.org/index.asp?PageID=687 (accessed October 2009).

Roberts ID, Cohen M, Benbow W (2007). The non-invasive or minimally invasive autopsy. In: Underwood J, Pignatelli M (eds) *Recent Advances in Histopathology*, Vol. 22, pp. 181–98. London: Royal Society of Medicine Press.

Schumacher R, Seaver LH, Spranger J (2004). *Fetal Radiology: A Diagnostic Atlas*. London: Springer.

Siebert JR (2007). Perinatal, fetal, and embryonic autopsy. In: Gilbert–Barness E (ed.) *Potter's Pathology of the Fetus, Infant and Child*, Vol. 1, pp. 695–739. London: Mosby Elsevier.

Singer DB, Macpherson TA (1998). Fetal death and the macerated stillborn fetus. In: Wigglesworth JS, Singer DB (eds) *Textbook of Fetal and Perinatal Pathology*. Oxford: Blackwell Science.

Wigglesworth JS (1998). Causes and classification of fetal and perinatal death. In: Wigglesworth JS, Singer DB (eds) *Textbook of Fetal and Perinatal Pathology*. Oxford: Blackwell Science.

Chapter 14

THE MATERNAL AUTOPSY

G Harry Millward-Sadler

Introduction

A maternal death is frequently unexpected and converts an anticipated happy event into a tragedy. The natural father and family are often asking 'why?', and in many cases a carefully conducted autopsy will contribute evidence of the diagnosis and its causes and so help answer their question.

Most pathologists will have no experience of the maternal death autopsy, and it is preferable wherever possible that the autopsies should be performed by one of a small number of pathologists in a particular region so that a quality autopsy and report can be produced. Nonetheless the requirements necessary to achieve a good standard are simple: the autopsy should assess and address the clinical issues, and it should be conducted to the latest standards recommended by the Royal College of Pathologists (RCPath, 2004). For some specific deaths there are particular additional points that have been summarised in the College guidelines (RCPath, 2005). These in turn, for maternal deaths, have drawn on the recommendations in the pathology chapters of the Confidential Enquiries 1997–99, 2000–02 and other publications (Millward-Sadler, 2001, 2003, 2004). See also Box 14.1.

Definitions, classification and incidence

A *pregnancy-related death* is one that occurs during pregnancy or within 6 weeks of parturition. It may be *direct*, *indirect* or *coincidental*. A *maternal death* is death when pregnant or within 6 weeks of termination or delivery from any cause related to – or exacerbated by – the pregnancy or its management. It does not include coincidental deaths.

- A *direct maternal death* is one that is a consequence of pregnancy in a previously healthy woman.
- An *indirect maternal death* is one where pre-existing disease is adversely influenced by the pregnancy.
- A *coincidental maternal death* is one where the cause of death is not known to be related to, or influenced by, the pregnancy. 'Coincidental' is the preferred term of the aforementioned Confidential Enquiry reports, but the international definition uses the slightly incongruous term 'Fortuitous'.
- A *late maternal death* occurs more than 6 weeks, but less than 12 months, after the end of pregnancy and is subcategorised as direct or indirect.

The classification is sometimes illogical. For instance, a peri-partum cardiomyopathy is classified as an indirect maternal death along with the other cardiac deaths. Also, the most recent Confidential Enquiries have identified a subset of 'coincidental' and sometimes late suicidal deaths that appear to be related to the post-partum pregnant state. The latest Enquiry Report for 2003–05 has therefore proposed

Box 14.1 Recommendations for pathologists

Clinical history
- Carefully review the medical records and correlate the autopsy findings with their findings.
- For community deaths in particular, it may be necessary to identify the previous obstetric history.

The autopsy
- Carefully note the external features, including height and weight. For perioperative deaths, note the position of the endotracheal tube. For sepsis, note skin discolouration and/or evidence of haemolysis in skin veins and venules. For road traffic deaths, look for evidence that the seat belt was correctly worn – above and below, not across, the bump.
- Perform the internal examination to the standards recommended by the Royal College of Pathologists. Seek expert advice/support particularly for cardiac or central nervous system deaths. If in doubt, the local Regional Pathology Assessor may be able to help.

Notes on specific direct causes
- *Thromboembolus:* history including family history; source of emboli; distribution and evidence of previous episodes.
- *Hypertensive disease:* review of fluid balance, especially in adult respiratory distress syndrome (ARDS); histological confirmation of pre-eclamptic toxaemia (PET) – lungs, liver, kidneys, brain, and placental bed-site.
- *Haemorrhage:* careful examination of the genital

tract for placental abruption or accreta, genital tract trauma; exclude causes of disseminated intravascular coagulation (DIC) – pre-eclamptic toxaemia (PET) and amniotic fluid embolus (AFE) in particular; review of surgically resected tissues.
- *Sepsis:* source and nature of infection; search for precipitating causes in the genital tract.
- *Early pregnancy:* site and size of ectopic with estimate of blood loss; abortions, medical and otherwise; evidence of perforation of uterus or bowel; retention of products; culture of tissues.
- *Amniotic fluid embolism:* examination of genital tract for trauma or tears; histological confirmation using immunocytochemistry, if in doubt (cytokeratin antibodies LP34 or AE1/2 recommended).
- *Anaesthetic death:* position of endotracheal tube; search for aspiration of gastric contents; toxicology to exclude inadvertent drug administration.

Notes on indirect deaths
- *Cardiac and central nervous system deaths:* seek specialist advice and support wherever possible; exclude pre-eclamptic toxaemia, particularly for cerebral haemorrhage; examine the dural sinuses.
- *Cardiac deaths:* detailed histology of heart and lungs and for aneurysms, arteries; consider tissue sampling for genetic analysis.
- *Epileptiform deaths:* toxicological analysis of anti-epilepsy medicines; exclude eclampsia as cause of fits.

that the next revision of the International Classification of Diseases (ICD-11) should reclassify peripartum cardiomyopathy, ovarian hyperstimulation syndrome (OHSS) and suicide from puerperal psychoses as *direct* maternal deaths.

Maternal deaths are very rare in the UK and the vast majority are a consequence of natural causes. The mortality rate for 2003–05 calculated for direct and indirect maternal deaths was 14 per 100 000 maternities; in absolute terms this was approximately 100 deaths a year throughout the UK. When coincidental and late maternal deaths are included there have been only approximately 200 deaths per year. When adjustments are made for the different ways in which various countries collect and analyse their maternal death data, the UK rate is among the lowest in the world.

Despite this, the Confidential Enquiries have consistently identified factors in the diagnosis and clinical management of the cases under scrutiny that significantly contributed to – or failed to prevent – death. In the most recent report (Lewis, 2007) there was a major deficiency in 55 per cent of all 'direct' and 28 per cent of all 'indirect' deaths for that triennium. Such analysis of course is dependent on an accurate diagnosis of the cause of death and its precipitating pathological processes, and knowledge of the key events. By providing a careful review of the clinical sequence of events, establishing an accurate diagnosis and determining the underlying pathological processes, the autopsy and its report can make a significant contribution to improving the quality of care for other mothers.

Quality of the autopsy

Analysis of the direct and indirect maternal deaths in the Confidential Enquiries from 1997 to 2005 inclusive has identified that 93 of the 535 autopsy reports were of poor quality or worse (Millward-Sadler, 2001, 2004, 2007). The major and most common failings were a lack of correlation of the clinical history with the pathological findings, and just determining the immediate cause of death. There were several instances where the cause of death was simply given as cerebral haemorrhage without establishing whether this was due to hypertension, pre-eclamptic toxaemia (PET), vascular malformation or cerebral vein thrombosis. But there were also cases demonstrating the value of pursuing the cause of the cerebral haemorrhage.

Clinical History

A first-time mother had a family history of two closest female relatives dying from brain haemorrhage in the latter half of their pregnancies. A thrombophilia screen of unknown detail was negative. She was admitted in the third trimester with vomiting, weakness and loss of balance. CT imaging showed brain swelling due to cerebral haemorrhage and, despite intensive treatment, she died. At autopsy the cerebral haemorrhage was secondary to cerebral vein thrombosis deep in the thalamostriate vein. The superficial venous sinuses were patent, confirming the imaging findings, and there was no histological evidence of PET. Review of the autopsy material from one of the relatives confirmed that cerebral venous thrombosis and not cerebral haemorrhage was also the cause of her death.

(Millward-Sadler, 2007)

As a result of this autopsy it was recommended that other family members be referred for detailed haematological investigation. The autopsy also raises the question of how many pregnancy-related cerebral haemorrhages are actually secondary to thrombosis in deep cerebral veins.

Retention of histological material

The legalities of the autopsy examination are addressed in Chapter 4. There are few direct or indirect maternal deaths that can be adequately assessed without histological examination of some tissues. The example of cerebral haemorrhage has already been cited, but even with massive pulmonary thromboembolus there can be some justification. The clinical history, for example, may refer to medical consultations for breathlessness in the days or weeks prior to death but diagnosed as anxiety or normal for pregnancy. Histological examination of the lungs could provide evidence of thromboembolic episodes preceding death. There are also sporadic cases in the Confidential Enquiry reports of undiagnosed choriocarcinoma presenting as massive pulmonary thromboembolus, and another where a lobectomy was performed for a pulmonary abscess attributed to bronchiectasis that was actually secondary to pulmonary artery embolus of undiagnosed choriocarcinoma. The patient did not know she was 'pregnant' but her beta-HCG levels were very high and she had missed one period 3 months earlier: treatment was successful and so a maternal death was avoided (Millward-Sadler, 2003).

For non-medicolegal autopsies, consent is either explicitly given or denied. If the latter, then this should be clearly stated in the report. For medicolegal cases conducted under the auspices of HM Coroner or the Procurator Fiscal, there is only authority to take tissue samples to establish the cause of death and there is no authority to retain those samples without further written signed consent once the coroner or fiscal has completed the investigation. However, there is variation in how establishing the cause of death is interpreted by different coroners: some permit histology to define parts 1b and 1c of the death certificate; a few (in the author's experience) do not. In reviewing the UK maternal death autopsy reports over the last 10 years, the absence of histology seems to be strongly associated with a poor description of the macroscopic findings, suggesting that the absence of permission is a convenient smokescreen for a hurried and poorly performed autopsy. It would be helpful if coroners were empowered to authorise a detailed autopsy for those deaths whose investigation also falls within the remit of a national audit or survey such as the maternal death or the national perioperative death enquiries. Even if this were to transpire, permission to retain histological material as part of the autopsy record should be obtained whenever possible.

Causes of maternal death

The maternal death rate in the last triennial report for 2003–05 (Lewis, 2007) was 6.24 per 100 000 maternities for all 'direct' causes and 7.71 per 100 000 for all 'indirect' ones. The rates have changed very little for 'direct' causes over the past 20 years but have increased for the 'indirect' causes – largely because of improved case ascertainment methods employed for the four reports from 1994 onwards. In comparison, internationally the World Health Organization estimated that globally there were 400 deaths per 100 000 maternities in the year 2000 (Lewis, 2004).

The major causes for the years 2000–05 are given in Table 14.1. However, in each of these categories there are also underlying themes increasing the likelihood of death. The more significant are increasing maternal age, social deprivation, obesity and immigrant status.

Table 14.1 Numbers of UK maternal deaths by specific cause

Cause of death	2000–02	2003–05
Thromboembolism/thrombosis	30	41
Pre-eclampsia	14	18
Haemorrhage	17	17
Amniotic fluid embolism	17	5
Early pregnancy	14	15
Genital tract sepsis	18	11
Anaesthesia	6	6
Other 'direct'	4	0
Cardiac	48	44
Psychiatric	19	16
Other 'indirect'	86	90

Derived from Lewis (2007) with permission.

Maternal age

In the period 2003–05, 19 per cent of all maternities occurred in women over the age of 34, compared with just fewer than 8 per cent for the period 1985–87. Although the death rate per 100 000 maternities has fallen in this age cohort since 1985–87, almost halving in the over-40 age group, the current rate is still more than double that found in the under-25 cohort.

Social deprivation

Socio-economic data are difficult to identify in the information provided to the Confidential Enquiry, but the death rate for women whose partners were known to be unemployed or where there was no identifiable partner was over seven times higher than for women with partners in known employment. Similarly, if death rates for deprived areas (derived from postcode analysis) are compared with those for least deprived, there is a five-fold increase.

Obesity

The body mass index (BMI) is defined as weight in kilograms divided by height in metres squared: 25–29.9 is overweight, 30–34.9 is obese, 35–39.9 is very obese, and 40+ as morbidly obese. Although not all BMIs were recorded, over a quarter of all patients who died as a result of 'direct' and 'indirect' causes where the information was available had a BMI greater than 30. The risks appeared to relate to cardiac disease, pre-eclampsia, thromboembolism, gestational diabetes, post-partum haemorrhage, and infections – particularly following caesarian section.

Ethnicity

The ethnicity data are incomplete; but, compared with white women, most ethnic groups seem to have a higher relative risk of maternal death. This is particularly so for black Africans, who have a five-fold increase in their relative risk rates. The reasons are multiple, but poor access to antenatal clinics, previous ill-health (particularly in recent immigrants) and language problems are some of the related factors.

Clinical History

A non-English speaking woman had recurrent vaginal bleeding from a known cervical fibroid. Heavy bleeding occurred in the 2nd trimester but her husband failed to take her to hospital as promised. She required emergency admission next day at which time she was unconscious. Her wrists were noted to be grazed and bandaged and a partially organised retroplacental clot was found at hysterotomy. She had severe disseminated intravascular coagulation (DIC) and a CT scan showed cerebral contusions associated with non-displaced fractures of her temporal and frontal bones. In the autopsy report there was no mention of her wrist injuries, no reference to her DIC or its possible causes and no examination of the skull. The report did identify a swollen brain with no signs of raised intracranial pressure.

(Millward-Sadler, 2007)

The clinical history

The importance of knowing and understanding the clinical history has been repeatedly stressed in all recent pathology chapters of the triennial reports (Millward-Sadler, 2001, 2004, 2007), and other publications (Rushton and Dawson, 1982; Millward-Sadler, 2003), and should be obvious from the above vignette. The clinical history can also influence the conduct of the autopsy. It is unlikely that air embolism as a cause of death is routinely excluded by opening the heart and pulmonary trunk under water, but this should be performed if there is sudden death during intercourse in the immediate post-partum period.

For thromboembolism there may be a family history of clotting disorders or even a previous history of deep vein thrombosis. An increased risk of idiopathic thromboembolus has also been described in patients taking antipsychotic drugs (Zornberg and Jick, 2000). There is sometimes a history of episodic shortness of breath that had been dismissed as normal for pregnancy or even anxiety and precedes the catastrophic final collapse by days or weeks. Unfortunately only rarely is there any attempt by the pathologist to identify whether these symptoms were the consequence of less catastrophic emboli

that with correct diagnosis may have resulted in successful therapy. In pre-eclampsia, adult respiratory distress syndrome was the cause of death in over a third of cases in 1985–90 but has caused only one death in 2000–05. This striking reduction has been attributed to more careful fluid management of these patients, so careful review of the fluid balance charts may be necessary. It is unlikely that the pathologist will be completely abreast of modern obstetric and anaesthetic practice, such as the interpretation of fetal monitoring records or detailed knowledge of the drugs and fluids used in the management of pregnancy, labour and anaesthesia, so close liaison with the relevant clinicians is essential. In the writer's experience, the involved clinical staff are only too willing to help and will even attend the autopsy.

Even with a death in the community conducted under the authority of the coroner or fiscal, there could be additional information that is relevant but not included in the coroner's officer's report. For example, in a death from epilepsy there could have been reluctance to take anti-epileptic drugs during pregnancy because of the risk of fetal malformations. For suicides there is now evidence that pregnancy is protective but not in the 12-month post-natal period. There is obviously a cohort of suicidal deaths – particularly in those with preceding history of depression or bipolar disorder – where the death is 'coincidental', but another cohort with a large proportion of 'late' deaths has recently been identified and separated out from these 'coincidental' deaths. In this cohort the most likely mode is not by drug overdosage but by more violent methods – hanging, jumping off tall buildings or under trains, throat cutting etc. The history of an earlier pregnancy may not have been considered relevant by the reporting officer and should be sought.

External examination

The external examination can direct the autopsy in a specific direction or provide supportive evidence for the internal findings. There are the obvious points about the presence and siting of vascular access, endotracheal tubing and surgical incisions following medical interventions. The calf diameters may differ in cases of pulmonary thromboembolism, and petechial haemorrhages may indicate DIC. Given the higher risk of maternal death in obese patients, the BMI should be recorded. If accurate body mass cannot be given, then some surrogate marker such as depth of subcutaneous fat at the umbilicus should be provided. Much of this should be part of standard autopsy procedure, but perhaps the condition most specific to a maternal death is the rapid onset of blotchy skin erythema with 'marbling' due to prominent skin veins in streptococcal septicaemias.

Autopsy of 'direct' deaths

As is probably apparent from the multiple possible causes of a maternal death, the autopsy should be detailed and thorough. If performed to the autopsy standards recommended by the Royal College of Pathologists, these criteria should be met. Most pathologists, however, will not be accustomed to the anatomical changes of pregnancy. It is not possible to be comprehensive in this chapter but salient points are covered below.

Thromboembolism

The cause of death is usually obvious, but there should also be a careful search for the source. The pelvic veins are much more frequently involved than in non-pregnancy deaths from emboli. There should also be a careful search for evidence of preceding thromboembolic episodes. Not all emboli arise from venous thrombus. Excluding amniotic fluid emboli, there have been recorded deaths and near misses from metastasising choriocarcinoma masquerading as emboli (Millward-Sadler, 2003) and it was histological examination of the thrombus that revealed the diagnosis.

Pre-eclampsia

Pre-eclampsia may be a very easy and obvious diagnosis to make, especially if there is the classic clinical history of hypertension with proteinuria arising in the last trimester, but it can sometimes be very difficult. Occasionally, it may arise in the immediate post-natal period, or it may have a fulminant onset. In the latter instance it may arise and cause death from a haemorrhagic stroke or even a ruptured liver with no clinically documented features of the disorder when last reviewed by clinical staff. It can also be superimposed on pre-existing hypertensive disease, and differentiating the relative roles of the two processes is difficult. Careful histology looking for DIC, multifocal periportal hepatic necrosis, the 'tramlining' of the basement membrane in glomeruli, and the acute atherosis of intrauterine arteries with failure of the normal endovascular trophoblast to extend beyond the decidual–myometrial junction within the placental bed-site should be helpful (Millward-Sadler, 2003).

Haemorrhage

There are many potential causes of death from obstetric haemorrhage. First-trimester ruptured ectopic pregnancy is usually categorised with the early pregnancy deaths, but sometimes the ectopic is not tubal but ovarian or even peritoneal, and survival into the second trimester or even later can occur before the fatal haemorrhage arises. Otherwise most cases of haemorrhage arise in four categories: placental abruption, placenta praevia, post-partum haemorrhage, and genital tract trauma. For these deaths it is important to record the location of the placenta and its appearance and to search carefully for signs of genital tract trauma. In placenta praevia it is helpful to know whether this was percreta or accreta and the nature of the underlying tissues especially in relation to previous surgical scars. The most difficult category is the post-partum haemorrhage as there are multiple predisposing causes that can masquerade as uterine atony. These include amniotic fluid embolus, sepsis, PET, DIC, and prolonged shock from any cause. Frequently an emergency hysterectomy has been performed in an attempt to control bleeding. If so, then the appearance and histology of the surgical specimen should be incorporated into the autopsy report and correlated with the other findings.

Amniotic fluid embolus

Amniotic fluid embolus (AFE) can be a very simple diagnosis to establish at autopsy, but there are situations where this is difficult and sometimes impossible to confirm or exclude. In addition, the quality of the autopsy has in some cases been poor so that apparently clear-cut clinical cases of AFE have not been confirmed but simply ascribed to, for example, post-partum haemorrhage. For these reasons, deaths from AFE based on firm clinical criteria have been accepted by the Confidential Enquiries since 1991. In the last report (Vlies, 2007) there were 19 reported deaths from AFE. There was full clinical and pathological correlation in 11 of these, and amniotic fluid embolism was identified in two deaths with atypical clinical presentations. Of the remainder there was no autopsy in one case, the autopsy report and investigations were inadequate in three cases, and there was prolonged survival in intensive care prior to death in two cases.

The findings at autopsy are not macroscopically specific but include wet and relatively airless lungs often with pleural petechial haemorrhages indicative of DIC. There may be tears in the placental bed, which should be carefully searched for, but failure to find the entry site is common and does not preclude the diagnosis. The finding is usually confirmed by demonstrating the presence of fetal squames or mucin or lanugo hairs in the maternal pulmonary circulation. The squames can readily be seen in routine histological stains when in large numbers, but immunocytochemistry for cytokeratins may be necessary. The high-molecular-weight cytokeratin antibodies LP34, AE1/2 or 34BE12 are most useful as few other lung epithelial cells positively react. There are some factors to be considered when interpreting the findings, especially if the numbers of demonstrable squames are small.

- Fetal squames have been found in pulmonary artery catheter blood from mothers not suffering clinically from AFE. This suggests that there is a threshold trigger of unknown quantity or quality to be achieved before onset of symptoms.
- The survival time of fetal squames in the maternal circulation is unknown. This may be critical when considering death after a prolonged stay in intensive care.
- Squames may be only a surrogate morphological marker for AFE, with other amniotic fluid components having a more significant pathogenetic role. For instance, an immunological reaction to the fetal sialyl Tn antigen has been demonstrated in cases of presumed AFE (Benson et al., 2001).

Genital tract sepsis

More than 150 years after the classical studies of Semmelweiss into puerperal sepsis, there were eight deaths from group A beta-haemolytic streptococcal infections in the last triennial report (Harper, 2007), of which three were classical puerperal sepsis and the portal of entry could not be defined in the others. The onset is often insidious but rapidly becomes fulminating, and the mother may become moribund within hours of the first non-specific symptoms. The diagnosis can often be suspected on the mortuary table prior to the start of the autopsy when there is haemolytic staining outlining the peripheral skin veins; sometimes a skin erythema is detectable. The source of infection – genital or non-genital – should be sought and the organism confirmed by taking samples for microbiological culture.

Other deaths were caused by Escherichia coli and by Pseudomonas species, but these often followed or complicated a procedure – miscarriage with retention of products, cervical sutures for recurrent or threatened miscarriage, prolonged intrauterine death etc. Following the Abortion Act 1967, infection arising from criminal abortion is now very rare, but occasional deaths do still occur. Therefore, not only should the putative organism be isolated and identified, but a careful inspection of the genital tract is necessary to identify or exclude the reason for the infection.

Anaesthetic death

Often the death is metabolic or therapeutic so that there is little to find at autopsy. Nonetheless, carefully documented and detailed negative findings can be of great value in evaluating the events prior to death; and, conversely, a poorly documented autopsy leaves possible alternatives open. In particular, the autopsy should establish the siting of the endotracheal tube, exclude as far as possible inhalation of gastric contents, and through toxicological analysis ensure that there has been no inadvertent error of drug administration.

It is of interest that in the last triennial report (Cooper and McClure, 2007) there were six deaths directly attributed to anaesthetic management. Of these six, four subjects were obese and two of these four were morbidly obese.

Other 'direct' deaths

There are many other rare or even esoteric direct causes of maternal death and even esoteric presentations of rare causes. Choriocarcinoma and hydatidiform mole are potential causes, but because of the effective treatment regimes now available these only rarely cause death. Four deaths from choriocarcinoma occurred in the 3 years to 2005, but they illustrate the value of vigilance, histology and timely communication.

> Following an intrauterine death at term, an externally normal infant was found to have haemoperitoneum with a massive liver tumour. This was a choriocarcinoma. There was no trace of the tumour in the placenta. There was delay in conveying the findings to the mother's clinicians; the mother was subsequently admitted with a brain haemorrhage from metastatic choriocarcinoma and, despite treatment, she died.
>
> (Millward–Sadler 2007)

The other condition is fatty liver of pregnancy, which can be difficult to differentiate from the HELLP syndrome (haemolytic anaemia + elevated liver enzymes + low platelet count) that complicates PET. The incidence of fulminating cases of fatty liver in pregnancy has been estimated at 1 per 6000–7000 births, but there may be many milder cases. A high proportion of mothers are heterozygous for deficiency of a long-chain hydroxyacyl-coA dehydrogenase mitochondrial enzyme and seem to develop the condition when bearing children also carrying the trait (Ibdah *et al.*, 1999). The disease usually affects primigravid women

in the third trimester but can occasional arise in the second trimester. At autopsy the liver is pale from the fatty change, which is also evident on histology, but on careful examination there is also considerable loss of hepatocytes that is masked by the steatosis. There have been only four recorded deaths from this condition in the 6 years up to 2005.

Autopsy of 'indirect' deaths

Cardiac deaths

Cardiac deaths are one of the most common causes of maternal death and are second in numbers reviewed in the recent triennial reports only to psychiatric deaths. As the physiological effects of pregnancy place an increased workload on the heart this is not surprising. The recorded cardiac deaths for 2003–05 are given in Table 14.2. Some may have occurred anyway, but it is worth noting that in one study 40 per cent of family members had cardiac abnormalities when the index case died unexpectedly of cardiac disease (Tan *et al.*, 2005).

Table 14.2 Causes of maternal death from cardiac disease in the UK, 2003–05

Type and cause of death	Indirect	Late
Acquired		
Aortic dissection	9	0
Myocardial infarction	12	4
Ischaemic heart disease	4	0
Sudden adult death syndrome (SADS)	3	9
Peri-partum cardiomyopathy	0	12
Cardiomyopathy	1	4
Myocarditis or myocardial fibrosis	5	0
Mitral stenosis or valvular disease	3	0
Infectious endocarditis	2	2
R or L ventricular hypertrophy or hypertensive heart failure	2	1
Congenital		
Pulmonary hypertension	3	0
Congenital heart disease	3	2
Totals	47	34

Reproduced with permission from Nelson–Piercy (2007).

As might be expected the range of cardiac diseases largely reflects the spectrum of cardiac disease to be found in a relatively young population which includes a recent immigrant population. Consequently death from rheumatic fever-induced mitral stenosis was recorded in the last report. The exception is the increasing rate of death from myocardial infarction/ischaemic heart disease, which has increased from 0.24 per 100 000 maternities in the period 1997–09 to 0.57 per 100 000 in 2003–05. This is partly a reflection of the increasing maternal age as the mean age of maternal death in this category was 35 years. Apart from this there are two categories that are more specific to pregnancy: aneurysms (particularly of small muscular arteries) and peripartum cardiomyopathy.

Aneurysms

Dissecting aortic aneurysm was the cause of death in 19 pregnancies in the last two triennial reports and has been one of the major causes of 'indirect' cardiac death. Frequently there was a history of crushing chest pain, and this may have been investigated as suspected pulmonary thromboembolus some days before the final collapse but without a definitive diagnosis. The autopsies often provided evidence that dissection had started some days earlier as there was organising blood clot within the wall of the aorta on histology. Not all patients have Marfanoid features, though the presence or absence of these should be noted in the external description of the body. In the last triennial report (Nelson-Piercy, 2007) there were eight aortic dissections: only two had Marfanoid features, although a third death had a family history of aortic dissection. Two other women were morbidly obese. Approximately three-quarters of patients fulfilling the Ghent diagnostic criteria for Marfan's syndrome have a mutation in the fibrillin-1 gene, and this can be identified in post-mortem tissues if appropriate samples are submitted for analysis (Halliday et al., 2002).

Dissecting aneurysms of small muscular arteries are almost as common as aortic dissection in pregnancy. The coronary, splenic and adrenal arteries are most frequently affected, but in the last report there were also deaths from a ruptured basilar and from a ruptured external iliac artery. The latter was unusual in that the surgeon commented on the extreme friability of the tissues when operating and this was separately noted by the pathologist during the autopsy. Histology was normal but no tissue was submitted for genetic analysis so that the possibility of Ehlers–Danlos syndrome remains unproven. As might be expected, dissection of a coronary artery presents clinically as myocardial infarction whereas those of intra-abdominal arteries present as severe but obscure blood loss with abdominal pain. If laparotomy has been undertaken, the relevant source of bleeding may have been resected (e.g. splenectomy for splenic artery rupture). It is important to retrieve and review such specimens to complete the clinicopathological correlation.

Histologically the accumulation of acid mucopolysaccharides in the media of muscular and elastic arteries (cystic medial necrosis) is common in pregnancy, but histology should be undertaken to determine its severity and extent. Consideration should also be given to submitting tissue samples for genetic analysis as the autopsy may provide the best opportunity for the diagnosis of an inherited abnormality and hence for counselling of relatives.

Cardiomyopathy

All causes of cardiomyopathy may precipitate death during pregnancy, particularly in the last trimester and during labour. Their diagnosis and investigation is dealt with elsewhere (Sheppard, 2003) and does not differ significantly because of the pregnancy. One of the anomalies of the international definition of maternal deaths is that it is restricted to death in pregnancy or within 42 days, yet a peripartum cardiomyopathy can by definition arise within 5 months of delivery. Even if it arises within the internationally defined period there is often survival beyond the time limits. Of the 13 recorded deaths from peri-partum cardiomyopathy in the 3-year period up to 2005, only one died within 6 weeks of delivery. Three had presented antenatally and a further six within the 6-week post-partum period. It follows that comparison of rates with international data are not valid. Because of these data, the Confidential Enquiry has recommended that the next revision of the ICD–11 should include all deaths from peri-partum cardiomyopathy at any point after childbirth, and that they should be categorised as 'direct deaths'.

At autopsy the features are macroscopically indistinguishable from those of a dilated cardiomyopathy, and it may be, in some instances, that pregnancy has exposed an underlying but asymptomatic cardiomyopathy. Nonetheless, a dilated cardiomyopathy diagnosed in association with pregnancy must be regarded as a peri-partum cardiomyopathy until proved otherwise. There is a family history in approximately one-third of patients with non-puerperal dilated cardiomyopathy and several genetic mutations have been found. Similar information is not available for peri-partum cardiomyopathy and is needed. Histology of the heart is required to exclude a myocarditis masquerading as a peri-partum cardiomyopathy, although interpretation is difficult as an inflammatory infiltrate has been found in three-quarters of cases diagnosed as peri-partum cardiomyopathy in one series (Midei et al., 1990). Wherever possible, therefore, an expert cardiac pathological opinion should be sought.

Central nervous system

The major causes are subarachnoid and intracerebral haemorrhages, cerebral thrombosis and epilepsy. Very few cases come to autopsy (six of the 17 intracerebral haemorrhage deaths in the last triennial report), as the haemorrhage is frequently diagnosed on CT scan. The immediate cause of death is thus known but possible antecedent causes are not necessarily excluded. Even in the absence of pre-existing hypertension, PET, primary erythrocytosis or vascular malformation – all of which have been documented in the triennial reports – there is still an unexplained increased risk of post-partum haemorrhage or stroke (Witlin et al., 2000; Geocadin et al., 2002). As the vignette cited on page 205 demonstrates, it is also possible that thrombosis in a deep cerebral vein such as the thalamostriate can be diagnosed clinically, and on imaging, as a haemorrhage.

It might also be expected that, with the increased risk of arterial dissections in pregnancy, there would be an enhanced risk of rupturing a berry aneurysm, particularly during labour. However, of the 28 deaths attributed to subarachnoid haemorrhage in the 6-year period 2000–05, only one had its onset during labour. Again, few of these deaths came to autopsy so that the proportion of ruptured Berry aneurysms is unknown and antecedent or contributory morphological causes unascertained.

The typical pregnancy-related cerebral thrombosis involves the large dural sinuses and is classified as a direct maternal death. It is normally grouped with thromboembolic diseases as the antecedent causes are identical. There were eight deaths between 2003 and 2005, and again obesity is a factor. Weight is not recorded in all these deaths, but at least two patients were morbidly obese and another two obese. Four of the eight deaths arose in the first trimester. As the pregnant state may be unknown or even concealed, it should therefore be carefully excluded in any woman with cerebral sinus thrombosis who is of child-bearing age.

As so few cases come to autopsy, it is recommended that the whole brain should be fixed and a neuropathological opinion should be sought whenever possible.

Epileptiform deaths

The influence of pregnancy on epilepsy is unpredictable. Some women enjoy a considerable reduction in the frequency and/or severity of fits, others have more and some are unchanged. However, what is known is that some patients reduce or omit their anti-epileptic medication for fear of fetal abnormalities. Seven of the 10 deaths from 2003 to 2005 were classified as SUDEP (sudden unexpected death in epilepsy). Toxicological analysis of anti-epileptic drug levels was not undertaken in four of the deaths. It is not known whether pregnancy is a risk factor for SUDEP. One reason is that there is only limited information on drug compliance, so toxicology should be performed in all these epileptiform deaths.

Psychiatric deaths

Suicide deaths were previously considered to be relatively rare and coincidental to the pregnancy. With the recent ability of the Office for National Statistics (ONS) to link mothers' deaths within 1 year to recorded births, this view has been revised.

Psychiatric disorders during pregnancy and post-partum are common with both new episodes and recurrence of pre-existing illnesses. It is estimated that four women per 1000 will be admitted to a psychiatric unit each year, and half of these will have puerperal psychosis (Oates, 1996). While suicide *during* pregnancy is uncommon, and overall may not be substantially increased in the post-partum period compared with matched controls, there is a subgroup with severe illness for which the relative risk is substantially increased. The last triennial report (Oates, 2007) divided suicide deaths into either 'coincidental' or 'indirect': 33 suicide deaths were then categorised as 'indirect' and of these 21 were 'late indirect'.

A significant characteristic of these deaths is the high proportion committing suicide by violent methods – hanging, jumping from a height or under a train etc. Given that these are community deaths and that for many the history of preceding pregnancy will not be given, it is important that the pathologist seeks the information when presented with a violent suicidal death in a young female.

Other 'indirect' deaths

These are innumerable and cannot be comprehensively covered in this chapter. Every organ system is affected: the UK deaths from non-cardiac and non-suicide deaths from 1999 to 2005 are tabulated in the triennial report for 2002–05 (de Swiet, 2007) (Table 14.3).

Including disorders of the central nervous system, there are approximately 30 deaths each year from these causes. The causes range from common to esoteric. For instance, air embolism following sexual intercourse in the immediate post-partum period has occasionally been identified. Of note is that sometimes a relatively mild stable asthmatic may die with severe mucus plugging of airways; this may be consequent on stopping steroid therapy to minimise

Table 14.3 Causes of other indirect deaths in the UK, 2000–05

Cause	2000–02	2003–05
Central nervous system	40	37
Subarachnoid haemorrhage	17	11
Intracerebral haemorrhage	3	11
Cerebral thrombosis	4	2
Epilepsy	13	11
Other	3	2
Infectious diseases	14	16
Human immunodeficiency virus	4	5
Bacterial infection	6	5
Other	4	6
Respiratory system	10	5
Asthma	5	4
Other	5	1
Endocrine, metabolic, immunity	7	5
Diabetes mellitus	3	1
Other	4	4
Gastrointestinal system	7	9
Intestinal obstruction	2	0
Pancreatitis	1	2
Other	4	7
Haematological	2	4
Circulatory disorders	3	6
Renal system diseases	3	1
Cause unknown	4	4
Totals	90	87

Adapted from de Swiet (2007).

the risk of fetal abnormalities. In other instances pregnancy may expose a latent condition. In complete lipoprotein lipase deficiency – a rare autosomal recessive disorder associated with elevated triglyceride levels from birth – pregnancy can induce a severe pancreatitis.

Autopsy of 'coincidental' deaths

Internationally these deaths are categorised as *fortuitous*, but the Central UK Assessors prefer to use the term *coincidental*. It is difficult to estimate the numbers, but there are still important medical and public health issues that arise from these deaths to which the pathologist can make a significant contribution. Previously, suicide deaths were considered to be coincidental, but as has been demonstrated some are now considered indirect. In road traffic deaths there is concern that seat belts may not be correctly positioned, and there is evidence that domestic violence has been ignored by healthcare professionals; some of these cases have been *sub judice* because of murder. Although non-gestational cancer is regarded as fortuitous, some – breast and cervix in particular – may have been accelerated by the increased hormonal stimuli of pregnancy. Finally, particularly with these rare cases of cancer, investigations may have been inappropriately deferred or even not performed because of concerns about the risks to the fetus.

Conclusion

The value of the autopsy was recognised in the 1973–75 Confidential Enquiry report when the Chief Medical Officer wrote:

Postmortem examinations have been carried out in 344 of the 390 deaths investigated, but the authors and regional assessors have all expressed concern that the reports available were not as helpful as they might have been.

(Millward-Sadler, 2004).

Despite the improvement in the range of clinical investigative techniques and expertise available today, a well-conducted and thorough maternal death autopsy still adds considerable value to the audit and evaluation of these tragic deaths.

References

Benson MD, Kobayashi H, Silver RK *et al.* (2001). Immunological studies in presumed amniotic fluid embolism. *Obstet Gynecol* **97**:510–14.

Cooper G, McClure J (2007). Anaesthesia. In: Lewis G (ed.) *Saving Mothers' Lives: Reviewing Maternal Deaths to Make Motherhood Safer, 2003–5*. London: Confidential Enquiry into Maternal and Child Health (CEMACH).

de Swiet M (2007). Other indirect deaths. In: Lewis G (ed.) *Saving Mothers' Lives: Reviewing Maternal Deaths to Make Motherhood Safer, 2003–5*. London: Confidential Enquiry into Maternal and Child Health (CEMACH).

Geocadin RG, Razumovsky AY, Wityk RJ *et al.* (2002). Intracerebral haemorrhage and postpartum vasculopathy. *J Neurol Sci* **205**:29–34.

Halliday DJ, Hutchison S, Lonie L *et al.* (2002). Twelve novel FBN1 mutations in Marfan syndrome and Marfan-related phenotypes test the feasibility of FBN1 mutation testing in clinical practice. *J Med Genet* **39**:589–93.

Harper A (2007). Genital tract sepsis. In: Lewis G (ed.) *Saving Mothers' Lives: Reviewing Maternal Deaths to Make Motherhood Safer, 2003–5*. London: Confidential Enquiry into Maternal and Child Health (CEMACH).

Ibdah JA, Bennett MJ, Rinaldo P *et al.* (1999). A fetal fatty-acid oxidation disorder as a cause of liver disease in pregnant women. *N Engl J Med* **340**:1723–31.

Lewis G (2004). The international context. In: Lewis G (ed.) *Why Mothers Die, 2000–2*. London: Confidential Enquiry into Maternal and Child Health (CEMACH).

Lewis G (2007). Which mothers died, and why. In: Lewis G (ed.) *Saving Mothers' Lives: Reviewing Maternal Deaths to Make Motherhood Safer, 2003–5*. London: Confidential Enquiry into Maternal and Child Health (CEMACH).

Midei MG, DeMent SH, Feldman AM *et al.* (1990). Peri-partum myocarditis and cardiomyopathy. *Circulation* **81**:1154–6.

Millward-Sadler GH (2001). Pathology. In: Lewis G, Drife J (eds) *Why Mothers Die, 1997–9*. London: Royal College of Obstetrics and Gynaecology.

Millward-Sadler GH (2003). Pathology of maternal deaths. In: Kirkham N, Shepherd NA (eds) *Progress in Pathology*, Vol. 6. London: Greenwich Medical Media.

Millward-Sadler GH (2004). Pathology. In: Lewis G (ed.) *Why Mothers Die, 2000–2*. London: Confidential Enquiry into Maternal and Child Health (CEMACH).

Millward-Sadler GH (2007). Pathology. In: Lewis G (ed.) *Saving Mothers' Lives: Reviewing Maternal Deaths to Make Motherhood Safer, 2003–5*. London: Confidential Enquiry into Maternal and Child Health (CEMACH).

Nelson-Piercy C (2007). Cardiac disease. In: Lewis G (ed.) *Saving Mothers' Lives: Reviewing Maternal Deaths to Make Motherhood Safer, 2003–5*. London: Confidential Enquiry into Maternal and Child Health (CEMACH).

Oates M (1996). Psychiatric services for women following childbirth. *Int Rev Psychiatry* **8**:87–8.

Oates M (2007). Deaths from psychiatric causes. In: Lewis G (ed.) *Saving Mothers' Lives: Reviewing Maternal Deaths to Make Motherhood Safer, 2003–5*. London: Confidential Enquiry into Maternal and Child Health (CEMACH).

Royal College of Pathologists (2004). *Guidelines for Post-mortem Reports*. London: RCPath (www.rcpath.org/publications).

Royal College of Pathologists (2005). *Guidelines on Autopsy Practice: Best Practice Scenarios*. London: RCPath (www.rcpath.org/publications).

Rushton DI, Dawson IMP (1982). The maternal autopsy. *J Clin Pathol* **35**:909–21.

Sheppard MN (2003). Sudden adult death and the heart. In: Kirkham N, Shepherd NA (eds) *Progress in Pathology*, Vol. 6. London: Greenwich Medical Media.

Tan HL, Hofman N, van Langen IM *et al.* (2005). Sudden unexplained death: heritability and diagnostic yield of cardiological and genetic examination in surviving relatives. *Circulation* **112**:207–13.

Vlies R (2007). Amniotic fluid embolus. In: Lewis G (ed.) *Saving Mothers' Lives: Reviewing Maternal Deaths to Make Motherhood Safer, 2003–5*. London: Confidential Enquiry into Maternal and Child Health (CEMACH).

Witlin AG, Mattar F, Sibai BM (2000). Postpartum stroke: a twenty-year experience. *Am J Obstet Gynecol* **183**:83–8.

Zornberg GL, Jick H (2000). Antipsychotic drug use and risk of first-time idiopathic venous thromboembolism: a case–control study. *Lancet* **356**:1219–23.

Chapter 15

TOXICOLOGICAL AND BIOCHEMICAL ANALYSES

Alexander RW Forrest

Introduction

The living human body can be considered as a complex assembly of dynamic chemical systems. Maintaining the integrity of these systems requires the constant expenditure of energy. Once death takes place, the supply of energy from metabolic processes is dramatically reduced. The integrity of the different compartments within the body breaks down at differing rates. Complex molecules tend to break down to their simpler subunits and to move down concentration gradients that were maintained in life by the expenditure of metabolic energy. Obviously, these processes do not all occur at once. Thus, for a variable length of time after death the analysis of appropriate samples may yield useful information about the metabolic state of the deceased in the period immediately before death.

Once death has taken place many drugs are released from their binding sites in tissue as pH decreases on death and as the processes of autolysis proceed. Where drugs have been bound to tissues in life, as they are released into the blood so there can be dramatic increases in the concentration of these drugs locally. For example, the release of tricyclic antidepressants from lung tissue leads to very high concentrations of these drugs in left ventricular blood samples. These phenomena can make the interpretation of drug levels after death less than straightfor-

ward. Equally, conventional clinical chemistry analyses can hardly be expected to yield 'normal' results on post-mortem samples. Haemolysis and the movement of ions and small molecules down concentration gradients are the least of the problems. Nonetheless, much useful information can be obtained by the careful analysis of samples obtained at post-mortem and the thoughtful interpretation of the results obtained. An individualised and informed approach to sample collection, analysis and the interpretation of results is needed in every case.

Sample collection

General principles

Interpretation of toxicological analyses is difficult enough under the best of circumstances, so as little variation as possible in the results should be introduced by the manner in which the samples are collected. Apart from the submission of samples appropriately labelled with the name of the deceased, the nature of the sample, the site from which the sample was collected and the date and time of sampling, the most important items that should be sent to the laboratory are properly completed request forms. Give the name and age of the deceased and an estimate of the time at which death took place and time at which the post-mortem examination was carried out, together with an account of the final illness or circumstances of the death and a list of all the drugs to which the deceased had access. This includes drugs prescribed to or used by the other family members.

The laboratory and the analyses it uses must be fit for purpose. Accreditation to ISO 17025 standard or equivalent should be required. While immuno-chemical methods may be suitable for screening analyses, confirmations and quantitative analyses should be carried out by hybrid methods such as gas chromatography/mass spectroscopy (GC/MS) or liquid chromatography with diode array detection (LC/DAD). A useful guide for the commissioner, be they coroner or pathologist, of post-mortem toxicology services is to ask the laboratory how well they comply with the Society of Forensic Toxicologists and American Academy of Forensic Sciences Guidelines for forensic toxicology laboratories.

In any case where toxicological investigations are indicated, the pathologist should always bear in mind the possibility that a criminal investigation leading to a prosecution may arise out of the death. Issues of the duty of care of those around the deceased and injection of the lethal drug dose may not arise until some time after the initial post-mortem. If the autopsy has not been performed and documented to a high standard and appropriate samples have not been collected, documented and sent to a competent laboratory, the pathologist may be subject to criticism.

It is important that, when biochemical analyses – normally carried out on serum or plasma – are indicated, the blood sample obtained at autopsy is centrifuged and the serum separated as soon as possible. In practice, by the time the autopsy is performed, it will not be possible to obtain haemolysis-free blood; for analyses such as urea and creatinine, vitreous humour or cerebrospinal fluid may be useful substitutes. If there is any possibility that the red cells may be usefully analysed – for example in the investigation of haemoglobinopathies or for the determination of glycated haemoglobin – then either they should not be disposed of after centrifugation or a separate sample should be taken.

Ideally, the decision to take samples for toxicological and/or biochemical analyses should be made before the post-mortem knife touches the skin of the body. A few minutes spent studying the case notes or the Police Sudden Death Report before the autopsy is started is time well spent.

Blood

Blood samples are best obtained from the femoral vein by puncture after exposing the vein by dissection and clamping or ligating it proximal to the collection site. Use a 30 or 50 mL syringe with a wide-bore needle. Aim to collect at least 20 mL of blood. However, for many analyses a smaller volume may be adequate. Most of the sample is placed in a fresh (not reused) glass screw-top universal container filled up to the brim and sealed with aluminium foil-lined caps. A sample should also be placed in tubes containing fluoride oxalate preservative to reach a final concentration of 1% by weight. Conventional grey-top Vacutainers° do not contain sufficient fluoride. The septum-sealed vials used by police surgeons for collecting blood samples for blood alcohol assays do contain sufficient fluoride. However, it is undesirable to fill a septum-sealed vial with potentially infected blood using a needle and syringe. There is still a pressing need for a commercially available screw-top vial containing an anti-coagulant and fluoride preservative to a concentration of at least 1%, made of amber glass to inhibit photo-degradation. The collection of a sample that is adequately preserved with fluoride is particularly important if samples are being collected for alcohol, nitrazepam or cocaine analyses. If there is any possibility that a second post-mortem may be required, take duplicate samples. Carefully label the sample with the name of the deceased, the time of collection and the sample site. Specify from which side of the body the sample has been taken – for example, 'left femoral vein blood'.

Ideally, blood should not be 'milked' from a limb. This process can engender significant changes in the concentrations of critical analytes in the expressed blood. If this is the only way to obtain a peripheral blood sample, this should be documented and the laboratory informed. Cardiac blood is not generally a suitable sample for quantitative toxicological analyses. While there is no problem in carrying out the analyses, interpreting the results can be extremely difficult. If cardiac blood is submitted to the laboratory then it should be identified as such. Blood collected from the paracolic gutter after evisceration is a less than suitable sample for most investigations; it may well be contaminated with gut contents, urine or other body fluids. Unless no blood from any other site is available – as, for example, might be the case in a second post-mortem or the autopsy of a decomposed body – its use should be avoided. When it is possible to obtain only a small amount of peripheral blood, paracolic gutter blood or heart blood can then be used for the identification of the drugs present, followed by quantitative measurement of the drugs of interest in the peripheral sample.

Because of the very great variations in the concentrations of drugs that can be found in blood samples taken from different sites in the same body, it is important that sample collection be standardised so that the results obtained can be meaningfully interpreted by comparison with the databases that are being developed incorporating the results of the analysis samples of blood collected by a uniform technique at post-mortem. Many of the compendiums that purport to provide therapeutic, toxic and lethal concentrations of drugs in post-mortem blood samples are misleading because they incorporate therapeutic ranges for drugs measured in plasma in samples collected in life and post-mortem samples collected from unspecified body sites. Useful collections of data are emerging, particularly from northern Europe, derived from the measurement of drug blood concentrations by validated methods, with the blood samples being collected following standard protocols. The results are categorised taking into account the history and pathological findings. Such collections are invaluable, and useful databases can be developed locally where pathologists and toxicologists work together.

One point that has emerged from the increasing degree of uncertainty in the way in which post-mortem toxicological results can be interpreted is that in very many cases it is not possible to estimate the amount of the drug that may have been taken from the application of the pharmacokinetic calculations that might have been applicable in life.

Simply multiplying the volume of distribution of the drug as determined in life by the post-mortem blood concentration can produce a result for the amount of drug in the body that is wrong by as much as a factor of 100. Although the volume of distribution in life is not a parameter that has any validity after death, drugs that have a high volume of distribution in life tend to show both post-mortem redistribution, with increases in concentration in blood generally after death, as well as site dependency, where the extent of the increase in post-mortem drug concentration depends on the site from which the sample is collected. In short, in most cases, you cannot answer without equivocation the question so often asked by the coroner, 'How many tablets did she take?', on the basis of the drug concentration in even a properly collected post-mortem blood sample.

Urine

Urine is best obtained by direct puncture of the exposed bladder with a needle and syringe, once the abdomen has been opened. It may also be obtained by the insertion of a urethral catheter before the start of the autopsy. A common practice is to obtain urine by aspiration without a needle, once the dome of the bladder has been opened in the course of the post-mortem. If this technique is used then great care should be taken to ensure that blood or other fluids do not contaminate the urine sample. When the patient has been catheterised shortly before death then high concentrations of lignocaine (lidocaine), derived from the catheter lubricant gel, may be present in the urine.

Vitreous humour

Vitreous humour is obtained by needle puncture of the eyeball. A 19 gauge needle attached to a 5 mL syringe is suitable. The eyelid should be firmly retracted (Fig. 15.1) and the sclera punctured at a latitude of about 30–40 degrees, taking the pupil as the North Pole. The needle should be directed towards the centre of the eyeball (Fig. 15.2). Gentle aspiration will usually yield 2–3 mL of vitreous humour. Once the sample has been obtained, the syringe should be detached from the needle, leaving

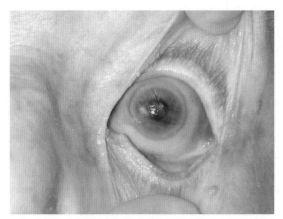

Figure 15.1 To aspirate the vitreous humour, the eyelids are first retracted to expose the globe.

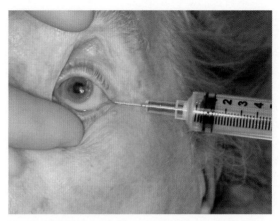

Figure 15.2 Vitreous humour is aspirated from the eye using a needle inserted at a latitude of about 30 degrees and aiming for the centre of the globe

the needle in place and a volume of water or physiological saline equal to the amount of vitreous removed should be slowly injected to achieve cosmetic restoration. A portion of the sample aspirated should be preserved with fluoride, with an aliquot also being collected into a tube without added preservative or anticoagulant. Before collecting a vitreous humour sample always consider the possible need for histology of the eyeball.

Cerebrospinal fluid

Cerebrospinal fluid (CSF) is difficult to collect at post-mortem by conventional lumbar puncture. However, it is relatively easy to obtain by cisternal puncture. With the the body lying prone and the neck flexed, palpate the atlanto-occipital membrane in the midline (Fig. 15.3) and, using a needle and syringe, gently introduce a disposable spinal needle through the skin at that point, directing the needle towards the bridge of the nose (Fig. 15.4). In thin individuals a 21 gauge (green) hypodermic needle is adequate. As the atlanto-occipital membrane is punctured at a depth of approximately 2 cm, loss of resistance will be felt, following which CSF can be aspirated (Fig. 15.5). As an alternative, CSF can be aspirated anteriorly, after evisceration, by introducing a needle into the spinal theca via the spinal foramina between the first and second lumbar vertebrae.

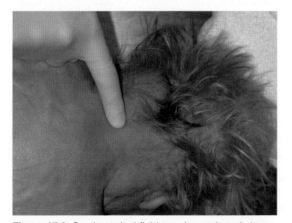

Figure 15.3 Cerebrospinal fluid may be aspirated via a cisternal puncture. With the body prone, the atlanto-occipital membrane is first palpated in the midline.

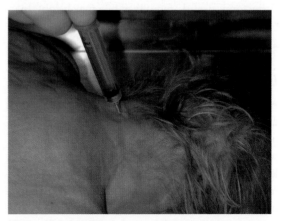

Figure 15.4 A needle is inserted through the foramen magnum, aiming towards the bridge of the nose.

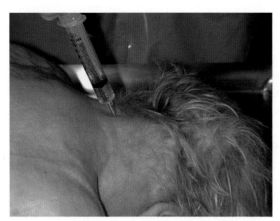

Figure 15.5 The needle is advanced approximately 2 cm and cerebrospinal fluid can be aspirated.

Bile

The toxicological analysis of bile can be extremely useful in some cases of overdose. For example, high concentrations of paracetamol (acetaminophen) and its metabolites may occasionally be found in bile aspirated from the gallbladder after the paracetamol concentration in the blood has fallen to relatively inconsequential levels. It may also be useful in cases of opiate overdose. Bile is easily aspirated from the gallbladder before abdominal evisceration. Alternatively the gallbladder can be dissected free from the liver and its contents gently squeezed into a clean specimen container, taking care not to contaminate the sample with blood. If the patient has had a cholecystectomy, useful amounts of bile may be obtained by aspiration of the common bile duct with a needle and syringe.

Gut contents

A stomach content sample is best obtained by either clamping or applying ligatures to the lower end of the oesophagus and the pylorus before the stomach is dissected free. The stomach should then be held over a large container while it is opened and the contents removed. If an attempt is made to make a small opening in the stomach and then to pour the contents into a honey pot or similar sized container there is a significant risk of loss of stomach contents by spillage. If cyanide poisoning is suspected, the stomach should be opened in a fume cupboard. Ideally the total stomach contents should be submitted to the laboratory, but if that is not done then a note of the total volume of the stomach contents should accompany the sample that is submitted. If only a small sample of the total stomach contents is sent then there is a risk of a sampling error. Be aware that the toxicologist is likely to homogenise the stomach contents in a blender before analysis. This will render it unsuitable for microscopic analyses to determine the nature of the last meal, if that is subsequently requested. If a representative sample of the stomach contents is analysed, then the total amount of drug in the stomach contents can be estimated from the volume of the stomach contents multiplied by the drug concentration. The analyst will usually report the drug concentration as the free base (e.g. as morphine free base), while the pharmaceutical preparation may be measured out as the salt (e.g morphine sulphate). This needs to be taken into account when making such calculations.

In some circumstances, samples of the lower bowel contents can usefully be submitted for analysis. This can be particularly useful where a modified-release formulation of, for example, morphine has been taken.

Faeces may occasionally be useful, principally if porphyria is suspected.

Tissues

Tissue samples can be useful. In decaying, exhumed or embalmed bodies submit about 50 g of quadriceps muscle. In cases where the cause of death is not immediately apparent at autopsy, it is appropriate to take tissue samples in case the necessity for toxicological analysis becomes apparent at a later stage in the investigation. Normally samples of about 50 g are adequate for most toxicological analyses. In most cases only liver and muscle are needed in addition to the usual fluid samples. The samples should be placed in new glass containers and should under no circumstances be placed in fixative. Care should be taken to avoid contaminating the liver sample with bile. Try to take the sample from the right lobe of the liver away from the stomach and gallbladder. If an inborn error of metabolism is suspected as the cause of death, then the advice of the local reference laboratory as to which samples may be required should be sought as soon as possible, and in any case before the autopsy is commenced. They may well ask for skin to be used as a source of hopefully viable fibroblasts for cell culture.

In cases where it appears likely that the death has been associated with volatile substance abuse, then often blood and urine will suffice. If lung is taken, seal about 50 g into a nylon (not polythene) bag. Polythene bags allow the volatiles in the sample to escape. Nylon bags such as are used for the collection of arson scene debris are suitable. The nylon bags sold in supermarkets for roasting poultry can also be used. When investigating a death that may be associated with volatile substance abuse, do not collect blood samples into containers that may contain volatiles themselves (e.g. gel tubes as used for clinical chemistry). It is worthwhile sending an empty container to the laboratory with the specimen, as this will help in the investigation of the possibility of contamination if aberrant results are obtained.

When the possible circumstances of the death might relate to long-term drug use, if multiple surreptitious administration is suspected, or if it would be useful to confirm or exclude the possibility that the deceased was a naive opioid user, then hair or possibly fingernail samples may be useful. Analysis of hair for markers of alcohol misuse can be helpful in some cases. Hair samples should be obtained by plucking rather than trimming with scissors. Take a clump of hair about the thickness of a pencil and bind it together with an elastic band. If the samples are obtained by trimming with scissors then the proximal end of the hair sample must be clearly identified. The hair should be taken before the body is opened. Body fluids containing drugs can soak into the hair and confound the interpretation of the analyses despite decontamination of the hair sample in the laboratory.

Sample analysis and interpretation

The ability of cells to maintain the concentration gradient of electrolytes between the intra- and extracellular environment is energy dependent. Once death has taken place these concentration gradients can no longer be maintained and there is a rapid flux of the smaller molecules down the appropriate concentration gradients. The most immediate effect is that there is a very rapid rise in the serum potassium in the first minutes after death. Within an hour or so the post-mortem serum level, even in the absence of haemolysis, is at least six times that of the ante-mortem level. This occurs even in the absence of post-mortem haemolysis. Serum potassium determinations in post-mortem samples are thus of no probative value.

Serum sodium concentrations tend to decrease after death but rather more slowly than the serum potassium concentration increase. The decrease is variable from subject to subject and it is unlikely that much useful information can be obtained from analysis of post-mortem serum sodium concentrations, although very high or very low values found in samples collected within a few hours may be helpful. The special case of apparent drowning is discussed below.

Glucose concentrations in post-mortem blood samples are of little value unless they are high. Glycolysis continues after death and the blood glucose concentration falls extremely rapidly. The finding of high blood glucose concentrations in a post-mortem sample by a specific analytical method, such as the hexokinase method, is a useful reflection of post-mortem hyperglycaemia. Blood collected from the inferior vena cava may have a high blood glucose concentration due to autolysis of the liver with the associated breakdown of glycogen. The measurement of glycated haemoglobin is useful when death due to diabetes mellitus undiagnosed in life is suspected. In the course of the laboratory examination of post-mortem samples, often the first clue that otherwise unrecognised diabetes mellitus is present is a large acetone peak found when carrying out an assay for ethanol by head-space gas chromatography. β-Hydroxybutyrate can be measured in post-mortem blood by conventional clinical laboratory methods after perchloric acid precipitation and can also usefully indicate ante-mortem ketosis. High concentrations of β-hydroxybutyrate are also found in alcoholic ketoacidosis. In such cases the acetone concentration is not grossly elevated as it is in diabetic ketoacidosis. The blood glucose concentration is not elevated. Alcoholic ketosis cannot be diagnosed by using dipsticks or tablets for detecting ketones. These screening tests depend on the presence of aceto-acetate in urine. In alcoholic ketosis the principal ketone body present is β-hydroxybutyrate. (See Chapter 20 for a further consideration of ketoacidosis.)

Urea, creatinine and urate in post-mortem serum samples appear to be stable for at least 48 hours, although there may be a slight rise in the urea and urate.

The major problem in the analysis of post-mortem blood samples for biochemical parameters is that haemolysis appears to take place relatively quickly *in vitro* unless the sample is promptly centrifuged. By the time the sample has reached the clinical chemistry laboratory, it may be so haemolysed as to be unsuitable for analysis. Vitreous humour is often of more use for biochemical analyses than blood. Although vitreous humour tends to be more viscous than normal human serum, most multichannel analysers will analyse samples of vitreous humour satisfactorily. Such samples should be centrifuged before being presented to the analyser and care must be taken that the analyser probe does not short sample the specimen. Microfiltration of vitreous humour using a Centrifree cone increases the reproducibility of results.

For many analytes, vitreous humour can be regarded as an ultrafiltrate of blood. Because vitreous humour is low in protein, which is positively charged at physiological pH, the chloride concentration is about 10–20 per cent higher than that found in serum. It has been suggested that the potassium concentration in vitreous humour is a useful marker of the time of death, said to increase by roughly 1.7 mmol/L per hour in the first 12 hours after death. However, the rate of increase in practice is variable. Such data should be interpreted with extreme caution. The urea and creatinine concentrations in vitreous humour are a reasonable guide to the concentrations at the time of death. It should be noted that vitreous humour has much lower non-Jaffé chromagen concentrations than does serum. Thus the vitreous creatinine corre-

lates more closely with serum creatinine as measured by specific methods such as high-performance liquid chromatography (HPLC) or creatininase-based assays than by conventional picrate-based chemistries. Typically the 'normal' post-mortem vitreous creatinine concentration, measured by a picrate-based chemistry, is about 40 μmol/L.

The glucose concentration in vitreous humour tends to fall very quickly after death and a low vitreous humour glucose concentration in no way indicates ante-mortem hypoglycaemia. A normal or high vitreous glucose concentration usually can be taken to imply that hyperglycaemia was present at the time of death. An exception is where the body is rapidly chilled after death. Under such circumstances the vitreous humour glucose concentration may be of the same order as that found during life. High vitreous glucose concentration may be a resuscitation artefact, particularly if glucose, adrenaline or glucagon have been used during resuscitation. This is seen particularly in deaths in childhood, where paediatricians often take a vitreous humour sample immediately after attempts at recuscitation cease.

Bicarbonate concentrations are usually low in post-mortem vitreous humour. This may in part be artefact, rather than a reflection of peri- and post-mortem acidosis, since it is usual for the laboratory to be sent 1–2 mL of vitreous humour sloshing around in a 20 mL universal container. This gives a significant dead space for carbon dioxide to be lost from the sample, with a consequent reduction in the total bicarbonate concentration. To avoid this dead-space effect, small sample tubes should be used for vitreous humour. Lactic acid can be measured in vitreous humour, with high concentrations being associated with a prolonged agonal period. It is rarely useful. The present author has not found it helpful to attempt to back-calculate the glucose concentration in life from the lactate concentration in vitreous by assuming that the vitreous glucose is converted to lactate after death.

Large molecules, particularly protein-bound ones such as cholesterol and most hormones, cannot be usefully measured in vitreous humour.

Vitreous humour can be useful for certain toxicological analyses. For example, concentrations of

6-monoacetylmorphine tend to be higher in vitreous humour than in post-mortem blood – where it is quite ephemeral – after death following heroin use. Measurement of the vitreous 6-monoacetylmorphine can thus be useful where it is desirable to confirm that death was associated with heroin use rather than morphine overdose.

A variety of other analytes can be measured in serum separated soon after collection of a blood sample within 48 hours of death. Cholesterol and lipoprotein electrophoresis can be particularly useful in demonstrating whether or not there are increases in the pre-beta or chylomicra fractions over and above those normally found in non-fasting samples. However, when a young person dies from coronary artery disease it is probably more important for serum lipids to be measured in members of the immediate family than attempting to characterise any disorder of lipoprotein metabolism that the deceased may have suffered from by post-mortem serum analyses.

Analysis of post-mortem serum and urine samples for cortisol can be worthwhile; very high concentrations may suggest a stressful agonal process and low concentrations may be associated with adrenal hypofunction. A steroid profile on the urine can be useful in a few, selected, cases. Urinary catecholamines can be difficult to interpret. Catecholamines are best measured in urine. If it is thought that measurement of catecholamines might be appropriate then an aliquot of the urine collected at post-mortem examination should be acidified to a pH of less than 2.0 by the dropwise addition of concentrated hydrochloric acid. High concentrations of catecholamines in urine have been reported in patients dying of hypothermia.

The determination of enzyme activity in post-mortem samples is not usually useful. Autolysis rapidly releases intracellular enzymes and other macromolecular markers of tissue damage into blood and makes the interpretation of enzyme activity in post-mortem specimens extremely difficult in practice. An exception to the general rule that post-mortem enzymology is unhelpful is that the vitreous humour and urine amylase activity may be elevated in deaths associated with hypothermia.

Putrefied or embalmed bodies
The putrefied body

Biochemical analyses have little to offer in the examination of the putrefied body. It is essential that the toxicologist be informed that the body was putrefied if samples are collected for toxicological analysis. Where no blood can be obtained, tissue samples, including a sample of skeletal muscle, may be of great value for toxicological analyses. Even bone marrow may be useful. When a body is partially skeletonised the process may be less advanced in the feet if they have been protected by substantial footwear. It may be possible to recover sufficient soft tissue from the foot for worthwhile toxicological analyses under such circumstances.

When assays for ethanol are carried out on blood removed from a putrefied body then questions inevitably arise as to the validity of the results obtained. The question obviously arises as to whether or not the ethanol present in the sample has arisen as a result of ante-mortem alcohol ingestion or post-mortem fermentation. Where the sample does not have an adequate amount of fluoride preservative added, then alcohol production can take place in the collection tube. If the alcohol analysis has been carried out by head-space gas–liquid chromatography and there are a number of peaks present on the tracing other than ethanol and the internal standard, the implication is that other volatiles are present. It is likely, when the sample has come from a putrefied body, that they are present as a result of post-mortem fermentation. Culture of the sample may reveal the presence of alcohol-producing organisms. A simpler technique may be simply to leave the sample at room temperature and to repeat the analysis a week later. If alcohol-producing organisms are present in the sample then the alcohol concentration will normally have increased in the interim. If blood samples are taken from multiple sites in the body and there is a discrepancy in their blood alcohol concentrations, then the implication that post-mortem fermentation is confusing the issue is an obvious one. The possibility that alcohol present in the stomach at the time of death might have diffused to the sampling sites should also be considered. Thus, if blood alcohol analyses are to be carried out on samples collected from a putrefied body, blood samples should be obtained from several sites, those sites being carefully specified on the sample tubes, the analyses should be carried out by head-space gas–liquid chromatography, and aliquots of the samples should be submitted for microbiological examination. Samples of vitreous humour can also assist in this situation. Markers of recent alcohol ingestion other than ethanol, such as ethyl glucuronide, ethyl sulphate and phosphatidylethanol, are becoming increasingly available and can be invaluable in helping to address the possibility of alcohol use when a body is showing signs of putrefaction.

In general, gas chromatographic rather than enzymatic methods should be used for ethanol assay on post-mortem samples, whether putrefied or not. If an enzymatic method without protein precipitation is used, falsely elevated concentrations of alcohol may be reported. Also, confidence that the result obtained is actually a reflection of the presence of ethanol in the sample is greatly enhanced by the use of a gas chromatographic assay.

The embalmed body

In the UK, most pathologists will be asked, from time to time, to examine an embalmed body that has been returned from abroad. The vitreous humour may, but not always, remain uncontaminated and is often available in reasonable amounts for toxicological analyses. Also submit a sample of the embalming fluid to the laboratory if at all possible.

Deaths in specific circumstances

Death due to drowning

When significant inhalation of water takes place in freshwater drowning there is often consequent dilution of the blood in the left ventricle with a reduction in the sodium and chloride concentration. Measurement of sodium and potassium in haemolysed blood samples such as commonly recovered when left and right blood samples are obtained from bodies recovered from water is not a trivial procedure for contemporary clinical laboratories. Sodium and potassium are not routinely measured by flame emission spectrophotometry but by ion-selective electrodes. Ion-selective electrodes, dedicated to analyses of normal clinical samples, are in general likely to produce less than reliable results when used to analyse post-mortem haemolysed samples. An additional problem is the possibility that products of putrefaction such as ammonia may confound the analyses. A simple alternative may be to estimate the water content of blood samples submitted for analysis by accurately dispensing about 1 g of blood into a weighing boat, weighing it on an analytical balance, drying the sample to constant weight in a laboratory oven at 70°C and noting the change in weight. High concentrations of magnesium may be found in the left ventricular blood from those who drown in seawater.

If examination for diatoms is thought to be useful, then the spleen, rather than the bone marrow, may be the best sample to take. Samples of the water in which the body was found should also be taken, care being taken to ensure that the water samples cannot contaminate the spleen or marrow samples during specimen collection or transport. Finally analysis of fluid for sodium and magnesium recovered from the supraorbital sinuses may be useful in the investigation of saltwater drowning.

Suspected non-therapeutic injection of insulin

When non-therapeutic intramuscular or subcutaneous injection of insulin is suspected, the prudent prosector will immediately seek the help of an experienced forensic pathologist. As well as peripheral blood samples, samples of tissue from the putative injection site(s) and a control should be collected. Unless blood and vitreous humour samples are collected within a very few minutes of death, the measurement of glucose in post-mortem samples is of no value in such cases – except, of course, that if it is not done, at some stage the question will be asked why it has not been done. If the death has taken place in hospital every effort should be made to retrieve ante-mortem samples, particularly if they have been appropriately preserved.

In addition to post-mortem peripheral blood samples, consideration should be given to collecting blood samples from the inferior vena cava. Concentrations of insulin and C-peptide will usually be higher in blood samples collected from the inferior vena cava than in peripheral blood samples. The samples should be centrifuged as soon as possible after collection, avoiding haemolysis if at all possible. Enzymes present in red cells are capable of reducing the disulphide bonds that maintain the secondary structure of insulin necessary for its immunological recognition by the antibodies used in immunoassays. Measurement of insulin by non-immunochemical techniques such as time-of-flight mass spectroscopy is a useful tool in forensic cases. It can even identify the type of insulin injected. Demonstration of the injection of insulin depends on the finding of high tissue concentrations together with a low tissue concentration of C-peptide at the putative injection site and low tissue concentrations of both insulin and C-peptide in the control tissue. It is supported by the finding of a high concentration of insulin in association with a low concentration of C-peptide in peripheral blood. Usually, death from insulin overdose will be associated with high blood cortisol concentrations, but this is a non-specific finding.

Once the possibility of death due to inadvertent or deliberate overdose of insulin has been raised it is important to seek specialist advice.

Carbon monoxide deaths

There should always be a high index of suspicion for carbon monoxide poisoning. Accidental CO poisoning may present in life in a variety of ways, including as a collapsed patient with an electrocardiogram suggestive of a massive myocardial infarction. Suicide with techniques such as lighting a disposable barbecue indoors may not immediately suggest CO poisoning to the inexperienced scene investigator. Normally, where there is a high prior probability that CO is implicated as a cause of death, measurement of carboxyhaemoglobin using a clinical co-oximeter is adequate. Where the prior probability of CO poisoning is low, and an analysis using a clinical co-oximeter produces a high result, the possibility of a false-positive result should be considered, and the result confirmed with an alternative technique such as molecular-sieve gas chromatography. This also applies where the result may be subject to legal challenge.

Conclusion

The key to the successful collection of suitable samples for post-mortem chemical analyses that yield useful data is to prepare oneself before the autopsy by reading all relevant papers, to have the necessary sample containers to hand, to ensure that the samples are adequately labelled, that the chain of evidence is properly maintained, and to submit all the samples to the laboratory without delay. In difficult cases, discussion with the analyst before the samples are collected is time well spent. In every case, a full account of the case should be submitted to the laboratory along with the samples. Two millilitres of unpreserved blood in an unlabelled bottle submitted a week after the autopsy, having been kept at room temperature in the interim, with a note that says 'Sudden death, ?cause' is unlikely to yield results of great value to anyone, and may facilitate undetected homicide.

Further reading

Coe JI (1993). Postmortem chemistry update. Emphasis on forensic application. *Am J Forensic Med Pathol* **14**(2):91–117.

Cook DS , Braithwaite RA, Hale JKA (2000). Estimating antemortem drug concentrations from postmortem blood samples: the influence of postmortem redistribution. *J Clin Pathol* **53**:282–5.

Drummer OH (2007). Post-mortem toxicology. *Forensic Sci Int* **165**(2/3):199–203.

Drummer O, Forrest ARW, Goldberger B, Karch SBG (2004). Forensic science in the dock. *Br Med J* **329**:636–7.

Flanagan RJ, Connally G, Evans JM (2005). Analytical toxicology: guidelines for sample collection postmortem. *Toxicol Rev* **24**(1):63–71.

Jonsson AK, Spigset O, Tjaderborn M, Druid H, Hagg S (2009). Fatal drug poisonings in a Swedish general population. *BMC Clin Pharm* **9**:7.

R v. Gemma Evans [2009] 2 Cr App R 10, [2009] EWCA Crim 650.

Reis M, Aamo T, Ahlner J, Druid H (2007). Reference concentrations of antidepressants: a compilation of postmortem and therapeutic levels. *J Anal Toxicol* **31**:254–64.

SOFT/AAFS Forensic Toxicology Laboratory Guidelines. www.soft-tox.org/docs/Guidelines%202006%20Final.pdf.

Zilg B, Alkass K, Berg S, Druid H (2009). Postmortem identification of hyperglycemia. *Forensic Sci Int* **185**(1/3):89–95.

Chapter 16

MICROBIOLOGY OF THE AUTOPSY

Elisabeth J Ridgway and David J Harvey

Introduction

At autopsy, infection may be suspected as a cause of death or may be an unexpected finding. Analysis of missed diagnoses has repeatedly shown that, along with pulmonary thromboembolism and acute myocardial infarction, infection is one of the most common unexpected findings at post-mortem examination (Landefeld *et al.*, 1988). Even when infection has been diagnosed during life, autopsy reveals that disseminated infection such as bacterial endocarditis and acute pyelonephritis is consistently under-diagnosed (Cameron and McGoogan, 1981). This chapter examines the evidence for the need to take microbiological samples at autopsy, the techniques used to take samples, how to get the most from the samples that have been taken, how to interpret the results, and the clinical conditions where microbiological investigations are considered important. The role of the autopsy in suspected bioterrorism is not covered, but has been dealt with elsewhere (Roy, 2004; Mazuchowski and Meier, 2005; Lucas, 2008).

Historical perspective

While in the early part of the twentieth century the practice of post-mortem bacteriology enjoyed considerable support, there followed a marked decline in interest in this field by clinicians and pathologists alike. Although the post-mortem examination often reveals the cause of death, the significance of the micro-organisms recovered at autopsy has been difficult to clarify and still remains controversial. Two theories have been proposed, each concluding that microbiological findings at autopsy should be regarded with a high index of suspicion.

Fredette (1916) suggested that 'agonal invasion' accounts for a large proportion of positive cultures recovered at autopsy. The hypothesis proposes that, for variable periods preceding death, a decline in cell structure, function and viability renders the dying person susceptible to disseminated infection from endogenous micro-organisms. It might be expected that any bacterial growth would be mixed and could comprise both commensals and potentially pathogenic species.

The counter theory proposed by Carpenter and Wilkins (1964) states that endogenous bacteria multiply and migrate throughout the body only after death, a phenomenon termed 'post-mortem invasion'. Carpenter and Wilkins retrospectively studied 2033 autopsies and found that the proportion of positive cardiac blood cultures increased linearly with the interval from death to the time of blood culture collection. However, other studies have failed to confirm this finding; nor have they found, as would be expected, that the number of micro-organisms per culture increases with the duration of the post-mortem interval (Wilson *et al.*, 1993; Hove and Pencil, 1998).

Currently, neither of these theories has been fully substantiated. The frequent finding of positive post-mortem cultures that have no apparent diagnostic significance has led to a widely held belief that post-mortem bacteriological data are unreliable.

Perhaps more importantly, given that it is largely preventable, is that samples may become contaminated during collection at the post-mortem examination. This is particularly important in sites that are relatively protected from bacterial invasion, such as the brain and meninges, where contamination has the potential to generate misleading results. Several approaches to reducing bacterial contamination have been attempted. Some authors have advocated the use of a sterile autopsy technique by modifying surgical techniques and employing a surgically clean post-mortem room (O'Toole *et al.*, 1965; Minckler *et al.*, 1966). Using this method the body is scrubbed for 5 minutes with povidone iodine, followed by a 5-minute rinse with 70% alcohol. All autopsy staff undergo routine scrubbing, gowning, gloving and masking. At least 1 g portions of each organ are obtained using a separate set of instruments for each sample. Under such stringent conditions, O'Toole *et al.* (1965) found that 324 of 440 (74 per cent) tissue samples were sterile, and Minckler *et al.* (1966) found sterile cultures for 45 per cent of lung and 75 per cent of kidney specimens. However, this complex technique is impractical for routine use and may be unnecessary to achieve reliable microbiological culture results. de Jongh *et al.* (1968) obtained similar results using much less elaborate methods.

Despite the controversies, the correct taking of autopsy specimens for microbiological examination may be of immeasurable value both in confirming a presumptive ante-mortem diagnosis and in highlighting an obscure and possibly unsuspected organism as the cause of a patient's illness (Moar and Millar, 1984; du Moulin and Patterson, 1985).

Collection of microbiology specimens

The interpretation of microbiological specimens taken at autopsy requires the expertise of an experienced medical microbiologist. However, on its own, correct microbiological interpretation is insufficient. In order to maximise the yield of useful information, a collaborative approach between the pathologist and microbiologist is needed. This will ensure that the correct specimens are collected, that they are appropriately processed, and that the clinical significance of subsequent microbiological results is accurately assessed.

General principles

To obtain good-quality microbiological specimens during routine autopsies, the following guidelines may be followed.

Principle 1

If infection is suspected as a cause of death, the case should be discussed with a microbiologist before commencing the autopsy. This will avoid the situation where the opportunity to collect appropriate specimens has been missed and will alert the laboratory that the samples are on their way. Discuss the need for specialised or extended culture (e.g. for fungi, *Mycobacterium tuberculosis*, *Legionella pneumophila*), toxin production (e.g. *Clostridium difficile*, Panton–Valentine leucocidin-producing *Staphylococcus aureus*), antigen detection (e.g. *L. pneumophila*), nucleic acid detection (e.g. *Neisseria meningitidis*, rotavirus, norovirus) and antibody tests, as well as the need for transport media, and the relative merits of different sample types that may be required to make a diagnosis. For example, in investigation of respiratory tract infection a nasopharyngeal aspirate plus nose and throat swab in viral transport medium is preferable to lung tissue for virus detection, whereas a bronchial swab and lung tissue is preferable for bacterial culture. Alerting the microbiology laboratory before samples arrive will ensure that appropriate identification, sensitivity testing, typing and storage of isolates can be performed to allow epidemiological investigation, should it be required.

Principle 2

Assemble the necessary sterile sample containers (e.g. universal or other screw-topped containers), blood culture sets and transport media before commencing the autopsy.

The microbial yield will be optimal if the autopsy is performed, and samples taken, as soon as possible after death. This is particularly important in order to retrieve fastidious organisms or those present in low numbers. Studies in guinea pigs indicate that, if bacterial counts are low at the time of death, organisms are eliminated from blood and muscle to the point of sterility at 24 hours. With higher counts, rapid multiplication begins within a few hours of death, especially at higher temperatures (Gill and Penney, 1979). This could yield misleading culture results or could compound the difficulty of retrieving a true pathogen present in low numbers, as it will be competed out by fast growers. However, there is no doubt that robust pathogens can survive after the death of the host as transmission of organisms to post-mortem room staff has been well documented, such as *Streptococcus pyogenes* (Hawkey *et al.*, 1980) *M. tuberculosis* (Lundgren *et al.*, 1987) and varicella zoster virus (Paul and Jacob, 2006). Fastidious organisms such as *Haemophilus influenzae*, *N. meningitidis* and *S. pneumoniae* can also be retrieved, although it should be noted that in one series the mean time from death to autopsy was only 5 hours (Sadler, 1998).

Principle 3

The body should be refrigerated as soon after death as possible and movement of the body strictly restricted. It would appear that, provided the body is refrigerated at 4–10°C, post-mortem invasion by micro-organisms can be delayed from 15 to 48 hours, and perhaps as long as 96 hours in the case of anaerobic organisms (Moar and Millar, 1984; du Moulin and Patterson, 1985). By limiting body movement, passive re-circulation of blood from contaminated areas such as the gut vasculature, and consequently the potential for false-positive blood cultures, is decreased.

Principle 4

The amount of care taken to prevent contamination when taking autopsy samples for cultures is a key factor in obtaining significant information. Contamination may be avoided by careful attention to technique and aseptic practice.

Principle 5

Once samples have been taken, they should be sent to the microbiology laboratory with the minimum delay. Refrigeration will kill some fragile organisms such as *S. pneumoniae* and *Neisseria gonorrhoeae*. Full clinical details should accompany the specimens to allow the microbiologist to make the correct interpretation. It is helpful to make a note of the death to autopsy time (in hours) on the request form and including the timing and method of sample collection.

Specimen collection

Blood

Ideally, blood cultures should be collected before the body is placed in refrigerated storage; failing this, they should be collected before the autopsy is commenced. Blood cultures are essentially an enrichment culture, so even small numbers of organisms will yield an apparently significant result. Consequently they are particularly prone to contamination if the sampling technique is substandard.

The classical method of autopsy blood culture, where blood is obtained during the autopsy from the right atrium after searing its surface with a heated spatula, is associated with a high contamination rate. In contrast, if blood is collected before the autopsy begins by large vein puncture, after careful skin preparation, the contamination rate can be reduced dramatically (Hove and Pencil, 1998). The skin should be cleaned with a 70% alcohol preparation (with or without povidone iodine or chlorhexidine), the excess wiped off and the skin allowed to dry. Using an aseptic technique and wearing sterile gloves, blood should be collected using a sterile needle and syringe from the neck or subclavian veins or by direct cardiac puncture through the fourth intercostal space. The femoral or intra-abdominal veins should not be used as blood collected from sites below the waist is much more likely to be contaminated. Inoculate the blood directly into blood culture bottles (the volume required will depend on the system in use), rather than into another sterile container, using the same aseptic technique as for samples collected from the living. Note that changing needles between blood culture bottles is not advisable because of the risk of inoculation injury (Saving Lives, 2007).

Blood for serological investigations or molecular antigen detection may also be collected before the autopsy but, as these techniques are much less susceptible to contamination, the site of blood collection is less critical and samples may be collected later in the procedure. One point to note is that, if samples are heavily haemolysed, analysis may not be possible. As each assay will vary, discussion with the laboratory will be required.

Cerebrospinal fluid

Cerebrospinal fluid (CSF) should be collected by cisternal or lumbar puncture (L4/L5). As for blood cultures, the skin should be cleaned with a 70% alcohol preparation (with or without povidone iodine or chlorhexidine), the excess wiped off and the skin allowed to dry. Using an aseptic technique and wearing sterile gloves, CSF should be collected using a sterile needle and syringe and collected in a sterile universal container (screw top).

Tissue and fluids

A variety of different tissues may be collected for microbiological examination depending on the suspected diagnosis or autopsy findings, such as heart valve, lung, meninges, brain, spleen and abscesses. Samples should be collected immediately after entering the body, and may be collected *in situ* or from an excised organ. All possible steps should be taken to minimise contamination. For example, the organ should be raised to prevent contaminated fluids from flowing across it, particularly once an area has been prepared for sampling. A section of the external surface of the organ (approximately 2 cm × 2 cm) should be sterilised by searing to dryness with a flat-faced soldering iron or a palette knife or new PM40 blade heated with a blowtorch. Alcohol or iodine cannot be used for this purpose as it may have a persistent antibacterial effect that could interfere with culture. Using a sterile scalpel and forceps, as generous a portion as possible (e.g. 1 cm³) should be removed for examination. A different set of instruments should be used for each site/culture. Alternatively, a sterile swab can be forced through the seared area or fluid aspirated using a sterile needle and syringe.

Specimens should be placed in a sterile container of appropriate size. Tissue fragments may be suspended in a small volume of sterile saline to prevent desiccation. Under no circumstances should containers that have held formalin be used, even if the formalin is discarded prior to use. Where there is a collection of pus, this should be aspirated and placed in an airtight sample container without delay as anaerobic organisms die rapidly on exposure to air; swabs should be sent only as a last resort. A wide-bore needle or irrigation syringe may be required to aspirate thick pus. If an abscess is present, part of the abscess wall should be sent for culture, as well as the contents. Attention should also be given to lymph nodes draining infected areas and samples sent as appropriate.

Fluids such as ascites, joint fluids and pleural fluid should be collected in an aseptic manner, as for blood cultures. A portion may be inoculated directly into blood culture bottles, which act as an enrichment broth and will also prevent the demise of fastidious organisms if there is a delay in processing. However, it essential that a plain sample is also sent (in a sterile universal container) so that Gram and Ziehl–Neelsen staining, direct culture (including specialised techniques and for mycobacteria) and molecular analysis can be performed if required. If the direct culture is negative, it raises the possibility that organisms isolated from the blood culture bottles are contaminants introduced at collection. If urine samples are taken, the urine should be aspirated directly from the bladder using an aseptic technique and sent promptly to the laboratory in a sterile universal container.

Diagnostic methods

A range of microbiological investigations may be performed on autopsy specimens (Table 16.1). Each varies in its usefulness depending on the clinical condition under investigation.

Traditional culture methods have refined over recent years. For example, continuously monitored

Table 16.1 Microbiological techniques routinely available for analysis of autopsy specimens

Method	Type	Examples and comments on use
Culture	Routine bacterial culture	Standard culture and sensitivity testing method
	Enrichment culture	Uses a broth to amplify low bacterial counts (including contaminants); e.g. blood cultures, pus, fluids, tissue
	Prolonged bacterial culture	*Legionella* sp., *Actinomyces* sp.
	Mycobacterial culture (routine or rapid liquid-based systems)	*M. tuberculosis* and non-tuberculous mycobacteria
	Viral culture	Herpes viruses, adenovirus, enteroviruses
	Fungal culture	Yeasts, moulds, dimorphic fungi
Microscopy	Light	Wet film for fungal elements, helminth ova and cysts
		Stained films, e.g. Gram stain, Ziehl–Neelsen, calcofluor white
	Fluorescent	Stained films, e.g. cryptosporidia, mycobacteria
		Immunofluorescence, e.g. *Pneumocystis carinii*, respiratory viruses
	Electron	Predominantly virus detection, e.g. SRSV, herpes viruses, enteroviruses, adenovirus
Serology	Enzyme immunoassay, complement fixation, particle agglutination, immunofluorescence	Archived sera may be available to allow comparison of titres; e.g. respiratory viruses, *Legionella*, *Chlamydia*, hepatitis viruses, CMV, EBV, measles
Antigen detection	Latex agglutination	*Meningococcus*, *Pneumococcus*, *Cryptococcus*
	Enzyme immunoassay	*L. pneumophila* (urine), rotavirus, *Chlamydia*, RSV, hepatitis B surface antigen, rotavirus
	Immunofluorescence	RSV, VZV, HSV, respiratory viruses
	Nucleic acid detection	*M. tuberculosis*, *Meningococcus*, *Aspergillus*, *Candida*, CMV, HSV and an increasing number of other organisms

CMV, cytomegalovirus; EBV, Epstein–Barr virus; HSV, herpes simplex virus; RSV, respiratory syncytial virus; SRSV, small round structured virus; VZV, varicella-zoster virus.

liquid culture for *M. tuberculosis* is now able to yield a positive culture result in 10–14 days, compared with 6–8 weeks for traditional Löwenstein–Jensen slope culture. Serological tests have become more sensitive, and specific and nucleic acid detection methods, such as the polymerase chain reaction (PCR), are being continuously refined with an increasing number of tests coming into routine diagnostic use. Nucleic acid detection methods can often detect specific microbial pathogens and antimicrobial resistance genes more rapidly and with greater sensitivity and specificity than conventional culture and susceptibility testing, and quantitative methods are now widely available. However, a recognised limitation of these methods is the difficulty of detecting the wide range of possible pathogens contained in a clinical sample and the lack of an isolate for definitive biochemical identification, sensitivity testing and typing – which may have clinical, epide-miological and public health significance. On the positive side, amplification technology brings welcome new possibilities for the rapid and sensitive detection of specific pathogens in a sample, including viruses, slowly growing bacteria, fastidious or uncultivable bacteria, fungi and protozoa. This may prove particularly useful in the diagnosis of conditions where serological tests are imperfect (e.g. aspergillosis); in immunocompromised patients who fail to mount a serological response (e.g. cytomegalovirus); where micro-organisms are difficult or dangerous to culture from autopsy samples (e.g. *Chlamydia pneumoniae*, *Yersinia pestis*, rickettsias); where culture methods are relatively slow (e.g. mycobacterial infection); and where diagnosis relies on examination of a blood film, the quality of which may be very poor in autopsy specimens (e.g. malaria).

Quantification of bacterial growth may be a way of differentiating between infecting and colonising flora. Knapp and Kent (1968) analysed cultures obtained from homogenates of peripheral lung tissue. They found that large numbers of organisms ($>10^6$ colony-forming units per cubic centimetre of tissue) correlated with histological evidence of infection, whereas contaminating organisms were present in much lower numbers ($<10^4/cm^3$). The problem that arises when tissue is homogenised for quantitative counts is that organisms contaminating the surface of the tissue become incorporated into the homogenate, giving false results. This is overcome if quantification is performed using impression cultures. In this instance, the cut surface of the tissue is pressed onto agar culture plates, allowing the quantity, types and distribution of bacteria to be determined. Surface contaminants are localised at the edges of the print, and friable tissues (e.g. lung) can be rapidly frozen to allow easier handling without interfering with the culture results. Using this technique, Zanen-Lim and Zanen (1980) found that large numbers of organisms, usually in pure culture, were associated with pulmonary infection in life. The techniques available in each microbiology laboratory will vary and will need to be discussed with the microbiologist.

Even when samples result in positive cultures, this may be insufficient to reach an overall diagnosis – and examination of tissue sections will often yield useful additional information. Haematoxylin and eosin (H&E)-stained sections can be useful in staining bacteria and fungi as well as some viral inclusion bodies, which can be further assessed with special stains. Silver impregnation stains blacken all bacteria non-selectively including *Legionella* species and non-Gram-staining bacteria such as the spirochaetes and *Bartonella* species. Gomori's methenamine silver (GMS) stain is the stain of choice for fungi. These stains may distort the normal morphology, but have the advantage of being more sensitive than tissue Gram stain, particularly with low numbers of organisms. If organisms are detected by silver impregnation stains, then further sections can be Gram stained to elucidate their morphology and Gram reaction. Mycobacterial species can be detected using acid-fast stains such as the Ziehl–Neelsen stain, or auramine–rhodamine fluores-

cence stains for greater sensitivity. Other stains include Giemsa for identification of protozoa, rickettsiae and chlamydiae, mucicarmine for *Cryptococcus neoformans*, and melanin for dematiaceous fungi (Mazuchowski and Meier, 2005).

These stains can be extremely useful but may still result in failure to detect an organism or result in ambiguous morphology. It is here that the use of immunohistochemical (IHC) techniques, in-situ hybridisation (ISH) techniques or molecular biological techniques such as PCR may clinch the diagnosis. ISH combines molecular biological techniques with histological and cytological analysis of gene expression. RNA and DNA can be readily localised in specific cells with this method. Recent developments in the applications of ISH involve in-situ PCR and in-situ reverse transcription (RT)-PCR, which can be used to detect very low levels of nucleic acids in tissues by taking advantage of the powerful amplification capacity of PCR. At present these are generally research tools, but they have been used successfully in the identification of emerging infectious agents, such as hanta virus, West Nile virus, severe acute respiratory syndrome (SARS) and influenza H5N1 (Gu *et al.*, 2007).

Interpretation of culture results

Interpretation of post-mortem cultures is not an exact science because there are many variables that need to be taken into account in interpreting results. This is particularly pertinent when assessing sites with a normal flora such as the respiratory, gastrointestinal and genitourinary tracts, as the microbial flora is readily deranged by illness and medical intervention and culture results can be misleading. As in life, the following factors should be considered: past medical history, including chronic co-morbidities, immunosuppression, medication, surgical procedures, presence of prostheses; travel history; occupation; contact with animals; place of residence (own home, nursing or residential home, no fixed abode); recent hospital admissions, including details of type of ward, admission to intensive care, use of peripheral cannulae or central venous lines, urinary

Table 16.2 Guide to interpretation of culture results from different anatomical sites

	Sterile site (e.g. CSF)	Protected site (e.g. lung)	Site with normal flora (e.g. skin/GI tract/upper respiratory tract)
Organism that acts as an unequivocal pathogen (e.g. *M. tuberculosis*)	Significant	Significant	Significant
Organism that acts as a coloniser and a pathogen (e.g. *S. aureus*, herpes simplex virus)	Significant	Could be significant Needs corroboration[a]	Could be significant Needs corroboration[a]
Organism that acts mainly as a coloniser, opportunist pathogen only (e.g. coagulase negative *Staphylococcus*)	Could be significant Needs corroboration[a]	Unlikely to be significant Needs corroboration[a]	Unlikely to be significant

[a] Corroboration by clinical history, results of other cultures, histology, consideration of how the sample was collected.
GI, gastrointestinal; CSF, cerebrospinal fluid.

catheterisation, endotracheal intubation and artificial ventilation; use of antimicrobial agents; and previous microbiology results.

In cultures from any site, consideration should be given to whether an organism is:

1. a true pathogen;
2. part of the normal flora that would be expected at that site;
3. present secondary to agonal spread of organisms (pre-mortem mucosal compromise or possibly arising from prolonged resuscitation);
4. present secondary to post-mortem translocation of organisms;
5. a contaminant that has been introduced during specimen collection at autopsy.

Careful correlation of the culture results from different sampling sites, and between ante-mortem and post-mortem samples, with the clinical history and gross and microscopic findings, plus an understanding of the behaviour of pathogens at different sites, will usually allow the microbiologist and pathologist to accurately assess their clinical relevance (Table 16.2).

Blood cultures

As with positive blood cultures taken in life, a distinction commonly needs to be made between a true positive and contamination, particularly if the organism is one that has the capacity to act as both a coloniser and a pathogen – such as *S. epidermidis*. This is also true in the post-mortem setting.

Although it is recommended that contamination rates should be below 3 per cent in diagnostic blood culture systems (Weinstein, 2003), they are often significantly higher than this (Madeo *et al.*, 2005). Consequently, it is inevitable that a proportion of blood cultures taken at autopsy will be contaminated. Generally the same principles applied in life can be used to interpret post-mortem blood cultures, in that a pure growth of a recognised pathogen is usually significant, and mixed cultures are typically contaminants. However, some caution is required as, although interpretation of organisms such as *N. meningitidis*, *H. influenzae*, *S. pneumoniae*, *Salmonella* spp. and *S. aureus* is straightforward, the significance of others such as *Enterococcus* spp., Enterobacteriaceae and other Gram-negative enteric organisms is more difficult. As the last group arise from the gastrointestinal tract and grow rapidly as contaminants, it may be necessary to seek supporting evidence such as multiple isolates of the same organism from different sites, histological appearance or a compatible clinical picture, before regarding them as pathogens. Coagulase-negative staphylococci are very commonly contaminants, but may be significant when associated with intravenous and prosthetic devices (Weinstein, 2003). As in life, a positive blood culture does not always correlate with symptomatic disease, so it may not indicate the cause of death. Mixed cultures in the post-mortem setting could arise from options 3–5 above, and are usually artefacts. Differentiating these from true polymicrobial bloodstream infections, which are not uncommon and which, in life, are usually confirmed by repeated isolation, is extremely difficult (Lee *et al.*, 2007).

In terms of determining how frequently contamination occurs, autopsy studies have found remarkable consistency. About 20 per cent of cultures have yielded a single pathogen that was compatible with the cause of death, while about 10 per cent yielded mixed cultures of doubtful significance and the remainder were sterile (Fredette, 1916; Adelson and Kinney, 1956; Carpenter and Wilkins, 1964; Pryce-Davies and Hurley, 1979; Morris *et al.*, 2006). This would suggest that, if contamination rates for autopsy blood cultures are comparable to those in life, agonal spread and post-mortem translocation appear to account for only a very small proportion of positive cultures. Further evidence that post-mortem invasion is negligible comes from studies where authors have found either no or only a weak association between the yield of cultures and time after death (Carpenter and Wilkins, 1964; Pryce-Davies and Hurley, 1979; Morris *et al.*, 2006).

Cerebrospinal fluid

Unlike blood cultures where agonal and post-mortem spread may account for a small proportion of positive results, this appears to be very uncommon in CSF. Most well-collected autopsy samples are sterile or yield a single, clinically relevant pathogen (Pryce-Davies and Hurley, 1979; Eisenfield *et al.*, 1983). The small number of samples that yield mixed cultures probably arise from contamination during collection. This suggests that the blood–brain barrier remains intact after death, preventing ingress of any bacteria that are present in the bloodstream (by whatever mechanism), and that CSF results at autopsy are reliable provided contamination is avoided. Sustained integrity of the blood–brain barrier within the first 24 hours after death is supported by the finding that CSF protein measurements are reliable during this period (Mangin *et al.*, 1983) and, as in life, this may be a useful adjunct when interpreting CSF culture results.

The value of the CSF white cell count as a marker for inflammation or infection depends greatly on the time after death. After death, the count increases substantially, predominantly due to an increase in mononuclear cells (Platt *et al.*, 1989) that probably detach from the meninges (Wyler *et al.*, 1994).

Although polymorphs are not seen in the absence of inflammation, they have a short half-life so may be absent if the autopsy is delayed (Morris *et al.*, 2006). It is important to remember that prior neurosurgery may have a significant impact on the CSF findings and interpretation of culture results.

Other samples

In the absence of evidence of local infection, positive cultures from normally sterile tissues can be interpreted in a similar fashion to blood cultures. Careful attention to preparation of the surface of the organ before sample collection will minimise the chances of contamination. Although, theoretically, organisms could penetrate into tissue from surface contamination, this is unlikely to be a problem in practice. Studies on muscle have shown that, although penetration into the interior depends on the bacterial species involved and the density of surface contamination, it is relatively slow and substantially reduced at refrigeration temperatures (Gill and Penney, 1977). Consequently, with adequate storage of the body and timely post-mortem examination it should not be an issue.

Interpretation of cultures of sites with a normal bacterial flora, such as the upper respiratory tract or gastrointestinal tract, is difficult unless an unequivocal pathogen (e.g. *M. tuberculosis*) is isolated. Many organisms that are able to act as pathogens are commonly found as incidental passengers in these sites, and clinical or pathological evidence of an infecting role is required. The diagnostic contribution of samples from non-sterile sites may, in reality, be limited. In a review of neonatal, infant and young childhood deaths, Sadler (1998) found that significant pathogens were often demonstrated by bacteriological culture of the cerebrospinal fluid, blood and trachea, whereas culture of swabs from the ears, nose and throat usually yielded insignificant commensals or contaminants.

Contribution of autopsy microbiology to the diagnosis of specific clinical conditions

Pneumonia

Community-acquired lower respiratory tract infection is an important clinical problem. It has been estimated that the incidence of community-acquired pneumonia (CAP) in adults ranges from 1 to 4.7 per 1000 adults annually, so that a million cases occur each year in western Europe alone. The impact on hospital practice is significant, as 7 per cent of all adult admissions are due to pneumonia and the overall mortality ranges from 3 to 11 per cent. Between 5 and 10 per cent of patients admitted to hospital with CAP are suffering from severe disease requiring management on the intensive care unit (ICU), and the mortality in such patients is high at about 33 per cent (MacFarlane, 1995).

Studies examining the causative pathogens in CAP have been remarkably consistent, even when patients treated in the community, hospital or ICU are compared. Notably, about one-third of infections are due to *S. pneumoniae*, with other organisms being relatively less important. In a large proportion of cases (up to 50 per cent in some studies) no pathogen could be identified despite extensive investigation, but it is likely that a large number of these are also pneumococcal.

When faced with a patient with pneumonia, problems arise in deciding the likely infecting agent, for several reasons. Despite the 'classical' presentations that have been associated with different infections, generally symptoms, signs and radiographic changes are not specific enough to make a diagnosis in an individual patient. Only about one-third of patients produce sputum; many patients have been on antibiotics in the community prior to admission; and laboratory diagnosis by culture is relatively insensitive. It is therefore perhaps unsurprising that in about 10 per cent of cases of bacterial pneumonia the diagnosis is missed during life and only made at autopsy (Landefeld *et al.*, 1988). With nosocomial pneumonia, the situation is even worse. It often occurs against a background of coexisting lung injury and adult respiratory distress syndrome (ARDS). In ventilated patients, it can be difficult to distinguish between bacterial colonisation and infection, and blood cultures are positive in only about 5 per cent of cases. In a necropsy study of 24 patients dying of ARDS, 14 had histological evidence of pneumonia, of which only nine (64 per cent) had been accurately diagnosed in life (Andrews *et al.*, 1981). In contrast, of the 10 non-pneumonia deaths, eight (80 per cent) were correctly diagnosed ante-mortem.

Even in apparently straightforward cases of pneumonia, lung samples should still be taken. This is because of the possibility that resistant organisms have caused treatment failure and so contributed to the fatal outcome. Resistance in pathogens causing CAP is increasingly prevalent (Klugman, 2007); and in ventilated patients, infection with multi-resistant pathogens is associated with substantially worse clinical outcome (Parker *et al.*, 2008).

Legionnaires' disease is another infection where treatment failure may appear to be due to antibiotic resistance. However, in this instance, the intracellular location of the bacterium leads to in-vivo resistance, even when in-vitro sensitivity tests suggest that the organism should respond to antimicrobials with good intracellular penetration such as ciprofloxacin and rifampicin. The mortality from legionellosis is significant: in 2006, 10 per cent of patients reported in England and Wales died (Health Protection Agency, 2008a). In the UK, just less than half the reported *Legionella* infections are acquired in the community, about the same proportion in association with foreign travel, and the remainder in hospital. Most cases are sporadic; but outbreaks are common, and clusters of cases have been reported in travellers returning from a wide range of countries, particularly Spain and Turkey. *L. pneumophila* may be difficult to diagnose in life, as culture is not routinely performed in most laboratories, the serological response may be slow, and urinary antigen becomes negative relatively early in the course of the illness. Isolation of the organism from autopsy material may not only give a clinical diagnosis but, by allowing speciation and typing, also permits the identification of environmental sources and epidemiological links during outbreaks. However, care in interpretation may be necessary, as shown by a report from Newcastle (Lightfoot *et al.*, 1991). These authors demonstrated the contamination of autopsy material by *L. pneumophila* serogroup 8, presumably from the hot water outlets in the post-mortem room, reinforcing the need for sterile techniques in obtaining such samples.

In the last few years, the importance of toxins in the pathogenesis of *S. aureus* pneumonia, specifically Panton–Valentine leucocidin (PVL), has become apparent. PVL is a toxin that destroys leucocytes by causing pore formation. Its significance lies in the fact that it causes a necrotising haemorrhagic pneumonia, which is often fatal in otherwise healthy young adults. Although the genes encoding the toxin are carried by fewer than 2 per cent of clinical *S. aureus* isolates, concern has arisen over the prospect of PVL production emerging in strains resistant to many of the antibiotic agents currently available. This has occurred in the USA300 clone, which is a PVL-positive meticillin–resistant *Staphylococcus aureus* (MRSA) strain currently spreading extensively through the community and hospitals in the USA (Francis *et al.*, 2005). Obtaining suitable post-mortem specimens (blood, lung tissue) will allow isolation of the organism and permit further toxin and susceptibility testing, as well as the use of newer techniques such as RT-PCR to look for co-infection with viruses such as influenza A or B (Francis *et al.*, 2005). This may provide information important in controlling spread and which may guide clinicians and public health officials in subsequent prophylaxis or decolonisation of close contacts (family members, healthcare workers, patients). It also highlights the need for close liaison between microbiology and histopathology departments.

Mycobacterial infection

In many parts of the world, mycobacterial infection is a significant cause of morbidity and mortality and is of great public health concern. The autopsy has an important contribution to make to the epidemiological control of tuberculosis (TB), to the management of the contacts of an individual case, and to the understanding of non-tuberculous mycobacterial disease. Many cases of TB are unrecognised during life and diagnosed only at autopsy – up to half of cases in a study from Hong Kong (Lee and Ng, 1990); and it has been calculated that in the USA about 0.1 per cent of all autopsies reveal TB not suspected in life (Juul, 1977). In most parts of the world the incidence of TB is increasing. In England and Wales, for example, the incidence has increased successively over the last two decades with over 8497 cases reported in 2006, a rate of 14 cases per 100 000 population. The London region accounted for the largest proportion of cases (40 per cent) and had the highest rate, 44.8 per 100 000 population (Health Protection Agency, 2007a).

Although TB may be suspected macroscopically at autopsy, and mycobacterial infection can be confirmed on later histological examination, it is important to send samples for culture. Because of the public health implications of both the diagnosis and resistance to antituberculous therapy (in particular multi-drug resistance), full speciation and sensitivity testing of the infecting organism is required. Resistance has been relatively stable in England and Wales since the mid-1990s with approximately 1 per cent of strains showing primary multi-drug resistance (MDR) (Health Protection Agency, 2007a). This is not the case in other countries, most notably the former Baltic states, where rates of primary multi-drug resistance approach 15 per cent. Placed in the context of an estimated incidence of TB of over 250 cases per 100 000 population in that region, this gives an incidence of MDR TB of 35 cases per 100 000 (Zager and McNerney, 2008). Extensively drug-resistant (XDR) strains – those resistant to most available agents – have recently emerged as a problem in South Africa in association with HIV infection, and with a uniformly fatal course. However, patients from areas not normally associated with XDR TB may present unexpectedly (Blaas *et al.*, 2008).

Mycobacteria other than *M. tuberculosis* have been recognised as a cause of human disease since the early 1950s. These strains have been variously referred to as atypical, non-tuberculous or environmental – but most act as opportunists and can be referred to as such. In general, disease requiring treatment occurs only in individuals with a predisposing condition such as chronic lung disease or impaired immunity, but they are an increasing clinical problem owing to rising numbers of immunocompromised and HIV-positive patients (García García et al., 2005). Four main types of disease arise due to infection with these organisms: pulmonary disease is the most common manifestation, but skin infection and local abscesses, cervical adenopathy, and disseminated infection also occur. In life there is a problem distinguishing between colonisation and infection with these organisms, especially for pulmonary disease, and uncertainty about the optimal treatment. In order to more precisely define the role of opportunistic mycobacteria, the American Thoracic Society has recommended that a lung biopsy should be taken from patients in whom the presence of pulmonary disease is in doubt, and this is essential in patients who apparently die of their infection (American Thoracic Society, 1997).

Fungal infections

Fungal infections in the immunocompromised are a significant cause of morbidity and mortality, and have been found to be one of the most common unexpected autopsy findings in this group of patients (Landefeld et al., 1988). Advances in the treatment of haematological malignancies and disorders, particularly allogeneic bone marrow and stem-cell transplants, has led to a sub-group of patients at particularly high risk of fungal infections. It is difficult to judge the true incidence of fungal infection, as they are often problematic to diagnose during life. Apart from a few well-characterised syndromes, the clinical picture is often unclear with non-specific symptoms, signs and radiological changes. In addition, cultures of readily obtainable specimens and serological tests are often negative, even in the presence of disseminated infection, and invasive sampling is usually hindered by thrombocytopenia or clotting abnormalities. To further complicate the picture, many immunocompromised patients are treated empirically with antifungals

without a firm diagnosis being made (Sipsas et al., 2005). Consequently, many infections remain undiagnosed and are discovered only if an autopsy is performed. In a study from Birmingham (Boon et al., 1991), 32 cases of invasive aspergillosis were identified from 2315 consecutive autopsies performed between 1980 and 1989 – an incidence of 1.4 per cent overall, but 10.7 per cent in immunosuppressed patients. Only eight of the cases (25 per cent) were diagnosed during life. In patients with haematological malignancy, another autopsy study found invasive fungal infection (IFI) in 314 of 1017 patients (Chamilos et al., 2006). Particularly high rates (30 per cent) were seen in patients who had received an allogeneic haemopoietic stem-cell transplant, with even higher rates (42 per cent) in patients with acute myeloid leukaemia. The difficulty of ante-mortem diagnosis was highlighted, with 77 per cent of the IFI thought to be related significantly to the patient's death, but only 25 per cent diagnosed as proven or probable IFI during life. Nonetheless, the rate of ante-mortem diagnosis of IFI did improve from 1994 to 2003, compared with 1989–1993, and this might reflect the use of more sensitive antigen detection and molecular tests.

One final point of interest was the observation of an increased number of uncommon moulds in patients who were splenectomised with otherwise low-risk malignancies (Chamilos et al., 2006). This study clearly illustrates the need for the empirical use of antifungal therapy in these patients and also highlights the value of necropsy. The association between demolition work, construction work and outbreaks of invasive aspergillosis in immunocompromised patients has been recognised since the 1980s (Weems et al., 1987). It is an association of which pathologists need to be aware, as, despite improvements in building design and ventilation and the use of antifungal prophylaxis, these infections still occur.

A wide range of fungal pathogens has been reported in immunocompromised patients (Chamilos et al., 2006). The most common causes of infection are Candida and Aspergillus species, but systemic infections are increasingly due to organisms previously considered as contaminants, colonisers, plant pathogens or environmental organisms. Within the last two decades, there has been a shift in the aetiology of invasive fungal infections in favour of non-albicans *Candida* species, non-*Candida* yeasts and non-*Aspergillus* moulds (Chamilos *et al.*, 2006). Currently, about 30–40 per cent of isolates from systemic yeast infections such as fungaemias, endophthalmitis and hepatosplenic infections are *Candida* species. Systemic infections are increasingly reported with *C. krusei, C. glabrata, C. parapsilosis, C. lusitaniae* and *C. tropicalis*. Among the non-*Candida* yeasts, organisms such as *Trichosporon beigelii, Malassezia furfur, Hansenula* and *Rhodotorula rubra*, which were previously not considered pathogenic for humans, are being reported. Mortality as high as 60–90 per cent for infection with *Trichosporon* species leaves no doubt that they can cause serious infection in humans (Krcmery, 1996). Disseminated infection with non-*Aspergillus* moulds has a significantly higher mortality than infection due to *Aspergillus* species. The latter has a mortality of 40–60 per cent, whereas disseminated zygomycosis or fusariosis approaches 100 per cent.

Many potential fungal pathogens are commonly found in the environment or as colonisers and the relevance of cultured fungi can be difficult to determine. An autopsy study of ICU deaths found that, of the six unexpected cases of invasive aspergillosis found at autopsy (representing 2.7 per cent of the total deaths), all had been culture positive in life but the *Aspergillus* had been dismissed as a coloniser (Dimopoulos *et al.*, 2003). The significance of fungi isolated from immunosuppressed patients is often different from when the same organisms are isolated from the immunocompetent.

Histological examination of tissue slides may help to confirm that such fungi are the agents responsible for the observed pathology. However, it may be impossible to speciate fungi in tissue sections, or even to identify them to the level of genus. The presence of septate hyphae may be due not only to *Aspergillus* species, but also to *Pseudallescheria boydii, Fusarium* species, zygomycetes and several less common fungi (Walsh *et al.*, 1995). Similarly, *Candida* species appear in tissue as blastoconidia,

pseudohyphae and hyphae. The relative proportions of these elements depend on local tissue conditions, exposure to antifungal agents and species, and speciation on the basis of histological appearance is unreliable. Thus, culture confirmation is essential in order to determine the identity of yeasts and filamentous fungi seen in tissue.

Endocarditis

Endocarditis may occur anywhere within the heart chamber but is usually located on the heart valves, whether native or prosthetic. The causal agents can be bacteria, fungi, rickettsiae or chlamydiae: consequently the term 'infective endocarditis' has replaced the older 'bacterial endocarditis'. The true incidence of endocarditis is unknown but it is currently estimated to be 30 cases per million population per year. This amounts to approximately one case per 1000 hospital admissions, so it is not a 'rare' condition (Pittet and Harding, 1998). Despite modern antibiotics and specialist surgery it remains a life-threatening illness and it is estimated that 20–40 per cent of patients die as a direct consequence of their infection. This is a considerable improvement on the early 1930s when endocarditis was universally fatal, but the mortality rate has barely altered in the last 50 years (Young, 1987). The continuing high mortality is probably in large part due to the failure to diagnose the condition during life.

Robinson *et al.* (1972) reviewed patterns of endocarditis seen at autopsy between 1965 and 1969 and found that endocarditis was present in 47 of 1881 patients (2.5 per cent). Among those patients with native valves, a clinical diagnosis of endocarditis was made in only 39 per cent of cases during life. Despite the institution of appropriate antibiotic therapy, 10 of the 12 patients had evidence of active infection at autopsy. Using a combination of blood culture, valve culture and examination of sections for the presence of bacteria, the infecting organism could be identified at autopsy in 94 per cent of patients with native valve infections – although in 20 per cent of cases it was only on the basis of identification of Gram-positive cocci in valve sections. In patients who had undergone valve replacement for rheumatic or calcific valvular disease and who had become infected postoperatively, the infecting organism was cultured in all cases. Zeien and Klatt (1990) have described a routine approach for pathologists performing autopsies on patients with valvular implants.

Streptococci are the most common aetiological agents of native valve endocarditis, particularly viridans-type streptococci including *S. mutans*, *S. sanguis* and *S. salivarius*. Such streptococci are responsible for about 45 per cent of endocarditis cases (Young, 1987). *S. aureus* causes about 15 per cent of cases and can cause rapid and severe destruction of the valve with a high mortality – up to 70 per cent of cases in some series. Coagulase-negative staphylococci, particularly *S. epidermidis*, account for up to 40 per cent of reported cases of prosthetic valve endocarditis but only 5 per cent of native valve infections. Prosthetic valve infections are more common in the first 60 days of the postoperative period, although nosocomial infections may not be evident until months or even years later. The risk of developing an infection is highest in the first 6 months after surgery, and then decreases to 0.5 per cent or less per year (Pittet and Harding, 1998). Other less common bacterial pathogens include *Haemophilus* species, *Actinobacillus* species, *Listeria monocytogenes* and *Cardiobacterium hominis*. Although Enterobacteriaceae commonly cause bacteraemia, they are seldom responsible for endocarditis, except in intravenous drug users (IVDUs) and patients with prosthetic valves. Fungal endocarditis is usually caused by *Candida* species; again this is more common in IVDUs and patients who have undergone cardiac surgery.

Vigilance and a high index of clinical suspicion is needed to avoid missing infective endocarditis in older patients, who may have other foci of infection and do not always present with classical signs.

Gastrointestinal infections

If gastrointestinal infection is considered to be a major cause or contributing factor of death, then attempts must be made to identify the infecting micro-organisms. Although *Salmonella* species are often thought to be the most common cause of food poisoning, *Campylobacter jejuni* is by far the most common food-borne infection. In 2005, over 46 000 cases of *Campylobacter* infection were notified to the Communicable Disease Surveillance Centre in England and Wales, compared with fewer than 12 000 cases of salmonellosis (Health Protection Agency, 2008b). Most deaths due to gastroenteritis are due to fluid loss, which affects the young and very old. However, if there is an associated septicaemia, particularly with *Salmonella*, then there is an associated mortality. In children, viruses such as rotavirus are the leading cause of gastroenteritis, though rarely fatal. However, a report from Toronto described 21 fatal cases in healthy children over a 5-year period, all dying from severe dehydration with marked hypernatraemia (Carlson *et al.*, 1978).

Bacterial, viral and parasitic enteric pathogens are readily detected in faecal specimens collected at autopsy. It is essential to indicate whether there is a history of foreign travel as exotic bacteria such as *Vibrio cholerae* and *V. parahaemolyticus*, which are not routinely cultured, can then be looked for. It is mandatory that all enteric bacterial isolates have antibiotic susceptibility tests performed because of the increasing numbers of resistant organisms being reported. Such reports have serious clinical implications.

Verocytotoxin-producing *Escherichia coli* (VTEC) serotype O157 was recognised as a human pathogen as recently as 1982. It is an escalating public health problem, and both sporadic and outbreak cases have seen a steady increase over the last two decades. It causes particular problems because of its infectiousness in humans (the infecting dose can be as low as 50 organisms), capacity to spread from person to person as well as by food and water, and the severity of its complications for which no specific treatments are available. Most infections are sporadic, but food-borne outbreaks have been reported in the UK, Europe and North America, often associated with beef and dairy produce. A huge outbreak occurred in Japan in 1996 when 6333 people were affected and there were 13 deaths. However, an outbreak in Scotland in 1996, although less extensive, had a much higher death rate. In all, 490 cases were reported and 18 people died (Lansbury and Ludlam, 1997). The organism causes a spectrum of gastrointestinal disease from mild diarrhoea to severe haemorrhagic colitis. Overall the case fatality rate is about 3 per cent, but, in some outbreaks, 50 per cent of elderly patients died (Wall et al., 1996). A proportion of patients, particularly pre-school children and the elderly, develop haemolytic uraemic syndrome (HUS), a triad of microangiopathic haemolytic anaemia, renal failure and thrombocytopenia. In outbreak cases in the UK between 1992 and 1994, approximately 20 per cent of patients developed HUS but in children this reached 45 per cent (Wall et al., 1996). HUS is the most common cause of acute renal failure in children in the UK and North America.

Clostridium difficile-associated disease (CDAD) ranges from a relatively mild diarrhoeal illness to a life-threatening pseudomembranous colitis with a mortality of up to 30 per cent. Those with underlying disease and the elderly, particularly those over 65 years old, are especially susceptible. The use of broad-spectrum antibiotics dramatically alters the normal bowel flora and appears to be an important trigger in CDAD. A critical 'mass' of environmental contamination with C. difficile spores may also be crucial for disease acquisition. CDAD is primarily a hospital-associated infection and can occur sporadically or in outbreaks that can be difficult to control. However, it is now becoming increasingly recognised as a community-associated disease. C. difficile infection has shown a steady and worrying increase in incidence over the last decade with approximately 18 000 cases reported in England and Wales in 1999, increasing to over 55 000 cases in 2006 (Health Protection Agency, 2007b). While the introduction of mandatory surveillance in January 2004 may account for some of this increase, it is the spread of virulent clones such as ribotype 027 that is of major concern. This clone appears to be associated with hyper-toxin production and more severe disease – increased severity, high relapse rate and significant mortality. Initially described in North America, it is rapidly spreading throughout hospitals in the UK and Europe (Kuijper et al., 2007). It was linked with recurrent C. difficile outbreaks at a UK hospital between 2003 and 2005 and probably contributed to the high associated mortality of approximately 13 per cent (Healthcare Commission, 2006).

Meningitis

In managing cases of meningitis, consideration needs to be given not only to the care of the patient but also to the management of their contacts. In N. meningitidis, H. influenzae and tuberculous infection, but not other types of bacterial meningitis (including S. pneumoniae), there are considerable infective risks to the patient's close contacts. The risk of invasive meningococcal infection is higher in close family contacts than in community controls and has secondary attack rates of approximately 2–4 per 1000 – a thousand-fold increase over the overall reported attack rate of meningococcal disease in adults (0.23 per 100 000) (Begg et al., 1999). Similarly, children below the age of 48 months who are in close contact with H. influenzae meningitis are at risk of invasive infection.

In both these infections and tuberculous meningitis, the risk may be reduced by formal identification of contacts and by offering them appropriate antibiotic prophylaxis or vaccination (Hib or Meningococcal A/C vaccine). Consequently, identification of the causative pathogen in cases of meningitis is particularly important. In patients who present to hospital early enough for specimens to be taken during life, this is not usually a problem as the pathogens are readily identified by culture and molecular methods. In cases of sudden death it falls to the pathologist to take the appropriate specimens at autopsy to make the microbiological diagnosis. As many patients presenting with meningitis have already received antibiotics for a number of reasons – for example because meningococcal sepsis had been diagnosed clinically by the general practitioner who had given parenteral penicillin – non-cultural diagnostic techniques such as PCR are becoming increasingly important. These lend themselves particularly well to autopsy specimens because non-viable organisms will still give positive results and the tests are not significantly influenced by the presence of contaminants. It is important to discuss possible cases of meningitis with the microbiologist prior to the autopsy so that appropriate specimens are taken and to ensure that the public health authorities are alerted to the diagnosis so that contact tracing may commence.

Table 16.3 Microbiology specimens that may be taken at autopsy in cases of bacterial and viral meningitis

	Microscopy	Direct antigen detection	Culture	PCR	Serology
Throat swab (a sweep over the pharyngeal walls and tonsils)	–	–	Bacteria Viruses	Meningococcal PCR possible but not routine	–
Blood	–	Serum or plasma *Meningococcus* *Pneumococcus* *Cryptococcus*	Bacteria Viruses	EDTA specimen *Meningococcus* *Pneumococcus* Enteroviruses	Serum or plasma *Meningococcus* Viral
Cerebrospinal fluid Pus Brain tissue	✓	CSF *Pneumococcus* *Meningococcus* *H. influenzae* *Cryptococcus*	Bacteria Mycobacteria Viruses	Viruses *Pneumococcus* *Meningococcus* Mycobacteria	CSF viruses
Skin rash or vesicle aspirate	✓	–	Bacteria Viruses	Meningococcal PCR possible but not routine	–
Urine	–	*Pneumococcus* *Meningococcus*	–	–	–
Middle ear Sinuses Lung	✓	–	Bacteria Mycobacteria Viruses	–	–
Faeces	–	–	Viruses	–	–

CSF, cerebrospinal fluid; EDTA, ethylenediaminetetraacetic acid; PCR, polymerase chain reaction.

An indication of the samples that may be taken in cases of bacterial and viral meningitis is given in Table 16.3. There are a number of points that should be noted.

Antigen tests on CSF and blood are not particularly sensitive, particularly for serogroup B meningococci, and are of similar sensitivity to the Gram stain. The yield of meningococci from aspirated skin lesions is reasonably good: about two-thirds of rash aspirates from patients with meningococcal sepsis have confirmatory Gram stain or culture results (Begg *et al.*, 1999) and prior antibiotics do not affect visualisation of the organisms. Blood cultures are positive in only about 50 per cent of patients with invasive meningococcal infection, even if they have not received prior antibiotics, and meningococci can be isolated from the nasopharynx of up to 50 per cent of patients even if they have. Although nasopharyngeal isolates of meningococci in individual patients are almost always identical to those from their blood or CSF, the possibility of asymptomatic and irrelevant carriage needs to be considered. The carriage rate of meningococci can be 30 per cent or more in teenagers, so the significance of solitary nasopharyngeal isolates may be uncertain. Nasopharyngeal carriage of pneumococci is even higher, and isolation of pneumococci from patients of any age may be of doubtful significance.

With the advent of effective vaccines against the primary pathogens causing meningitis (*N. meningitidis*, *H. influenzae* and *S. pneumoniae*) and their adoption into the routine vaccination schedules in many countries, the epidemiology of bacterial meningitis has changed significantly in both children and adults over the last few years (Davison and Ramsay, 2003; Gjini *et al.*, 2006).

Septicaemia and shock

Septic shock generally occurs in immunocompromised patients, the elderly, and patients undergoing procedures in which significant bacterial contamination can occur. It is also a primary cause of death in infants. It is the most common cause of death in medical and surgical ICUs.

The terms 'sepsis', 'severe sepsis' and 'septic shock' are used to identify the continuum of the clinical response to infection. Patients with sepsis present with evidence of infection and clinical manifestations of inflammation; severe sepsis is the subsequent development of hypoperfusion with organ dysfunction; and progression to persistent hypotension is termed septic shock. The mortality ranges from 16 per cent in patients with sepsis to 40–60 per cent in patients with septic shock (Astiz and Rackow, 1998). Bacterial infection is the most common cause of septic shock, although it is also seen in fungal, viral and protozoal infection, with most infections arising from the lungs, abdomen and urinary tract. Bacteraemia occurs in 40–60 per cent of patients, with the proportion of Gram-positive and Gram-negative infections being approximately equal. A rise in the number of Gram-positive infections has been seen over recent decades owing to an increased incidence of pneumonia and wider use of intravascular devices. In a significant proportion of sepsis cases (10–30 per cent), the causative organism may not be isolated from blood cultures, possibly because of prior exposure to antibiotics.

Life-threatening sepsis is a long-term risk after splenectomy, so guidelines exist for the prevention of infection in patients with an absent or dysfunctional spleen (Davies *et al.*, 2002). It is recommended that patients be educated about their condition, be given lifelong antibiotic prophylaxis with phenoxymethylpenicillin, and be vaccinated against *S. pneumoniae*, *H. influenzae* type B, *N. meningitidis* group C, and influenza. However, despite efforts to improve awareness, cases of overwhelming post-splenectomy infection (OPSI) continue to occur. It would appear that, despite the potential for prevention of infection with vaccination and antibiotics, patient education is a critical factor. A study of splenectomised patients over a 17-year period found that OPSI occurred in 18 of 318 patients (5.7 per cent), of whom three died. Overall, 25 per cent of patients had poor knowledge of the risks of splenec-

tomy and their prevention, and this group had a 16.5 per cent prevalence of OPSI compared with 1.4 per cent among those with good knowledge (El-Alfy and El-Sayed, 2004). From these findings, it is clear that there is enormous potential to improve the management of asplenic patients, of whom there are an estimated 40 000–50 000 in the UK (Waghorn and Mayon-White, 1997).

The autopsy has an important role to play in patients dying of sepsis by confirming the source of the infection, identifying risk factors such as asplenism, and by obtaining tissue samples from which the causative organism may be isolated. This is possible even in patients who have received antibiotics in life and allows identification of both unsuspected pathogens and of treatment failure due to antibiotic-resistant strains. Consequently, monitoring of the efficacy of empirical antibiotic treatment in serious infections is possible.

Conclusion

Interpreted correctly, post-mortem microbiology can be a useful and important part of the examination. Careful studies with standard techniques in conjunction with new nucleic acid detection methods can determine the aetiological agent of infection in cases where ante-mortem clinical studies are unclear. In some cases this will have a profound impact on the management of the patient's contacts and the public. In addition, the efficacy of any antimicrobial therapy received by the patient can be evaluated and patterns of resistance monitored. With careful attention to technique, specimen collection and follow-up, and above all an interested medical microbiologist, post-mortem microbiology has the capacity 'To speak for the dead, to protect the living' (Coroners Association of Ontario; Dalton, 1994).

References

Adelson L, Kinney ER (1956). Sudden and unexpected death in infancy and childhood. *Pediatrics* **17**:663–99.

American Thoracic Society (1997).Diagnosis and treatment of disease caused by nontuberculous mycobacteria. *Am J Resp Crit Care Med* **156**:S1–25.

Andrews CP, Coalson JJ, Smith JD, Johanson WG (1981). Diagnosis of nosocomial bacterial pneumonia in acute, diffuse lung injury. *Chest* **80**(3):254–8.

Astiz AM, Rackow EC (1998). Septic shock. *Lancet* **351**:1501–5.

Begg N, Cartwright KAV, Cohen J *et al.* (1999). Consensus statement on diagnosis, investigation, treatment and prevention of acute bacterial meningitis in immunocompetent adults. *J Infect* **39**:1–15.

Blaas SH, Mutterlein R, Weig J *et al.* (2008). Extensively drug resistant tuberculosis in a high income country: a report of four unrelated cases. *BioMed Central Infect Dis* **8**:60.

Boon AP, O'Brien D, Adams DH (1991). Ten-year review of invasive aspergillosis detected at necropsy. *J Clin Pathol* **44**:452–4.

Cameron HM, McGoogan E (1981). A prospective study of 1152 hospital autopsies. II. Analysis of inaccuracies in clinical diagnosis and their significance. *J Pathol* **133**:285–301.

Carlson JA, Middleton PJ, Szymanski MT *et al.* (1978). Fatal rotavirus gastroenteritis: an analysis of 21 cases. *Am J Dis Child* **132**:477–9.

Carpenter HM, Wilkins RM (1964). Autopsy bacteriology: review of 2033 cases. *Arch Pathol* **77**:73–81.

Chamilos G, Luna M, Lewis RE *et al.* (2006). Invasive fungal infections in patients with hematologic malignancies in a tertiary care cancer center: an autopsy study over a 15-year period (1989–2003). *Hematologica* **91**:986–9.

Dalton AJP (1994). To speak for the dead, to protect the living. *Lancet* **334**:1367–8.

Davies JM, Barnes R, Milligan D (2002). Update of guidelines for the prevention and treatment of infection in patients with an absent or dysfunctional spleen. *Clin Med* **2**:440–3.

Davison KL, Ramsay ME (2003). The epidemiology of acute meningitis in children in England and Wales. *Arch Dis Child* **88**:662–4.

de Jongh DS, Loftis JW, Green GS *et al.* (1968). Postmortem bacteriology: a practical method for routine use. *Am J Clin Pathol* **49**:424–8.

Dimopoulos G, Piagnerelli M, Berré J *et al.* (2003). Disseminated aspergillosis in intensive care unit patients: an autopsy study. *J Chemother* **15**:71–5.

du Moulin GC, Patterson DG (1985). Clinical relevance of postmortem microbiologic examination: a review. *Hum Pathol* **16**:539–48.

Eisenfield L, Ermocilla R, Wirtschafter D, Cassady G (1983). Systemic bacterial infections in neonatal deaths. *Am J Dis Child* **137**:645–9.

El-Alfy MS, El-Sayed MH (2004). Overwhelming postsplenectomy infection: is quality of patient knowledge enough for prevention? *Hematol J* **5**:77–80.

Francis JS, Doherty MC, Lopatin U *et al.* (2005). Severe community-onset pneumonia in healthy adults caused by methicillin-resistant *Staphylococcus aureus* carrying the Panton–Valentine leukocidin genes. *Clin Infect Dis* **40**:100–7.

Fredette JW (1916). Bacteremias in the agonal period. *J Lab Clin Med* **2**:180–8.

García García JM, Palacios Gutiérrez JJ, Sánchez Antuña AA (2005). Respiratory infections caused by environmental mycobacteria. *Arch Bronconeumol* **41**:206–19.

Gill CO, Penney N (1977). Penetration of bacteria into meat. *Appl Environ Microbiol* **33**:1284–6.

Gill CO, Penney N (1979). Survival of bacteria in carcasses. *Appl Environ Microbiol* **37**:667–9.

Gjini AB, Stuart JM, Lawlor DA *et al.* (2006). Changing epidemiology of bacterial meningitis among adults in England and Wales 1991–2002. *Epidemiol Infect* **134**:567–9.

Gu J, Xie Z, Gao Z *et al.* (2007). H5N1 infection of the respiratory tract and beyond: a molecular pathology study. *Lancet* **370**:1137–45.

Hawkey PM, Pedler SJ, Southall PJ (1980). Streptococcus pyogenes: a forgotten occupational hazard in the mortuary. *Br Med J* **281**:1058.

Healthcare Commission (2006). *Investigation into Outbreaks of* Clostridium difficile *at Stoke Mandeville Hospital, Buckinghamshire Hospitals NHS Trust.* London: Commission for Healthcare Audit and Inspection.

Health Protection Agency (2007a). *Tuberculosis in the UK: Annual Report on Tuberculosis Surveillance and Control in the UK*. London: HPA Centre for Infections.

Health Protection Agency (2007b). *Surveillance of Healthcare Associated Infections*. London: HPA Centre for Infections.

Health Protection Agency (2008a). *Legionnaires Disease in Residents of England and Wales: Cases and Deaths by Sex, 1980–2007*. Available at www.hpa.org.uk/webw/HPAweb&HPAwebStandard/HPAweb_C/1195733778196?p=1191942128217 (accessed 13 July 2009).

Health Protection Agency (2008b). *Epidemiological Data on Gastrointestinal Infections*. Available at www.hpa.org.uk/webw/HPAweb&Page&HPAwebAutoListName/Page/1191942150126?p=1191942150126 (accessed 13 July 2009).

Hove M, Pencil SD (1998). Effect of postmortem sampling technique on the clinical significance of autopsy blood cultures. *Hum Pathol* **29**:137–9.

Juul A (1977). Clinical underdiagnosed active tuberculosis: experience from autopsy material. *Acta Med Scand* **202**:225–9.

Klugman KP (2007). Clinical impact of antibiotic resistance in respiratory tract infections. *Int J Antimicrob Agents* **29**(suppl. 1):S6–10.

Knapp BE, Kent TH (1968). Postmortem lung cultures. *Arch Pathol* **85**:200–3.

Krcmery V (1996). Emerging fungal infections in cancer patients. *J Hosp Infect* **33**:109–17.

Kuijper EJ, Coignard B, Brazier JS et al. (2007). Update of *Clostridium difficile*-associated disease due to PCR ribotype 027 in Europe. *Euro Surveil* **12**:E1–2.

Landefeld CS, Chren MM, Myers A et al. (1988). Diagnostic yield of the autopsy in a university hospital and a community hospital. *N Engl J Med* **318**:1249–54.

Lansbury LE, Ludlam H (1997). *Escherichia coli* 0157: lessons from the past 15 years. *J Infect* **34**:189–93.

Lee A, Mirrett S, Reller B, Weinstein MP (2007). Detection of bloodstream infections in adults: how many blood cultures are needed? *J Clin Microbiol* **45**:3546–8.

Lee JK, Ng TH (1990). Undiagnosed tuberculosis in hospitalized patients: an autopsy survey. *J R Soc Health* **110**:141–3.

Lightfoot NF, Richardson IR, Shrimanker J, Farrell DJ (1991). Post-mortem isolation of *Legionella* due to contamination. *Lancet* **337**:376.

Lucas S (2008). Bioterrorism. In: Rutty G (ed.) *Essentials of Autopsy Practice: Topics, Trends and Developments*. London: Springer.

Lundgren R, Norrman E, Asberg I (1987). Tuberculosis infection transmitted at autopsy. *Tubercle* **68**:147–50.

MacFarlane J (1995). The clinical impact of pneumococcal disease. In: Mayon-White RT (ed.) *The Clinical Impact of Pneumococcal Disease and Strategies for its Prevention* (International Congress and Symposium Series 210). London: Royal Society of Medicine Press.

Madeo M, Jackson T, Williams C (2005). Simple measures to reduce the rate of contamination of blood cultures in Accident and Emergency. *Emerg Med J* **22**:810–11.

Mangin P, Lugnier AA, Chaumont AJ et al. (1983). Forensic significance of postmortem estimation of the blood cerebrospinal fluid barrier permeability. *Forensic Sci Int* **2**:143–9

Mazuchowski EL, Meier PA (2005). The modern autopsy: what to do if infection is suspected. *Arch Med Res* **36**:713–23.

Minckler TM, Newell GR, O'Toole WF et al. (1966). Microbiology experience in collection of human tissue. *Am J Clin Pathol* **45**(1):85–92.

Moar JJ, Millar SD (1984). The value of autopsy bacteriology. *S Afr Med J* **66**:192–3.

Morris JA, Harrison LM, Partridge SM (2006). Postmortem bacteriology: a re-evaluation. *J Clin Pathol* **59**:1–9.

O'Toole WF, Saxena HM, Golden A, Ritts RE (1965). Studies of postmortem microbiology using sterile autopsy technique. *Arch Pathol Lab Med* **80**:540–7.

Parker CM, Kutsogiannis J, Muscedere J et al. (2008). Ventilator-associated pneumonia caused by multidrug-resistant organisms or *Pseudomonas aeruginosa*: prevalence, incidence, risk factors, and outcomes. *J Crit Care* **23**:18–26.

Paul N, Jacob ME (2006). An outbreak of cadaver-acquired chickenpox in a health care setting. *Clin Infect Dis* **43**:599–601.

Pittet D, Harding I (1998). Infective endocarditis and glycopeptides. *J Infect* **37**:127–35.

Platt MS, McClure S, Clarke R et al. (1989). Postmortem cerebrospinal fluid pleocytosis. *Am J Forensic Med Pathol* **10**:209–12.

Pryce-Davies J, Hurley R (1979). Infections and perinatal mortality. *J Antimicrob Chemother* **5**(suppl. A):59–70.

Robinson MJ, Greenberg JJ, Korn M, Rywlin AM (1972). Infective endocarditis at autopsy: 1965–1969. *Am J Med* **52**:492–8.

Roy MJ (2004). *Physician's Guide to Terrorist Attack*. New York: Humana Press.

Sadler DW (1998). The value of a thorough protocol in the investigation of sudden infant deaths. *J Clin Pathol* **51**:689–94.

Saving Lives (2007). *Taking Blood Cultures: A Summary of Best Practice. Reducing Infection: Delivering Clean and Safe Care*. London: Department of Health.

Sipsas NV, Bodey GP, Kontoyiannis DP (2005). Perspectives for the management of febrile neutropenic patients with cancer in the 21st century. *Cancer* **103**:1103–13.

Waghorn DJ, Mayon-White RT (1997). A study of 42 episodes of overwhelming post-splenectomy infection: is current guidance for asplenic individuals being followed? *J Infect* **35**:289–94.

Wall PG, McDonnell RJ, Adak GK *et al.* (1996). General outbreaks of Vero cytotoxin producing *Escherichia coli* 0157 in England and Wales from 1992 to 1994. Communicable Disease Report. *CDR Rev* **6**:R26–33.

Walsh TJ, Lyman CA, Pizzo PA (1995). Laboratory diagnosis of invasive fungal infections in patients with neoplastic diseases. In Meunier F (ed.) *Invasive Fungal Infections in Cancer Patients*. Baillière's Clinical Infectious Diseases, Vol. 2, No. 1. London: Baillière Tindall, 25–70.

Weems JJ, Davis BJ, Tablan OC *et al.* (1987). Construction activity: an independent risk factor for invasive aspergillosis and zygomycosis in patients with hematologic malignancy. *Infect Control* **8**(2):71–5.

Weinstein MP (2003). Blood culture contamination: persisting problems and partial progress. *J Clin Microbiol* **41**:2275–8.

Wilson SJ, Wilson WL, Reller LB (1993). Diagnostic utility of postmortem blood cultures. *Arch Pathol Lab Med* **117**:986–8.

Wyler D, Marty W, Bär W (1994). Correlation between the post-mortem cell content of cerebrospinal fluid and time of death. *Int J Legal Med* **106**:194–9.

Young SEJ (1987). Aetiology and epidemiology of infective endocarditis in England and Wales. *J Antimicrob Chemother* **20**(suppl. A):7–14.

Zager EM, McNerney R (2008). Multidrug-resistant tuberculosis. *BioMed Central Infect Dis* **8**:10.

Zanen-Lim OG, Zanen HC (1980). Postmortem bacteriology of the lung by printculture of frozen tissue. *J Clin Pathol* **33**:474–80.

Zeien LB, Klatt EC (1990). Cardiac valve prostheses at autopsy. *Arch Pathol Lab Med* **114**:933–7.

Chapter 17

INVESTIGATING POSSIBLE ANAPHYLACTIC DEATHS

Richard SH Pumphrey and Ian SD Roberts

Introduction

Anaphylaxis is an uncommon but under-recognised cause of death. Acute allergic reactions can kill quickly, presenting as sudden unexpected death and leaving no specific macroscopic findings at autopsy. The reported incidence of negative findings must be an underestimate as many cases with no specific changes at autopsy will not be certified as due to anaphylaxis. Sudden death is not uncommonly attributed to other coexisting pathology such as coronary artery atherosclerosis and, unless anaphylaxis is considered, the true cause of death will be overlooked (Pumphrey and Roberts, 2000). Careful review of the previous medical history and the events leading up to death may alert the pathologist to the possibility of anaphylaxis. In such cases, analysis of blood samples taken at autopsy or retrieved from laboratory investigations before death is essential and can provide data that may support or contradict anaphylaxis as a cause of death.

This chapter aims to provide a framework of knowledge, derived from a study of fatal allergic reactions, that will help the pathologist recognise when anaphylaxis is a possible cause of death, and to assist in the selection of helpful immunological investigations. Findings that may suggest the treatment given for anaphylaxis contributed to death will also be discussed. Abbreviated guidelines for the

autopsy approach to potential anaphylactic deaths, based in part on the authors' experience, are available on the Royal College of Pathologists' website (RCPath, 2005).

There are many potential triggers of anaphylactic reactions. The common allergens can be divided into three main groups: insect venom, foods and drugs. All may cause reactions that result in sudden death without classical features of an allergic response. The last group is the most common encountered in hospital deaths, with antibiotics and drugs used at induction of anaesthesia being the most frequent allergens in this group (Roberts and Pumphrey, 2001). While a detailed clinical history prior to autopsy is essential, to provide evidence of an allergic reaction at the time of death and also a history of previous reactions, absence of a suggestive history does not exclude anaphylaxis. For example, a reaction to a food allergen ingested during an evening meal may result in a delayed death, the presenting history being 'found dead in bed'. The majority of patients suffering fatal iatrogenic reactions do not have a documented allergy, and fewer than half of cases of fatal insect sting anaphylaxis have a history of previous sting reactions (Pumphrey, 2004; Golden, 2007).

Many anaphylactic deaths are avoidable, but improved management of patients at risk of life-threatening reactions will depend on better pathological diagnosis of the cause of death (Pumphrey and Davis, 1999). These deaths are certainly more common than mortality statistics would lead one to believe (Pumphrey, 2000; Pumphrey and Roberts, 2000; Pumphrey and Gowland, 2007). The exact incidence is uncertain, but elevated serum tryptase levels, indicative of mast cell degranulation, have been reported in 40 per cent of sudden unexplained adult deaths, compared with only 11 per cent of deaths with a known non-allergic cause (Edston and van Hage-Hamsten, 1998).

There is confusion about what constitutes an anaphylactic death. Some of this confusion stems from ignorance of basic immunological pathology, some from the alternative mechanisms that a single agent may trigger in different individuals. This chapter also aims to provide the knowledge necessary for accurate classification of these deaths.

More sinister than ignorance is the effect of pressures on the pathologist not to diagnose an anaphylactic death; alternative causes of death may cause fewer difficulties. An inquest may be needed if the death was due to injection or ingestion, rather than, for example, asthma. Furthermore, there is often no autopsy if the death was thought due to asthma because this is regarded as a 'natural' disease and, therefore, the death is not reported to the coroner. The small cost of the tests necessary to support a diagnosis of anaphylactic death has also been used as a reason not to investigate. Anaphylactic deaths are uncommon; these pressures should be resisted, and an attempt should be made to provide an accurate diagnosis.

What is anaphylaxis?

Anaphylactic reactions are usually defined as *severe, generalised, acute allergic reactions that may be fatal.* These are IgE-mediated reactions in which there is massive mast cell activation when allergen-specific IgE antibodies, bound to the high-affinity IgE receptor on the mast cells, are linked by the allergen. Activation causes the mast cells to release stored mediators such as histamine and tryptase, and synthesise and secrete other mediators such as leukotrienes and prostaglandins (Simons, 2008).

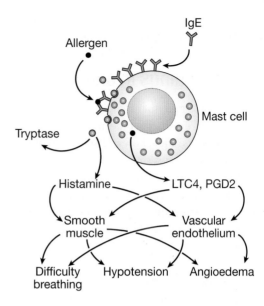

Figure 17.1 Scheme highlighting the main features of an anaphylactic reaction. Binding of allergen causes bridging between adjacent IgE molecules, attached to the surface membrane of the mast cell via the high-affinity IgE receptor (FcεRI). This leads to externalisation of the mast cell granules in the vicinity of the bridged receptors; thus major activation in an anaphylactic reaction will cause degranulation of the whole cell. Arachidonic acid is then released from the nuclear membrane by phospholipase A2 and converted to prostaglandin and leukotrienes (LTC4, PGD2), which are then secreted. These mediators then act on their respective receptors on smooth muscle, endothelial cells, secretory cells and so on to cause the clinical features of an anaphylactic reaction.

These mediators act on specific receptors in tissues throughout the body to cause the observable features of an anaphylactic reaction (Fig. 17.1).

Animal studies have demonstrated alternative pathways to anaphylaxis but their role in human disease is unclear. These include IgG-mediated reactions involving macrophages and basophils and antibody-independent mechanisms involving the innate immune system (Finkelman, 2007).

Any proof that an allergic reaction has been the cause of death is often missing in deaths certified as due to anaphylaxis. Though formal proof is commonly not possible, evidence indicating the most probable cause can usually be discovered by the pathologist by careful interpretation of the macroscopic and histological autopsy findings, and by utilising the appropriate laboratory investigations.

Autopsy findings in anaphylaxis

The macroscopic and microscopic autopsy findings in anaphylactic deaths have been reviewed (Pumphrey and Roberts, 2000; Low and Stables, 2006). An important conclusion is that in a high proportion of cases there are no specific features, especially in death following anaphylactic shock (Table 17.1). Asphyxial anaphylactic reactions generally result in positive macroscopic findings, but these are often classified as asthma and the trigger is then overlooked.

Non-specific pulmonary congestion and oedema is the most frequent macroscopic finding, reported in 73 per cent of cases (Pumphrey and Roberts, 2000). Features suggesting an allergic reaction include cutaneous erythema and urticaria, upper airway oedema and changes of acute asthma (Fig. 17.2). These findings are more common in reactions to food than to venom or iatrogenic causes (100, 67 and 37 per cent of cases, respectively, in the study of Pumphrey and Roberts, 2000). In one reported case, angioedema, cyanosis and laryngeal oedema were

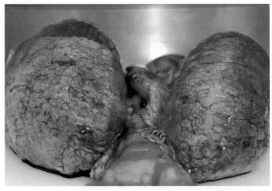

(a)

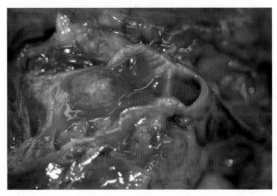

(b)

Figure 17.2 Pulmonary changes in a 72-year-old woman who died suddenly following the first dose of a course of a cephalosporin. An asthmatic mode of death is indicated by (a) hyperinflated lungs that did not collapse on removal from the chest, and (b) mucus plugging of bronchi – mucus expelled from lobar bronchi after compression of the lungs.

Table 17.1 Frequency of negative autopsy findings

Trigger	Total cases	No. of specific findings (%)	Reference
Venom	15	5 (33%)	Pumphrey and Roberts, 2000
Venom	8	3 (38%)	Schwartz et al., 1986
Venom	6	3 (50%)	Hoffman et al., 1983
Food	5	1 (20%)	Yunginger et al., 1988
Food	13	0	Pumphrey and Roberts, 2000
Iatrogenic	2	1 (50%)	Fisher et al., 1991
Iatrogenic	11	7 (63%)	Pumphrey and Roberts, 2000
Iatrogenic	43	22–32 (51–74%)	Delage and Irey, 1972

Adapted from Roberts and Pumphrey (2001).

noted at the time of cardiac arrest but not observed at subsequent autopsy, suggesting that oedema may occasionally resolve during the post-mortem period (Riches et al., 2002). The identification of a known allergen, such as nuts, in the stomach is infrequently reported in food-associated reactions. In delayed deaths, features of anaphylaxis are absent and changes reflecting the final mode of death will be seen. These include brain swelling, reflecting cerebral hypoxia, and bronchopneumonia following a period of ventilation.

Coexisting conditions are frequently found at autopsy and may contribute to death in some cases.

In an unselected series of 25 anaphylactic deaths with a mean patient age of 59 years, Greenberger *et al.* (2007) identified significant co-morbid disease in 22 of the cases. Coexisting coronary artery atherosclerosis, in particular, is a frequent finding with moderate or severe disease being reported in 44 per cent of anaphylactic deaths in a recent series (Low and Stables, 2006). This suggests that pre-existing coronary artery disease may render individuals more vulnerable to the hypotension and hypoxia associated with anaphylaxis, increasing the likelihood of a fatal outcome. It has also been proposed that the increased load of myocardial mast cells observed in various cardiac diseases contributes to a fatal outcome in anaphylaxis (Mueller, 2007).

In asphyxial deaths, histology of the upper airway mucosa may demonstrate oedema and an infiltrate of mast cells and eosinophils. Similarly, in those cases with an asthmatic component, there will be oedema of bronchial mucosa with eosinophilia, mucus plugging and epithelial sloughing. Histology of other organs may reveal evidence of previous episodes of anaphylactic shock. In one case from the authors' practice, a 40-year-old woman was prescribed a course of a cephalosporin. She took the first dose in the evening and, feeling nauseated and dizzy, went to bed. She took the second dose the following morning and suffered a fatal anaphylactic reaction. Post-mortem histology revealed massive necrosis within the liver with a dense neutrophilic infiltrate, indicating severe shock with tissue ischaemia following the first dose of the antibiotic 12 hours prior to death.

Immunological tests

Which serum sample to be analysed?

The two routine tests supporting or refuting the diagnosis of anaphylactic death, mast cell tryptase and specific IgE antibodies, depend on having a serum sample from the deceased. Often blood tests are taken during the reaction and these will be better preserved and more likely to provide positive results than samples taken at autopsy, particularly if death is delayed. An urgent search should be made for any serum or plasma samples remaining in the laboratories, which should be retrieved before they are jettisoned – usually around the time the autopsy is performed. A sample of blood from the femoral vein should be taken at autopsy before the removal of the intestines; ideally this should be separated and frozen if not tested immediately. The common practice of storing unseparated blood samples at 4°C as for toxicology is not suitable for immunological tests. Samples from sites other than the femoral vessels have varying probability of contamination by tryptase released after death from mast cell-rich organs (Edston and van Hage-Hamsten, 1998). Cardiac and other central sites should particularly be avoided.

Mast cell tryptase

Mast cell β-tryptase is a mast cell-specific enzyme that is stored in the granules and released along with histamine during allergic reactions (Hogan and Shwartz, 1997). Mast cell α-tryptase is secreted by resting mast cells and the level is raised in mastocytosis (Schwartz *et al.*, 1995). The assay for mast cell tryptase most commonly used in the UK since 1997 does not distinguish between these two forms: a raised level may therefore be due to mastocytosis or a generalised allergic reaction. In living patients, the level during a reaction can be compared with a later sample after recovery, and, after a fatal reaction, the absence of mastocytosis can be established histologically following autopsy.

Mast cell tryptase is a relatively stable protein and a raised level may be detectable for a few days in post-mortem blood. Schwartz *et al.* (1989) reported that more than 50 per cent of tryptase could still be detected in serum after incubation at 22°C and 37°C for 4 days. Furthermore, there appears to be no correlation between serum tryptase levels and interval between death and autopsy, or specimen storage condition (Schwartz, 1990; Edston and van Hage-Hamsten, 1995, 1998). The half-life of mast cell tryptase during life is around 2 hours (Schwartz *et al.*, 1989) and so tests for this protein should be performed on samples taken during or shortly after the reaction. In a third of fatal anaphylactic reactions, the patient is resuscitated following the reaction but

Table 17.2 Mast cell tryptase levels in serial blood samples taken during life, demonstrating normalisation within 24 hours of an anaphylactic reaction

Time of blood sample following reaction	Mast cell tryptase level (normal 0–16 µg/L)
Day 0 (shortly after reaction)	59.3
Day 1	13.7
Day 4	8.74

dies later (1 hour to 30 days, mode 60 hours), commonly from the effects of cerebral anoxia (Pumphrey, 2000). If death is delayed more than a few hours, tryptase levels measured in post-mortem blood will not be helpful; samples from the time of the reaction should be retrieved and tested. This is illustrated by a recent case from the authors' practice (Table 17.2).

> **Clinical History**
>
> The patient was a 75 year-old woman, known to be allergic to penicillin, who suffered a cardiac arrest following an intravenous dose of ceftriaxone. Resuscitation was performed but there was severe anoxic brain injury. She never regained consciousness but was ventilated for 4 days prior to death. Autopsy showed no specific features of anaphylaxis, and the diagnosis was therefore based on the clinical history and tryptase levels in ante-mortem blood.

Care must be taken when interpreting reports based on older studies of mast cell tryptase. A commonly used assay for β-tryptase, with an upper limit of normal of 1 ng/mL, was based on an antibody that did not react with the native form of the protein (Schwartz, 1990; Schwartz et al., 1994). The conversion from native to detectable caused a delay in the peak level; results therefore peaked 30 minutes to 6 hours after the reaction and a raised level might not be found in serum taken immediately following the reaction (Ordoqui et al., 1997). This is not the case with the Pharmacia Cap assay, the most commonly used assay in the UK at present (upper limit of normal, 13–16 µg/L), in which the antibody reacts with the native form of β-tryptase; this is detectable as soon as it is released (Schwartz et al., 1994). In addition, some reports of tryptase levels in autopsy blood do not specify the site from which the blood was taken, and there is the possibility that any raised tryptase levels were due to contamination by post-mortem release into the central vessels; other studies specifically sampled from the heart.

With this caveat in mind, the following conclusions may be drawn.

- Tryptase is a sensitive measure of mast cell activation and high levels will be found after severe anaphylactic reactions, especially those causing severe shock. Levels are not raised in local allergic reactions such as rhinitis and may not be significantly elevated in purely asthmatic reactions (Salkie et al., 1998); such normal levels may be more common for food-allergic reactions than for stings and iatrogenic reactions (Edston and van Hage-Hamsten, 1998; Pumphrey and Roberts, 2000).
- Tryptase levels may be raised in non-anaphylactic deaths, up to 50 ng/mL (Randall et al., 1995; Edston et al., 2007; Edston and van Hage-Hamsten, 1998). This may result from disruption of tissues containing mast cells, particularly in deaths due to trauma, non-anaphylactic mast cell degranulation by opioids (e.g. morphine given for cardiac pain or heroine overdose), or from post-mortem release, contaminating blood samples from central sites such as cardiac or portal blood (Yunginger et al., 1991; Holgate et al., 1994; Edston and van Hage-Hamsten, 1998).
- Unless grossly elevated, a high tryptase level in post-mortem serum should, therefore, be interpreted with some caution if there is no suggestion in the clinical history of an allergic reaction. However, in the presence of a suggestive history, and a lack of specific autopsy findings, elevated serum tryptase may be used as confirmatory evidence of an anaphylactic death.

Specific IgE antibodies

Specific IgE antibodies are stable for weeks even at room temperature and may be measured after death (Yunginger et al., 1991). Many different assay sys-

Table 17.3 Allergens associated with fatal anaphylactic reactions

Allergen	Availability of specific IgE	UK fatal reactions (Pumphrey, 2000)	Measurement in fatal cases
Venoms			
Insect venom (*Apis, Bombus, Vespula, Vespa, Polistes*)	Routine	25.2% (mostly *Vespula* spp.)	Yunginger *et al.*, 1991 Hoffman *et al.*, 1983 Schwartz *et al.*, 1986 Schwartz *et al.*, 1984 Prahlow and Barnard, 1998
Foods			
Nuts (peanut, brazil nut, walnut, pecan, hazelnut, almond, pistachio, cashew)	Routine	18%	Yunginger *et al.*, 1988 Boyd, 1989
Milk Fish Shellfish Other foods (peach, banana, chickpea)	Routine Routine Routine Available	10.1%	Pumphrey and Nicholls, 2000
Iatrogenic			
Beta-lactam antibiotics	Available for penicilloyl (V and G), amoxycilloyl, ampicilloyl, cefaclor	9.4%	Hoffman *et al.*, 1989
Other antibiotics	nga	2.2%	
Muscle relaxants	Available for thiocholine ester; others nga	Majority of anaesthetic induction reactions (19.4%)	Assem and Ling, 1988
Other anaesthetic agents	nga		Fisher *et al.*, 1991
Antisera Enzymes Other drugs	nga nga nga	7.9%	
Protamine	Available	1.5%	Sharath *et al.*, 1985
Contrast media	nga	5.8%	

nga, not generally available.

tems are used to measure specific IgE antibodies. The most common system used in the UK at the time of writing is the Pharmacia Cap assay, and levels given here refer to this type of assay. Levels below 0.35 kUA/L are taken as negative.

For some allergens, laboratory measurement of specific IgE antibodies is less sensitive than a skin prick test (SPT), and patients may be found who have negative specific IgE but positive SPT; such patients may have a history of reactions to the allergen and a positive response to a challenge test. Conversely, some patients may have positive specific IgE antibodies and not react to the allergen; this is particularly common for patients with eczema. Exceptionally, patients may have high levels of specific IgE (>500 kUA/L) without clinical sensitivity. In general, however, the presence of specific IgE antibodies correlates well with allergy,

and can be used after death to investigate possible allergies in life (Yunginger *et al.*, 1991).

Routine tests for specific IgE antibodies are available for many but not all reported causes of fatal anaphylactic reactions (Table 17.3).

Fatal reactions to foods have occurred almost exclusively in atopic individuals who may have specific IgE antibodies to many allergens. The finding of high levels cannot by itself implicate any allergen; however, known consumption of food containing an allergen to which specific IgE can be detected does raise the possibility of an allergic reaction. Sting allergy is not associated with atopy and the finding of elevated specific IgE to bee and wasp venom in postmortem sera from victims of sudden unexpected death has raised the possibility that some may have been due to anaphylaxis (Schwartz *et al.*, 1988). Such arguments, however, require careful consideration of the prevalence of these antibodies in the population (Herbert and Salkie, 1982; Zora *et al.*, 1984), and this will vary from one place to another.

Other tests less generally applicable

Passive cutaneous anaphylaxis

An interesting case report from the archives raises the possibility of using passive cutaneous anaphylaxis to test for allergic sensitivity after death (Lund and Hunt, 1941). In the original case report, a volunteer was given a subcutaneous injection of serum from the deceased with the intention of passively sensitising the cutaneous mast cells. Subsequent positive response to skin prick tests at the site of injection but not elsewhere was taken as evidence of allergic antibodies in the injected serum. This test could conceivably be used now with a higher primate recipient instead of a human volunteer for allergens where in-vitro measurement of specific IgE antibodies posed insuperable problems.

Histamine

Although histamine is one of the principal mediators of anaphylactic reactions (White, 1990), its use in the diagnosis of anaphylaxis is limited by its short half-life within the serum. Methyl histamine is a more stable metabolite of histamine and may be detected in the first urine voided following a reaction, but the validity of this assay at autopsy has not been established.

Complement levels

Some anaphylactoid reactions (see below) are associated with complement activation. Post-mortem blood samples are not suitable for assays of complement activation. If EDTA plasma or serum samples were collected during the reaction, measurement of complement levels may provide evidence of activation that might support the diagnosis of anaphylactoid reaction.

Leukotriene levels

Cysteinyl leukotrienes are important mediators of asthmatic reactions (Leff, 1998). Many studies have examined the levels of these mediators in the blood and urine following asthmatic reactions and found raised levels (O'Sullivan *et al.*, 1998). Such assays could potentially be used to investigate a sudden unexpected death where an anaphylactic reaction may have caused fatal asthma without a significant rise in the tryptase level; but the need for rapid analysis following the reaction is likely to reduce the applicability in this situation. No studies have reported this use of urinary leukotrienes following fatal reactions.

Conclusions from consideration of autopsy findings, laboratory results and history

Asthma or anaphylaxis?

The most common diagnosis offered as an alternative to anaphylaxis is asthma. Many anaphylactic reactions have a dominant asthmatic component that may be the only part of the reaction evident at autopsy. When asthma is identified as a cause of death, the pathologist should consider whether the asthma was due to a specific allergic cause, and whether this was purely a local reaction to inhaled antigen or part of a systemic allergic response.

What, then, should lead to the diagnosis of anaphylaxis rather than asthma as the cause of death? The clinical history and circumstances of the death are clearly important. Most pathologists would be happy to diagnose anaphylaxis if the asthma attack started suddenly a few minutes after a wasp or bee sting, even when there was no history of previous allergic reactions to stings. Asthma resulting from a sting on the foot is clearly part of a generalised allergic reaction. Specific IgE to bee or wasp venom can readily be measured and, if looked for, will be found in those dying from sting anaphylaxis. Mast cell tryptase levels will be elevated, except possibly in purely asthmatic reactions.

Reactions to food allergens are less clear-cut and acute asthma after eating a food that might have caused the attack is commonly not diagnosed as anaphylaxis. The previous medical history may encourage a diagnosis of asthma, as the majority of fatal acute allergic reactions to food are asthmatic reactions occurring in asthmatic individuals. In 48 out of the last 50 fatal reactions identified as due to food allergy in the UK, the patient took daily treatment for asthma (Pumphrey: unpublished data from the fatal anaphylaxis register). In all 50, difficulty breathing was a major component of the fatal reaction; for only five was this due entirely to upper airway occlusion by angioedema. Some of the remaining deaths were given an autopsy diagnosis of asthma, even when there had been other features of an acute allergic reaction such as urticaria, angioedema, vomiting, diarrhoea or sneezing, and even though the deceased had a history of previous acute allergic reactions to food. Surely, if asthma is the result of ingestion of a food to which the deceased was allergic, this was part of a generalised allergic reaction and was therefore due to anaphylaxis.

Detailed studies comparing the pathological changes in anaphylactic reactions with an asthmatic component to pure asthma are lacking, but a recent report suggests that there may be differences in the histology of the bronchi in fatal anaphylaxis and asthma. In an autopsy study of nine patients dying as a result of anaphylaxis and 10 as a result of acute asthma, Perskvist and Edston (2007) reported that bronchial mast cells were more numerous in anaphylaxis whereas there were greater numbers of bronchial eosinophils in asthma. The characteristic airway changes of asthma, such as basement membrane thickening and muscular hypertrophy (Sidebotham and Roche, 2003), are commonly absent in anaphylaxis.

The post-mortem diagnosis then depends on answers to the following questions.

- Was the deceased allergic to an ingredient of the food that is thought to have caused the reaction? Routine tests are available for specific IgE antibodies to all the food components that commonly cause anaphylaxis, and these tests can be performed on post-mortem serum samples.
- Was that ingredient present in the food eaten before the reaction that proved fatal? The quantity of allergen required to trigger a reaction, however, is so minute that the absence

of traces in the gastric contents cannot disprove exposure. Enquiry into the events leading up to the fatal reaction is more likely to reveal the possibility of exposure.
- Is there any evidence that an acute allergic reaction took place? A raised serum tryptase level immediately following the reaction is a helpful supporting finding, but tryptase levels may not be significantly raised in purely asthmatic reactions. Such reactions will, however, leave macroscopic autopsy findings (Pumphrey and Roberts, 2000). A detailed clinical history is essential to reveal the presence of features, such as urticaria and gastrointestinal disturbance, that indicate a systemic rather than purely local allergic reaction (Rainbow and Browne, 2002).

Anaphylaxis may also result from the inhalation of an allergen. This has occasionally been diagnosed as anaphylaxis in fatal cases. There has usually been autopsy evidence of asthma with changes of chronic asthma, and emergency treatment is effective in treating urticarial rashes and angioedema, even when it fails to overcome the effects of the bronchospasm. Even when there have been symptoms or signs of a generalised reaction, death is usually due to the local allergic reaction in the lungs. When shock is recorded in such reactions, it may be difficult to tell whether it is part of the generalised allergic reaction or whether it is secondary to anoxia resulting from the bronchospasm. Fatal anaphylactic reactions have been recognised following close contact with horses. Other inhalant allergens that might cause anaphylaxis include house dust mite, grass pollen and mould spores. In one well-documented case of fatal anaphylaxis associated with house dust mite allergy, there was a history of airway symptoms, hypotension, nausea and diarrhoea after going to bed. Death was sudden, the 47-year-old man being found collapsed in his bathroom at around midnight. There were no specific findings at autopsy but tryptase was markedly elevated in post-mortem blood and there was a high level of allergen-specific IgE (Edston and van Hage-Hamsten, 2003). Anaphylactic reactions to these allergens are regularly encountered in the allergy clinic; as well as the dominant asthmatic or rhinitic component there may be urticaria, angioedema, vomiting and shock. Specific IgE can be measured to all these allergens in most immunology laboratories. More unusual cases, such as a boy who died following an acute asthma attack with anaphylactic symptoms that started immediately after he stroked a stuffed badger in a museum, may need more diligence to confirm whether there might be a connection between the supposed trigger and the asthma. This could be important, as it might lead to a verdict of misadventure or accidental death rather than natural causes. It may be helpful to enlist the assistance of an interested immunologist when analysing such cases, since non-routine investigations may be needed.

In conclusion, when asthma is identified as the cause of death, the pathologist should consider whether the asthma was a local reaction or part of a systemic response, and whether it was due to a specific allergic cause. If a specific cause for the fatal reaction is evident from the history and/or postmortem investigations, it will be helpful to include it in the certified cause of death.

Anaphylactic or anaphylactoid reaction?

Anaphylactoid reactions may broadly be described as similar in appearance to anaphylactic reactions but are due to some mechanism other than allergen binding to IgE on mast cells or basophils. Some agents commonly thought of as causing anaphylactoid reactions may also cause anaphylactic reactions.

Vancomycin will cause flushing and hypotension in anyone if given by overly rapid intravenous infusion. The mechanism is uncertain but does *not* involve the release of mast cell tryptase (Renz et al., 1998). A very high level of tryptase has been found following a fatal reaction to vancomycin, suggesting that anaphylactic reactions may also occur (Fisher and Baldo, 1998), and may be the typical cause of vancomycin-related fatalities rather than the anaphylactoid process that causes the 'red man' syndrome.

The pathophysiology of reactions to *contrast media* is contentious and incompletely understood (Idee et al., 2005; Morcos, 2005). Initial investigations of the cause of contrast media reactions led to the supposition that these were anaphylactoid with uncertain mechanism, possibly involving activation of complement (Westaby et al., 1985; Eloy et al., 1991) – although there may be another explanation for these findings (Mikkonen et al., 1997) – or the contact (bradykinin) system (Hoffmeister and Heller, 1996). Hyperosmolarity may also contribute to the stimulation of histamine release from basophils and mast cells. Subsequently, specific IgE to iodinated contrast medium (Laroche et al., 1998) and raised tryptase (Yunginger et al., 1991; Brockow et al., 1999) were found, suggesting that fatal contrast medium reactions involved mast cell degranulation and may have been anaphylactic. We have also seen patients in the allergy clinic with a history of contact urticaria to contrast media, strongly suggesting an IgE-mediated aetiology: if these agents were to be injected, such patients must be at risk of an anaphylactic reaction.

Fatalities following sudden hypotension or bronchospasm at induction of *anaesthesia* are most commonly associated with sensitivity to muscle relaxants. IgE antibodies (and, in non-fatal cases, positive skin prick test reactivity) can be demonstrated. Some anaesthetic reactions have also been thought to be anaphylactoid reactions to opioids, but proof is difficult, as opioids will cause release of histamine from cutaneous mast cells in most people. It is clearly possible that these two processes are synergistic in such reactions, which generally follow rapid injection of an opioid, a muscle relaxant and an anaesthetic induction agent, any of which might individually cause a reaction (Gueant et al., 1998).

Aspirin has been associated with both anaphylactic and anaphylactoid reactions. Aspirin-induced asthma (AIA) is a well-defined syndrome and is accompanied by nasal polyposis and sinusitis (Szczeklik and Stevenson, 1999). The mechanism is clearly related to the actions of aspirin and other non-steroidal anti-inflammatory drugs (NSAIDs) on the cyclic oxygenases, COX1 and COX2. In those with aspirin-induced asthma, NSAIDs cause overproduction of cysteinyl leukotrienes, which in turn leads to asthma. However, fatal reactions to aspirin or NSAIDs may occur in those without AIA, and may have features of more typical anaphylactic reactions (Bosso *et al.*, 1991). There is some evidence for IgE antibodies to aspirin (Zhu *et al.*, 1992) and true anaphylaxis cannot be ruled out. Aspirin may be a cofactor for anaphylactic reactions. For example, a patient with positive allergy tests suggesting the possibility of allergy to carrots could tolerate carrot juice unless she had recently taken an aspirin tablet (Schöpf *et al.*, 2000). Reactions such as this may be more common than has been reported because they are difficult to recognise and will commonly be interpreted as a reaction to aspirin.

Bone cement (methacrylate methylmethacrylate copolymer) may cause fatal shock without evidence of fat embolism immediately after insertion. Modestly raised serum tryptase and urinary methyl histamine have been found following such reactions but it seems unlikely that the mechanism was anaphylactic (Lamade *et al.*, 1995; Pumphrey, 2000; Pumphrey: unpublished data from the UK fatal anaphylaxis register).

Some reactions indisputably due to different mechanisms

- *Dextrans.* These may cause anaphylactoid reactions due to IgG antibodies (Ljungström *et al.*, 1988).

- *Cremophore.* This is the epoxylated castor oil solvent used as an excipient for various medicines such as vitamin K. It may cause anaphylactoid reactions that involve activation and consumption of complement (Watkins *et al.*, 1976).

- *Contaminated heparin.* Recently, clusters of reactions resembling anaphylaxis have been reported secondary to heparin contaminated with an over-sulphated form of chondroitin sulphate. A recent study has demonstrated that the contaminant activates the kinin–kallikrein pathway and leads to production of the anaphylotoxins C3a and C5a in human plasma (Kishimoto *et al.*, 2008).

- *Angiotensin-converting enzyme inhibitors.* ACE is a major factor in control of bradykinin activity. ACE inhibitors commonly cause mild symptoms due to increased bradykinin activity (Agostoni *et al.*, 1999). A few patients experience more severe symptoms with angioedema that may occasionally prove fatal if it affects the upper airway (Pumphrey, 2000). A case is illustrated in Fig. 17.3.

Non-iatrogenic anaphylactoid reactions

Sudden death from insect stings has been studied extensively (Parrish, 1963; James and Austen, 1964;

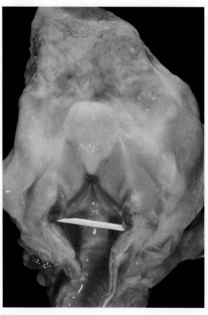

(a)

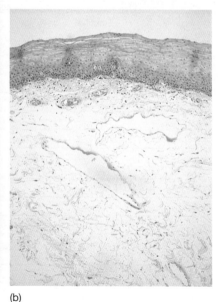

(b)

Figure 17.3 Fatal angioedema in a 62-year-old woman who died shortly after starting treatment with the ACE inhibitor lisinopril for hypertension. She collapsed suddenly having complained that it felt her throat was closing up with difficulty breathing. (a) At autopsy there was upper airway obstruction with marked oedema of the upper laryngeal and pharyngeal mucosa. (b) Histology of the larynx showed oedema only, with no significant infiltrate of mast cells or eosinophils.

Barnard, 1967, 1973; Hoffman *et al.*, 1983; Mosbech, 1983; Schwartz *et al.*, 1984, 1986, 1988; Lantner and Reisman, 1989; Yunginger *et al.*, 1991; Fernandez *et al.*, 1992; Ameno *et al.*, 1993; Ansari *et al.*, 1993; Wagdi *et al.*, 1994; Pumphrey and Roberts, 2000; Riches *et al.*, 2002).

Asphyxial death from insect stings can be due to pharyngeal oedema as part of a generalised anaphylactic reaction, or local swelling from a sting in the mouth or neck. The time from sting to asphyxial collapse may be a useful guide: allergic fatalities with raised mast cell tryptase have generally caused collapse within 30 minutes, whereas non-allergic swelling has commonly taken over 45 minutes (Mosbech, 1983).

Some deaths following massive bee sting envenomation resulting from swarm attacks may show features of anaphylaxis, with massive histamine release and shock, but do not involve an allergic mechanism. Venom contains vasoactive amines, melittin protein that hydrolyses cell membranes causing histamine release, and peptide 401 that triggers mast cell degranulation. The number of stings required to cause death without an allergic component is high – more than 500 stings in adults (Franca *et al.*, 1994; Vetter and Visscher, 1998). Severe reac-

tions to stings have also been associated with raised resting mast cell tryptase levels, and some patients with anaphylaxis have been found to have frank mastocytosis (Haeberli *et al.*, 2003; Brockow *et al.*, 2008).

Fatal amniotic fluid embolism shows some features of anaphylaxis, with elevated tryptase levels in post-mortem blood and increased numbers of pulmonary mast cells being reported (Fineschi *et al.*, 1998; Nishio *et al.*, 2002). It is likely, however, that other non-allergic mechanisms contribute to death, including complement activation (Nishio *et al.*, 2002).

Uncommon causes of fatal anaphylaxis

The range of agents that can cause anaphylaxis is vast, but reports of fatal reactions have attributed the reaction to a more limited list (Table 17.4).

When an agent not previously reported to cause anaphylaxis is implicated in the death, the diagnosis should be approached with caution. Occasionally deaths have been certified as due to anaphylaxis when some alternative explanation seems more likely. For example, following an intravenous injection of chlorpromazine, a 55-year-old woman with a history of brittle asthma and panic attacks devel-

Table 17.4 Uncommon causes of fatal anaphylaxis

Allergen	Availability of specific IgE	Reports
Latex	Routine	Ownby *et al.*, 1991 Martinez Jabaloyas *et al.*, 1995
Echinococcus (hydatid cyst rupture)	Available	Lande *et al.*, 1942
Camomile (enema)	nga	Jensen-Jarolim *et al.*, 1998
Mould in food	nga	Bennett and Collins, 2001
p-Phenylenediamine (hair dye)	nga	Belton and Chira, 1997
Platinum salts	nga	Zweizig *et al.*, 1994
Fluorescein (angiography)	nga	Fineschi *et al.*, 1999 Hitosugi *et al.*, 2004
Chymopapain (chemonucleolysis)	Available	Nordby *et al.*, 1996
Intravenous iron dextran	nga	Bailie *et al.*, 2005
Insulin	nga	Kaya *et al.*, 2007
Skin testing	Available	Blanton and Sutphin, 1949 Lockey *et al.*, 1987
Immunotherapy	Available	Lockey *et al.*, 1987

nga, not generally available.

oped progressive shock and died after 3 hours. There was no wheeze, rash, swelling or any other feature that might suggest an anaphylactic reaction; at autopsy there were no specific findings and death was certified as due to anaphylaxis (Pumphrey: unpublished data from the UK fatal anaphylaxis register). Chlorpromazine has never been recognised as a cause of an anaphylactic reaction, but it regularly causes cardiovascular side-effects that could explain the course of events in this case.

Was death due to the reaction or its treatment?

Epinephrine (adrenaline) is a potent hormone that has proved dangerous in overdose. Over-rapid intravenous administration may be fatal (Pumphrey, 2000). Doses as small as 1 mg, given as a bolus, have caused severe adverse reactions with permanent after-effects. When this has happened during the treatment of anaphylactic reactions, it has been possible to blame the injury on anaphylaxis rather than its treatment. There are also instances when bolus intravenous administration of epinephrine was given accidentally to patients with no anaphylactic symptoms. Adverse effects have been the same as during treatment of anaphylactic reactions, suggesting that the injury was due to the epinephrine. Doses over 1 mg have been followed by pulmonary oedema that, in some cases, was interpreted as a symptom of anaphylaxis, and more epinephrine given. Doses of 1–3.5 mg given as an intravenous bolus have caused fatal pulmonary oedema (Pumphrey, 2000).

Intravenous fluids are commonly given to patients with anaphylactic shock. Rare instances have been recorded where the patient has died from pulmonary oedema and analysis of the events leading up to the death suggest that fluid overload, probably in conjunction with epinephrine overdose, caused the pulmonary oedema (Pumphrey, 2000).

Intravenous hydrocortisone frequently causes unpleasant side-effects. Case reports of allergic reactions to steroids have recently been reviewed (Kamm and Hagmayer, 1999). Occasionally adverse effects following intravenous hydrocortisone have proved fatal: in one case studied by the authors the patient died following hypotension that became severe after an intravenous injection of hydrocortisone.

Conclusion

Sometimes acute allergic deaths will lead to specific macroscopic or microscopic findings at autopsy. In these cases, identifying the probable allergen and including this information with the certified cause of death will be helpful for those seeking to improve the management of allergic disease. Other acute allergic deaths – particularly those where death occurred rapidly or where resuscitation allowed any specific changes associated with the allergic reaction to resolve – may leave no reaction-specific visible change to find at autopsy. It is essential in such cases to be aware of the possibility of anaphylaxis and to study the clinical records carefully for clues about the cause of the reaction. Blood tests, preferably on samples from the time of the reaction, may help understand what happened.

References

Agostoni A, Cicardi M, Cugno M et al. (1999). Angioedema due to angiotensin-converting enzyme inhibitors. *Immunopharmacology* **44**:21–5.

Ameno S, Ameno K, Fuke C et al. (1993). *Hymenoptera* sting anaphylaxis: detection and clinical significance of individual bee and wasp venoms specific IgE and IgG4 antibodies. *Jap J Legal Med* **47**:207–12.

Ansari MQ, Zamora JL, Lipscomb MF (1993). Postmortem diagnosis of acute anaphylaxis by serum tryptase analysis: a case report. *Am J Clin Pathol* **99**:101–3.

Assem ES, Ling YB (1988). Fatal anaphylactic reaction to suxamethonium: new screening test suggests possible prevention. *Anaesthesia* **43**:958–61.

Bailie GR, Clark JA, Lane CE, Lane PL (2005). Hypersensitivity reactions and deaths associated with intravenous iron preparations. *Nephrol Dial Transplant* **20**:1443–9.

Barnard JH (1967). Allergic and pathologic findings in fifty insect-sting fatalities. *J Allergy* **40**:107–14.

Barnard JH (1973). Studies of 400 *Hymenoptera* stings in the United States. *J Allergy Clin Immunol* **52**:259–64.

Belton AL, Chira T (1997). Fatal reaction to hair dye. *Am J Forensic Med Pathol* **18**:290–2.

Bennett AT, Collins KA (2001). An unusual case of anaphylaxis: mold in pancake mix. *Am J Forensic Med Pathol* **22**:292–5.

Blanton WB, Sutphin AK (1949). Death during skin testing. *Am J Med Sci* **217**:169–73.

Bosso JV, Schwartz LB, Stevenson DD (1991). Tryptase and histamine release during aspirin-induced respiratory reactions. *J Allergy Clin Immunol* **88**:830–7.

Boyd GK (1989). Fatal nut anaphylaxis in a 16-year-old male: case report. *Allergy Proc* **10**:255–7.

Brockow K, Vieluf D, Püschel K, Grosch J, Ring J (1999). Increased postmortem serum mast cell tryptase in a fatal anaphylactoid reaction to nonionic radiocontrast medium. *J Allergy Clin Immunol* **104**:237–8.

Brockow K, Jofer C, Behrendt H, Ring J (2008). Anaphylaxis in patients with mastocytosis: a study on history, clinical features and risk factors in 120 patients. *Allergy* **63**:226–32.

Delage C, Irey NS (1972). Anaphylactic deaths: a clinicopathologic study of 43 cases. *J Forensic Sci* **17**:525–40.

Edston E, van Hage Hamsten M (1995). Immunoglobulin E, mast cell-specific tryptase and the complement system in sudden death from coronary artery thrombosis. *Int J Cardiol* **52**:77–81.

Edston E, van Hage-Hamsten M (1998). Beta-tryptase measurements post-mortem in anaphylactic deaths and in controls. *Forensic Sci Int* **93**:135–42.

Edston E, van Hage-Hamsten M (2003). Death in anaphylaxis in a man with house dust mite allergy. *Int J Legal Med* **117**:299–301.

Edston E, Eriksson O, van Hage M (2007). Mast cell tryptase in postmortem serum: reference values and confounders. *Int J Legal Med* **121**:275–80.

Eloy R, Corot C, Belleville J (1991). Contrast media for angiography: physicochemical properties, pharmokinetics and biocompatibility. *Clin Mater* **7**:89–97.

Fernandez J, Rodes F, Marti J, Blanca M (1992). Wasp sting anaphylaxis as a cause of death: a case report. *Allergol Immunopathol Madr* **20**:40–1.

Fineschi V, Gambassi R, Gherardi M, Turillazzi E (1998). The diagnosis of amniotic fluid embolism: an immunohistochemical study for the quantification of pulmonary mast cell tryptase. *Int J Legal Med* **111**:238–43.

Fineschi V, Monasterolo G, Rosi R, Turillazzi E (1999). Fatal anaphylactic shock during fluorescine angiography. *Forensic Sci Int* **100**:137–42.

Finkelman FD (2007). Anaphylaxis: lessons from mouse models. *J Allergy Clin Immunol* **120**:506–15.

Fisher MM, Baldo BA (1998). Mast cell tryptase in anaesthetic anaphylactoid reactions. *Br J Anaesth* **80**:26–9.

Fisher MM, Baldo BA, Silbert BS (1991). Anaphylaxis during anesthesia: use of radioimmunoassays to determine etiology and drugs responsible in fatal cases. *Anesthesiology* **75**:1112–15.

Franca FOS, Benvenuti LA, Fan HW *et al.* (1994). Severe and fatal mass attacks by 'killer' bees (Africanised honey bees – *Apis mellifera scutellata*) in Brazil: clinicopathological studies with measurement of serum venom concentrations. *Q J Med* **87**:269–82.

Golden DBK (2007). Insect sting anaphylaxis. *Immunol Allergy Clin North Am* **27**:261–72.

Greenberger PA, Rotskoff BD, Lifschultz B (2007). Fatal anaphylaxis: post-mortem findings and associated comorbid diseases. *Ann Allergy Asthma Immunol* **98**:252–7.

Gueant JL, Amoine Gastin I, Namour F *et al.* (1998). Diagnosis and pathogenisis of the anaphylactic and anaphylactoid reactions to anaesthetics. *Clin Exp Allergy* **28**(Suppl. 4):655–70.

Haeberli G, Brönnimann M, Hunziker T, Müller U (2003). Elevated basal serum tryptase and hymenoptera venom allergy: relation to severity of sting reactions and to safety and efficacy of venom immunotherapy. *Clin Exp Allergy* **33**:1216–20.

Herbert FA, Salkie ML (1982). Sensitivity to *Hymenoptera* in adult males. *Ann Allergy* **48**:12–13.

Hitosugi M, Omura K, Yokoyama T *et al.* (2004). An autopsy case of fatal anaphylactic shock following fluorescein angiography: a case report. *Med Sci Law* **44**:264–5.

Hoffman DR, Wood CL, Hudson P (1983). Demonstration of IgE and IgG antibodies against venoms in the blood of victims of fatal sting anaphylaxis. *J Allergy Clin Immunol* **71**:193–6

Hoffman DR, Hudson P, Carlyle SJ, Massello W (1989). Three cases of fatal anaphylaxis to antibiotics in patients with prior histories of allergy to the drug. *Ann Allergy* **62**:91–3.

Hoffmeister HM, Heller W (1996). Radiographic contrast media and the coagulation and complement systems. *Invest Radiol* **31**:591–5.

Hogan AD, Schwartz LB (1997). Markers of mast cell degranulation. *Methods* **13**:43–52.

Holgate ST, Walters C, Walls AF *et al.* (1994). The anaphylaxis hypothesis of sudden infant death syndrome (SIDS): mast cell degranulation in cot death revealed by elevated concentrations of tryptase in serum. *Clin Exp Allergy* **24**:1115–22.

Idee JM, Pines E, Prigent P, Corot C (2005). Allergy-like reactions to iodinated contrast agents: a critical analysis. *Fund Clin Pharmacol* **19**:263–81.

James LP, Austen KF (1964). Fatal systemic anaphylaxis in man. *N Engl J Med* **270**:597–603.

Jensen-Jarolim E, Reider N, Fritsch R, Breiteneder H (1998). Fatal outcome of anaphylaxis to camomile-containing enema during labour: a case study. *J Allergy Clin Immunol* **102**:1041–2.

Kamm GL, Hagmayer KO (1999). Allergic-type reactions to corticosteroids. *Ann Pharmacother* **33**:451–60.

Kaya A, Gungor K, Karakose S (2007). Severe anaphylactic reaction to human insulin in a diabetic patient. *J Diabetes Complic* **21**:124–7.

Kishimoto TK, Viswanathan K, Ganguly T *et al.* (2008). Contaminated heparin associated with adverse clinical events and activation of the contact system. *N Engl J Med* **358**:2457–67.

Lamade WR, Friedl W, Schmid B, Meeder PJ (1995). Bone cement implantation syndrome: a prospective randomised trial for use of antihistamine blockade. *Arch Orthop Trauma Surg* **114**:335–59.

Lande P, Courbin J, Dervillée P (1942). Sudden death of football player during game: intraperitoneal rupture of hydatid cyst of liver causing fatal anaphylactic shock revealed at autopsy. *J Med Bordeaux* **119**:580–3.

Lantner R, Reisman RE (1989). Clinical and immunologic features and subsequent course of patients with severe insect-sting anaphylaxis. *J Allergy Clin Immunol* **84**:900–6.

Laroche D, Aimoine-Gastin I, Dubois F *et al.* (1998). Mechanisms of severe, immediate reactions to iodinated contrast material. *Radiology* **209**:183–90.

Leff JA (1998). Leukotriene modifiers as novel therapeutics in asthma. *Clin Exp Allergy* **28**:147–53.

Ljungström KG, Revenäs B, Smedegård G *et al.* (1988). Histopathological lung changes in immune complex mediated anaphylactic shock in humans elicited by dextran. *Forensic Sci Int* **38**:251–8.

Lockey RF, Benedict LM, Turkeltaub PC, Bukantz SC (1987). Fatalities from immunotherapy and skin testing. *J Allergy Clin Immunol* **79**:660–7.

Low I, Stables S (2006). Anaphylactic deaths in Auckland, New Zealand: a review of coronial autopsies from 1985 to 2005. *Pathology* **38**:328–32.

Lund H, Hunt EL (1941). Postmortem diagnosis of allergic shock: the value of the Prausnitz–Küstner reaction. *Arch Pathol* **32**:664–9.

Martinez Jabaloyas JM, Broseta Rico E, Ruiz Cerda JL *et al.* (1995). Extracorporeal shockwave lithotripsy in patients with urinary diversion. *Acta Urol Esp* **19**:143–7.

Mikkonen R, Lehto T, Koistinen V *et al.* (1997). Suppression of alternative complement pathway activity by radiographic contrast media. *Scand J Immunol* **45**:371–7.

Morcos SK (2005). Acute serious and fatal reactions to contrast media: our current understanding. *Br J Radiol* **78**:686–93.

Mosbech H (1983). Death caused by wasp and bee stings in Denmark 1960–1980. *Allergy* **38**:195–200.

Mueller UR (2007). Cardiovascular disease and anaphylaxis. *Curr Opin Allergy Clin Immunol* **7**:337–41.

Nishio H, Matsui K, Miyazaki T *et al.* (2002). A fatal case of amniotic fluid embolism with elevation of serum mast cell tryptase. *Forensic Sci Int* **126**:53–6.

Nordby EJ, Fraser RD, Javid MJ (1996). Chemonucleolysis. *Spine* **21**:1102–5.

Ordoqui E, Zubeldia JM, Aranzabal A *et al.* (1997). Serum tryptase levels in adverse drug reactions. *Allergy* **52**:1102–5.

O'Sullivan S, Roquet A, Dahlen B, Dahlen S, Kumlin M (1998). Urinary excretion of inflammatory mediators during allergen-induced early and late phase asthmatic reactions. *Clin Exp Allergy* **28**:1332–9.

Ownby DR, Tomlanovich-M, Sammons-N, McCullough J (1991). Anaphylaxis associated with latex allergy during barium enema examinations. *Am J Roentgenol* **156**:903–8.

Parrish HM (1963). Analysis of 460 fatalities from venomous animals in the United States. *Am J Med Sci* **245**:129–41.

Perskvist N, Edston E (2007). Differential accumulation of pulmonary and cardiac mast cell-subsets and eosinophils between fatal anaphylaxis and asthma death: a post-mortem comparative study. *Forensic Sci Int* **169**:43–9.

Prahlow JA, Barnard JJ (1998). Fatal anaphylaxis due to fire ant stings. *Am J Forensic Med Pathol* **19**:137–42.

Pumphrey RS (2000). Lessons for management of anaphylaxis from a study of fatal reactions. *Clin Exp Allergy* **30**:1144–50.

Pumphrey RS (2004). Anaphylaxis: can we tell who is at risk of a fatal reaction? *Curr Opin Allergy Clin Immunol* **4**:285–90.

Pumphrey RS, Davis S (1999). Under-reporting of antibiotic anaphylaxis may put patients at risk [letter]. *Lancet* **353**:1157–8.

Pumphrey RS, Gowland MH (2007). Further fatal allergic reactions to food in the United Kingdom, 1999–2006. *J Allergy Clin Immunol* **119**:1018–19.

Pumphrey RS, Nicholls JM (2000). Epinephrine-resistant anaphylaxis. *Lancet* **355**:1099.

Pumphrey RSH, Roberts ISD (2000). Autopsy findings following fatal anaphylactic reactions. *J Clin Pathol* **53**:273–6.

Rainbow J, Browne GJ (2002). Fatal asthma or anaphylaxis? *Emerg Med J* **19**:415–17.

Randall B, Butts J, Halsey JF (1995). Elevated postmortem tryptase in the absence of anaphylaxis. *J Forensic Sci* **40**:208–11.

Renz CL, Laroche D, Thurn JD et al. (1998). Tryptase levels are not increased during vancomycin-induced anaphylactoid reactions. *Anaesthesiology* **89**:620–5.

Riches KJ, Gillis D, James RA (2002). An autopsy approach to bee sting-related deaths. *Pathology* **34**:257–62.

Roberts ISD, Pumphrey RSH (2001). The autopsy and fatal anaphylaxis. In: *Recent Advances in Histopathology*, Vol. 19. Edinburgh: Churchill Livingstone.

Royal College of Pathologists (2005). www.rcpath.org/resources/pdf/autopsyscenario4jan05.pdf.

Salkie ML, Mitchell I, Revers CW et al. (1998). Postmortem serum levels of tryptase and total and specific IgE in fatal asthma. *Allergy Asthma Proc* **19**:131–3.

Schöpf P, Ruëff F, Ludolph-Hauser D, Przybilla B (2000). Aspirin-dependent food allergy. *J Allergy Clin Immunol* **105**:S146 (abstract 444).

Schwartz HJ, Yunginger JW, Teigland JD et al. (1984). Sudden death due to stinging insect hypersensitivity: postmortem demonstration of IgE antivenom antibodies in a fatal case. *Am J Clin Pathol* **81**:794–5.

Schwartz HJ, Squillace DL, Sher TH et al. (1986). Studies in stinging insect hypersensitivity: postmortem demonstration of antivenom IgE antibody in possible sting-related sudden death. *Am J Clin Pathol* **85**:607–10.

Schwartz HJ, Sutheimer C, Gauerke MB, Yunginger JW (1988). Hymenoptera venom-specific IgE antibodies in post-mortem sera from victims of sudden, unexpected death. *Clin Allergy* **18**:461–8.

Schwartz LB (1990). Tryptase, a mediator of human mast cells. *J Allergy Clin Immunol* **86**:594–8.

Schwartz LB, Yunginger JW, Miller J et al. (1989). Time course of appearance and disappearance of human mast cell tryptase in the circulation after anaphylaxis. *J Clin Invest* **83**:1551–5.

Schwartz LB, Bradford TR, Rouse C et al. (1994). Development of a new, more sensitive immunoassay for human tryptase: use in systemic anaphylaxis. *J Clin Immunol* **14**:190–204.

Schwartz LB, Sakai K, Bradford TR et al. (1995). The alpha form of human tryptase is the predominant type present in blood at baseline in normal subjects and is elevated in those with systemic mastocytosis. *J Clin Invest* **96**:2702–10.

Sharath MD, Metzger WJ, Richerson HB et al. (1985). Protamine-induced fatal anaphylaxis: prevalence of antiprotamine immunoglobulin E antibody. *J Thorac Cardiovasc Surg* **90**:86–90.

Sidebotham HJ, Roche WR (2003). Asthma deaths; persistent and preventable mortality. *Histopathology* **43**:105–17.

Simons FER (2008). Anaphylaxis. *J Allergy Clin Immunol* **121**:S402–7.

Szczeklik A, Stevenson DD (1999). Aspirin-induced asthma: advances in pathogenesis and management. *J Allergy Clin Immunol* **104**:5–13.

Vetter RS, Visscher PK (1998). Bites and stings of medically important venomous arthropods. *Int J Dermatol* **37**:481–96.

Wagdi P, Mehan VK, Bürgi H, Salzmann C (1994). Acute myocardial infarction after wasp stings in a patient with normal coronary arteries. *Am Heart J* **128**:821–3.

Watkins J, Clark A, Appleyard TN, Padfield A (1976). Immune mediated reactions to althesin (alphaxolone). *Br J Anaesth* **48**:881–6.

Westaby S, Dawson P, Turner MW, Pridie RB (1985). Angiography and complement activation: evidence for generation of C3a anaphylatoxin by intravenous contrast agents. *Cardiovasc Res* **19**:85–8.

White MV (1990). The role of histamine in allergic diseases. *J Allergy Clin Immunol* **86**:599–605.

Yunginger JW, Sweeny KG, Sturner WQ *et al.* (1988). Fatal food-induced anaphylaxis. *JAMA* **260**:1450–2.

Yunginger JW, Nelson DR, Squillace DL *et al.* (1991). Laboratory investigation of deaths due to anaphylaxis. *J Forensic Sci* **36**:857–65.

Zhu D, Becker WM, Schulz KH, Schubeler K, Schlaak M (1992). The presence of specific IgE to salicyloyl and O-methylsalycoyl in aspirin sensitive patients. *Aspin Pacific J Allergy Immunol* **10**:25–32.

Zora JA, Swanson MC, Yunginger JW (1984). How common is unrecognized *Hymenoptera* venom allergy in the general population? *J Allergy Clin Immunol* **73**:139 (abstract).

Zweizig S, Roman LD, Muderspach LI (1994). Death from anaphylaxis to cisplatin: a case report. *Gynecol Oncol* **53**:121–2.

Chapter 18

PERIOPERATIVE AND POSTOPERATIVE DEATHS

Julian L Burton

Introduction

The autopsy examination of a patient who has died during an operative procedure or while recovering from one poses its own specific set of challenges. As for any autopsy, the pathologist called to undertake the examination must be satisfied that he or she will be competent to complete it. In addition, the pathologist should ideally be independent of the hospital and team that performed the operation, particularly if the instruction for autopsy comes from a medicolegal authority. This helps to prevent subsequent allegations of collusion between the pathologist and the operating team. Statements from the Coroner's Officer that the relatives of the deceased do not object to the autopsy examination being performed by a pathologist from the hospital in which the surgery took place should be viewed with caution and documented in the autopsy report. Only in exceptional circumstances should the pathologist and surgeon work for the same hospital; for example, when finding another pathologist would unduly delay the examination. The autopsy has a role to play in resolving conflicts between bereaved relatives (who may not believe the medical record) and the clinical team and may support the plaintiff or the surgeon in cases where malpractice is alleged (Juvin *et al.*, 2000).

However, the role of the autopsy in improving clinical practice is not fully appreciated owing to the low rate of autopsy examinations following a post-operative death (NCEPOD, 1992). There is clear regional variation in practice regarding the referral of these deaths to the coroner (NCEPOD, 1998), and the pathologist may have a role to play in encouraging clinicians to request hospital (consent) autopsies in patients dying after surgery where a coronial referral is not indicated (NCEPOD, 1997).

Why do patients die?

Most patients who die during or after surgery die from natural causes (Hickling *et al.*, 2007). Peri- and postoperative deaths may be the result of:

- the disease that brought the patient to the operating theatre (e.g. patients who die from bleeding oesophageal varices during an oesophagogastroduodenoscopy, or the patient who dies during an emergency repair of a ruptured atheromatous abdominal aortic aneurysm);
- a known co-morbidity unrelated to the disease for which the operation is being performed (e.g. a fatal infective exacerbation of chronic obstructive pulmonary disease in a patient undergoing a right hemicolectomy for carcinoma of the caecum);
- an unknown co-morbidity unrelated to the disease for which the operation is being performed (e.g. death due to unrecognised and

previously asymptomatic arrhythmogenic right ventricular cardiomyopathy in a patient undergoing excision of a hepatic cyst (Toh *et al.*, 2004);

- a recognised complication of surgery (e.g. bronchopneumonia or a pulmonary thromboembolism in a patient with reduced mobility following the elective replacement of a femoral head);
- a rare but avoidable surgical mishap (e.g. accidental trauma or ligation of major vessels, failure to remove all instruments from the body at the end of the operation, or failure to create a complete anastomosis);
- an anaesthetic event (e.g. an adverse drug reaction, prolonged hypoxia, or malignant hyperpyrexia);
- a hospital-acquired infection (e.g. meticillin-resistant *Staphylococcus aureus* or *Clostridium difficile*).

In a retrospective study of all 7379 operations performed in the main operating theatre at the University of Virginia Health Services Center in a 6-month period in 1999, Calland *et al.* (2002) found a patient death rate of 1.9 per cent. Procedures performed in the endoscopy suite, obstetrics operating theatres and the ambulatory surgery centre were excluded from the study. Of the 119 deaths, 72.3 per cent were attributed to the underlying natural disease and 19.3 per cent were considered suspicious of an adverse event, of which haemorrhage, infection, cardiovascular complications and stroke were the most common. In total, 12.6 per cent of the deaths (0.24 per cent of the surgical population) were deemed to be due to an error in care and potentially avoidable, and two patients died as a result of multiple errors. Errors associated with death occurred most often in the operating theatre and less commonly in the patient's room and the intensive care unit. It is likely that these data underestimate the true incidence of operative errors. The study was retrospective and, notably, makes no mention of autopsy findings.

As one might expect, postoperative mortality rates are higher in those undergoing emergency rather than elective surgery, presumably because the clinical condition of patients requiring emergency surgery is poorer (Seagroatt and Goldacre, 1994; Calland *et al.*, 2002). Death is also a more likely outcome when the patients are older than 70 years, have high American Society of Anesthesiologists (ASA) scores, and when surgery is performed at night or at the weekend (Calland *et al.*, 2002). This is worrying, given that the age of patients exposed to emergency surgery is rising and their preoperative condition is deteriorating (NCEPOD, 2001).

Curiously, the risk of death in the 90–364 days after an elective hip arthroplasty is lower than for the general population. This is likely to be a result of the selection criteria applied when scheduling patients for elective surgery. Cataract surgery also has a low standardised mortality ratio in the 30 days following surgery, but this effect is rapidly lost thereafter (Seagroatt and Goldacre, 1994). Five per cent of individuals undergoing cataract surgery are dead within a year, but this is comparable to the background population (Seagroatt and Goldacre, 1994). In contrast, there is a significant short-term rise in mortality among patients undergoing prostatectomy, cholecystectomy or hysterectomy, due either to the operative procedure or to the underlying disease (Lubitz *et al.*, 1985; Loft *et al.*, 1991; Seagroatt and Goldacre, 1994).

Although they are common procedures, surgery for squint correction, varicose veins, removal of the tonsils and adenoids, laminectomy, myringotomy, submucous resection of the nasal septum, vasectomy, female sterilisation, meniscectomy and termination of pregnancy have very low associated mortality rates. Seagroatt and Goldacre (1994) found no deaths in the 30 days following these surgeries. Consequently, they are not considered further in this chapter.

Autopsies are not performed on every patient who dies during or after surgery. The National Confidential Enquiry into Perioperative Deaths (NCEPOD) – later renamed the National Confidential Enquiry into Patient Outcome and Death – observed in 2001 that the autopsy rate had remained constant for these cases at 31 per cent, and that 95 per cent of such examinations were performed on the instruction of a medicolegal authority

(NCEPOD, 2001). NCEPOD reported that the overall autopsy rate in 1996/97 was 28 per cent (NCEPOD, 1998). Pathologists have been repeatedly criticised for the quality of the reports generated in perioperative and postoperative deaths. Common deficiencies are summarised in Box 18.1.

The procedures undertaken in a peri/postoperative death autopsy are broadly the same as those used in all examinations and are described in Chapters 8, 9, 10 and 11. This chapter deals with the specific considerations that arise following peri- and postoperative deaths. After a consideration of the general issues, deaths related to cardiovascular, thoracic, gastrointestinal, endoscopic, hepatic and pancreatobiliary and orthopaedic surgery are discussed.

Approaching the perioperative and postoperative autopsy

Clinical history

A detailed review of the deceased's clinical history is essential before examining the body. A short coroner's officer's report stating 'Died after a total hip replacement' is not sufficient and the pathologist must insist on access to the hospital records before proceeding (Suvarna, 2008). Careful attention should be paid to the (pre-) admission clerking, the operation note, the anaesthetic record, the medical and surgical notes and the nursing notes. If the deceased spent time in the intensive care unit, those notes (often kept in the department) must also be reviewed, if necessary with the help of an anaesthetist.

The dates on which drugs were prescribed, especially antibiotics and anticoagulants, are often of relevance and should be noted. Where tissue has been removed this should be either examined by the autopsying pathologist or the histopathology report of the specimen(s) reviewed. The pathologist should also ensure that he or she has all the results of any microbiological, biochemical or haematological investigations that were undertaken in life.

External examination

The external examination must be performed by the pathologist before the body is opened. NCEPOD has been critical of the fact that in 32 per cent of mortuaries surveyed it was not the standard practice for bodies to be examined by pathologists prior to evisceration (NCEPOD, 2006). Standard operating procedures should be in place to ensure that the bodies of all those who die following medical or surgical intervention are transported to the mortuary with all medical devices, including cannulae, catheters and drains, *in situ*. If the patient was ventilated via an endotracheal tube and the relatives wish to view the body prior to the autopsy, it is acceptable for the proximal portion of the tube to be removed and the remainder pushed into the mouth. The tube should then be left *in situ* to be examined by the pathologist. The site and nature of all medical devices should be recorded during the external examination.

The operative wound must be inspected and recorded. The location, orientation and length of the wound is noted, as is the state of healing, the method of wound closure (none, staples, sutures, buttress sutures, etc.) and the presence or absence of wound infection.

Initial specimen collection

Before proceeding to the evisceration, consideration is given to the collection of specimens, particularly for microbiological examination. The author has encountered cases where death was due to septicaemia from an operative wound infection or an infected pressure sore (decubitus ulcer). Wounds and pressure sores can be swabbed at this point for microbiological examination. The site and contents of any surgical drains should be similarly noted. Again, fluid within drains and catheter bags can be retained and submitted for microbiological examination at this point.

Blood should be retained for bacterial culture. This is obtained prior to opening the body, to reduce contamination of the specimen. The anterior neck should be swabbed with alcohol or a povidone iodine-containing antiseptic, which is allowed to dry. Blood is aspirated from the subclavian or jugular vein using a sterile 20 mL syringe and needle, and injected directly into blood culture bottles. The same needle is used to aspirate the blood and inject the culture bottles.

The tips of peripheral and central vascular access lines and of drains can be sent for culture in sterile universal containers, provided these have never contained formalin.

Evisceration

The body is eviscerated as described in Chapter 10. In the author's opinion, the evisceration of patients dying during or after surgery should never be delegated to an anatomical pathology technologist. Surgical anastamoses can be fragile and are easily damaged, producing severe problems with their interpretation.

The evisceration must include an assessment for the presence or absence of a pneumothorax (see Chapter 10), as this is a known complication of mechanical ventilation. In patients dying after abdominal surgery, consideration should be given to dissection of the anterior abdominal wall in layers, looking for haematomas and collections of pus. The author has dealt with cases where both of these were present and of relevance. If found, collections of pus must be sampled for microbiological examination.

Having opened the body cavities, all of the internal organs must be carefully inspected *in situ*. The presence or absence of abnormal collections of blood, effusions or pus in the pleural cavity, peritoneal cavity, paracolic gutters, subphrenic spaces and

pelvis is recorded. Failure to examine the paracolic gutters and subphrenic spaces at this point can result in significant collections being missed.

Any and all surgical anastamoses should now be examined prior to the removal of any of the internal organs. Anastomoses are fragile, especially if the interval between surgery and death was short, and these must be handled gently and with care. Anastamoses in blood vessels and the intestines are especially delicate. The surgeon and the coroner will want to know whether the anastamoses were patent and intact, and whether or not there were any associated leaks or tears.

Once any anastamoses have been examined, the placement of any devices should be noted. What devices are present, have they been correctly placed, and is there any associated organ damage?

Toxicology

Consideration of the need to retain samples for toxicological examination should be made before the internal organs are removed. Samples of blood and urine may be useful. In cases where the anaesthetic is suspected to be responsible for death, a lung may be removed and sealed in a nylon bag for gas analysis (see Chapter 15).

Dissection of the internal organs

When the organs have been examined carefully *in situ* and removed, they can be dissected as for any autopsy (see Chapter 11). Particular attention must be paid to the operative site, and a detailed account of this will be required in the autopsy report (see Chapter 23). Even if a cause of death is apparent in the torso, the brain should be examined (NCEPOD, 2006).

Further sampling

Deaths that occur during an operative procedure or the subsequent recovery period may generate complaints from relatives that ultimately result in civil or criminal legal proceedings against the clinician or the institution where the procedure was performed. It behoves the pathologist to exclude natural diseases

Table 18.1 Post-mortem samples to be retained[a]

Investigation	Organ or tissue	Comments
Histopathology	Brain	One block each of cerebellum, hippocampus and watershed cerebral cortex, to look for hypoxic damage
	Heart	Blocks of coronary arteries, left ventricular free wall, interventricular septum, right ventricle, atria
	Lungs	At least one block from each lobe
	Liver	One block
	Spleen	One block
	Pancreas	One block
	Kidney	One block, sampling both kidneys
	Any pathological lesion	Representative samples
Toxicology	Blood	Plain and preserved samples, from a peripheral vein
	Urine	Plain and preserved samples
	Gastric contents	Plain sample (record total volume of gastric contents)
	Vitreous	Plain and preserved samples
	(Lung)	Sealed in an impermeable nylon bag
Microbiology	Blood	Aerobic and anaerobic cultures
	Urine	
	Wound swabs	
	Lung tissue	Samples from each lung for bacteriology, looking for nosocomial pneumonia

[a] Samples of the liver and spleen can be combined in one block, or samples of the spleen and pancreas can be combined into one block. In cases where the deceased was the recipient of an organ transplant, that organ should be extensively sampled for histopathological evaluation, looking for disease recurrence and evidence of rejection.

that could account for the death, remembering that in the vast majority of cases the death will be due to a natural disease process rather than the medical or surgical intervention. Even where a natural cause of death is apparent, a thorough autopsy must be performed if the pathologist is not to be criticised.

All the major internal organs must be sampled for histopathological examination (Table 18.1). Any specimen that has been removed and submitted to a histopathological examination should be reviewed and the findings incorporated into the autopsy report.

Photography

Photography is an invaluable tool in peri- and postoperative death autopsies and all mortuaries should have a digital camera available. Modern digital cameras are inexpensive and allow multiple photographs of the operative site and any injuries to be taken and instantly reviewed. A scale should be included. The digital images can easily be annotated to indicate the anatomical orientation of the image and to highlight points of interest. The author has dealt with several cases where such photographs proved essential in the subsequent inquests (and this is particularly the case where the autopsy findings differ from the operative records) and the pathologist should be prepared to bring the photographs, in a sealed envelope, to the inquest.

Formulating the cause of death

The purpose of the autopsy will, in most cases, be to assist a medicolegal authority in determining the cause of death. At the end of the autopsy the pathologist must assimilate the results of the macroscopic examination, histopathology, surgical pathology, toxicology and microbiology into a report as described in Chapter 23.

A detailed discussion of the findings is required, and the cause of death should be formulated in Office of National Statistics (ONS) format. If the operative intervention has had a bearing on the death, this must be indicated in the statement of the cause of death (NCEPOD, 2006). The pathologist should concentrate on reporting the facts of the investigation and remember that it is not his or her role to apportion blame to an individual or institution.

Perioperative and postoperative deaths by operation type

The general considerations outlined above apply to all autopsies performed on patients dying during surgery or during the recovery period. Consideration of every operative procedure is beyond the scope of this chapter, but certain surgical procedures merit further discussion, either because they are common, or because complications are common, or because they pose specific difficulties.

Cardiac and vascular surgery

The autopsy of patients who die following cardiac surgery is a time-consuming process that poses a specific set of challenges and it is recommended that such examinations be performed by pathologists with a specific interest in postoperative pathology (Hickling et al., 2007). Pathologists who do not feel competent to perform these autopsies should request that they be referred to a specialist in cardiac pathology (Suvarna, 2008). The autopsy in such deaths is invaluable and can be expected to reveal findings in 5–10 per cent which, had they been known in life, would have affected management (Hickling et al., 2007) and to change the clinical diagnosis of the cause of death in 15 per cent (Lee et al., 1997). After coronary artery angioplasty, the autopsy reveals pathological findings different from the clinical impression in almost 25 per cent of cases (NCEPOD, 2000). Sadly, not all deaths following cardiac surgery are followed by an autopsy, even when the death is referred to a coroner, and the number of autopsies in patients dying following coronary artery bypass

grafting is declining (NCEPOD, 2008). Lee et al. (1997) report that the overall 30-day mortality rate for patients undergoing cardiac surgery is 4.4 per cent, but that it is much higher (18 per cent) in patients undergoing emergency surgery than in those who have elective procedures (2.6 per cent). There is no significant difference in the risk of postoperative death between men and women undergoing coronary artery bypass grafting (Aldea et al., 1999). Morbidity and mortality meetings (to which the autopsying pathologists are invited) should be held at least monthly (NCEPOD, 2008), although the author notes that he has never been invited to such a meeting, irrespective of whether death was perioperative or long-term postoperative. NCEPOD (2000) recommends that a copy of the autopsy report should always be sent to the clinicians (though this must take into account the appropriate coronial legislation).

Most patients who die during or after cardiac surgery die from cardiac disease (Lee and Gallagher, 1998). The incidence of postoperative complications in patients undergoing coronary artery bypass grafting is 94 per cent (NCEPOD, 2008). Common autopsy findings of significance include coronary artery bypass graft thrombosis, acute myocardial infarction, small bowel infarction, congestion and fatty change in the liver and pulmonary thromboembolus. With the exception of small bowel infarction and liver changes, which are indicative of multi-organ failure and poor perfusion, other abdominal complications are rare (Hickling et al., 2007). Atrial fibrillation is common postoperatively, more so in patients who undergo valvular repair than in those who have coronary artery bypass grafting. The development of atrial fibrillation postoperatively is associated with an increased risk of stroke and death (Gomes da Silva et al., 2004).

Initial dissection of the heart should be kept to a minimum (Lee and Gallagher, 1998). The degree to which the heart is dissected at the time of the autopsy will depend on the experience of the pathologist in many cases. Where the pathologist personally elects to dissect the heart, he or she should do so mindful of the protocols that have been developed for this, and do so in such a way that subsequent examination by a specialist in cardiac pathology, if needed, will not be hampered (Basso *et al.*, 2008; Suvarna, 2008).

The value of histology in these cases cannot be over-emphasised, but it is disappointing to note that it has been reported to be in decline (Lee and Gallagher, 1998; Hickling *et al.*, 2007). A representative slice through the ventricles should be sampled into mapped labelled cassettes as follows: left ventricular free wall (anterior, lateral and posterior), septum (anterior and posterior), right ventricle (anterior, lateral and posterior), atria (left and right), coronary arteries (most severe disease, and any distal graft anastamoses), and any focal lesion. Sampling of the other cardiac tissues including the conduction system may also be indicated. The collection and storage of tissues for future molecular testing is also advisable. Staining with haematoxylin and eosin and a connective tissue stain is standard, and further histochemical stains may be required (Basso *et al.*, 2008; Suvarna, 2008). Coronary arteries containing stents are best removed intact and fixed before being sent to a laboratory able to embed them in resin, and process and section them (Basso *et al.*, 2008; Suvarna, 2008). Retention of the brain for detailed neuropathological examination in patients dying perioperatively may also prove beneficial, and revealed significant pathology in almost 50 per cent of cases (Hickling *et al.*, 2007). Where present, pacemakers should be removed and returned to the local ECG or pacemaker department for testing (Suvarna, 2008).

It has long been known that the outcome of patients undergoing an aortic aneurysm repair is heavily dependent on whether the surgery is an elective or emergency procedure. The mortality rate is 4.0–6.2 per cent for elective surgery and 30–36 per cent for emergency surgery (Lausten and Engell, 1984; NCEPOD, 2005). Overall, the operative mortality rate is 5.6–13.4 per cent (Brady *et al.*, 2000; Kieffer *et al.*, 2008). Poor renal and lung function preoperatively, age greater than 70 years, coronary artery disease, and degenerative arterial disease are strongly associated with an increased risk of death (Brady *et al.*, 2000; Kieffer *et al.*, 2008). Causes of death include multiple organ failure, acute intestinal ischaemia, coagulation disorders, cardiac complications and stroke (Kieffer *et al.*, 2008).

In patients undergoing surgical repair of a dissecting aortic aneurysm, the risk of death from surgical complications is almost as great as the risk of death from rupture, at approximately 23 per cent. The risk of death increases as the number of arteries affected by the dissection and the number of abdominal organs with low CT-enhancement increases (Vernhet *et al.*, 2004).

Non-cardiac thoracic surgery

Lung resection for carcinoma has a postoperative mortality rate of 0.5–3.1 per cent, and this has been declining for the past three decades owing to earlier disease detection and improved patient selection for surgery. The risk of death is greater for men than for women, and increases with more extensive surgery (pneumonectomy versus bilobectomy or lobectomy) but is not related to the tumour type (Damhuis and Schütte, 1996; Watanabe *et al.*, 2004). Lung resection may be complicated by fatal pneumonia, adult respiratory distress syndrome (ARDS), bronchopleural fistula with empyema formation, and cerebrovascular or cardiovascular disease (Watanabe *et al.*, 2004). Pneumonia and ARDS have replaced bronchopleural fistula and empyema as the most common cause of death (Watanabe *et al.*, 2004), but the latter two still occur and are seen in autopsy practice.

Thorascopic pneumoplasty (pneumonoplasty) is a method of lung reduction that is used to provide symptomatic relief to patients with bullous and non-bullous emphysema. The procedure may be complicated by respiratory failure, tension pneumothorax, aspiration pneumonia and myocardial infarction. Overall, the in-hospital mortality rate is 4.1 per cent, the risk of death being greater in men than in women, in patients over the age of 65 years and in patients who require more than 24 hours of mechanical ventilation (Fujita and Barnes, 1996). In patients undergoing a bilateral procedure, the 4-year survival rate is 70 per cent for patients undergoing staged procedures and 81 per cent for those having a simultaneous procedure (Pompeo *et al.*, 2002).

Of all transplantation surgery, lung transplantation offers the greatest risks. Primary graft failure, infections (bacterial and fungal), airway dehiscence and haemorrhage account for most of the early deaths, whereas progressive respiratory failure due to bronchiolitis obliterans and infections account for most deaths in those who survive the initial 30-day post-transplant period (Pietrantoni *et al.*, 2003). A body mass index below the 25th percentile is a risk factor for death in the intensive care unit for those patients who require intensive care for more than 5 days (Plöchl *et al.*, 1996). Pietrantoni *et al.* (2003) observed that 10.5 per cent of patients died in the 30 days following surgery. Patients who survived at least 30 days after surgery but were then readmitted to the medical intensive care unit had a 22 per cent mortality rate, the risk of death being greater where the admission was for emergency treatment. The nature of the underlying disease which necessitated transplantation did not have a significant bearing on mortality rates. Concerns have been raised recently regarding the significance of *Burkholderia* species infections in the deaths of patients who undergo lung transplantation for cystic fibrosis. In general, infection with the different species of this organism has no bearing on mortality. However, patients who undergo lung transplantation because of cystic fibrosis who are infected with non-epidemic strains of *Burkholderia cenocepacia* have a significantly increased mortality rate compared with uninfected patients (Murray *et al.*, 2008). Given these considerations, transplanted lungs should be sampled widely at autopsy for histopathological and microbiological examination. If necessary, the histopathology of the lungs should be reviewed by a pathologist with an interest in pulmonary pathology and transplant rejection.

The author has dealt with one case in which a patient undergoing mediastinoscopy and biopsy of a mass in the superior mediastinum died during the procedure. The deceased was known to have prostate cancer with spinal metastases. Autopsy examination revealed a hard white tumour encasing the brachiocephalic artery. The biopsy procedure had perforated this artery, with resultant uncontrollable fatal haemorrhage. (Histopathological examination confirmed the presence of a metastatic carcinoma of the prostate.)

Endoscopic surgery

The mortality rates for upper and lower gastrointestinal tract endoscopy procedures are low, but these are widely used interventions.

The mortality rate following oesophagogastroduodenoscopy is 0.004–0.009 per cent (Sieg *et al.*, 2001; Thompson *et al.*, 2004) and death is directly due to the endoscopic procedure in 13 per cent of cases (Thompson *et al.*, 2004). The pathologist performing the autopsy in such a case should be aware that the potentially fatal complications include aspiration pneumonia, perforation of the oesophagus, stomach or duodenum, complications associated with sedation, cardiorespiratory complications and pancreatitis. Pancreatitis is a well-documented complication of endoscopic retrograde cholangiopancreatography (ERCP) (Thompson *et al.*, 2004). Death is more likely to occur when the patient has an ASA score of 3–5, when the gut is perforated, during over-sedation without giving oxygen therapy and without cardiac monitoring, when the procedure has been delayed or is performed by a junior endoscopist, and when complications are not recognised promptly (Quine *et al.*, 1994; Thompson *et al.*, 2004).

Percutaneous endoscopic gastrostomies (PEGs, feeding gastrostomies) are widely used to provide nutritional support to patients who are unable to eat, most commonly because of a neurological disorder such as dementia or stroke, but who have a functioning gut. The insertion of a PEG can be complicated by aspiration pneumonia, gastrostomy leakage, haemorrhage, tube migration, oesophageal perforation, wound infection and anaesthetic adverse effects, and the risk of death from these is increased by male sex, older age and diabetes mellitus (Abuksis *et al.*, 2000). The 30-day mortality rate associated with PEGs is greatest when they are inserted into hospitalised inpatients (29 per cent), compared with outpatients (4 per cent) (Abuksis *et al.*, 2000), and it has been recommended that they should not be inserted into patients suffering an acute illness. By multivariate analysis, Smith *et al.* (2000) found that the risk of death in hospitalised patients was increased if the patient was receiving mechanical ventilation, married or receiving dialysis. Each additional year of age adds a 1.9 per cent additional risk of dying following the insertion of a PEG while hospitalised. Patients with dementia also have a higher mortality than other subgroups, with a 54 per cent mortality rate at 1 month and a 90 per cent rate at 1 year (Sanders et al., 2000). It may be that some of the mortality associated with PEGs is due to poor patient selection, but the presence of numerous co-morbidities is also a factor (Stuart et al., 1993, Smith et al., 2000). NCEPOD (2004) considered that 19 per cent of all PEG procedures were futile or not indicated. It is notable that many of the patients dying after PEG insertion do not undergo an autopsy (Sanders et al., 2000).

Colonoscopy can result in death, and this may be due to over-sedation, mismanagement of ischaemic colitis due to traumatic instrumentation, or peritonitis due to perforation (Macrae et al., 1983). In addition, the procedure may be complicated by uncontrollable haemorrhage, septicaemia, pneumoperitoneum, volvulus, and minor complications including thrombophlebitis, abdominal distension and vasovagal episodes (Macrae et al., 1983). The mortality rate is 0.001–0.06 per cent (Macrae et al., 1983; Sieg et al., 2001; Viiala et al., 2003; NCEPOD, 2004).

In its 2004 report on endoscopy practice, NCEPOD noted that only 9 per cent of deaths resulted in an autopsy, the majority on the instruction of a coroner. Of those autopsies, 29 per cent were associated with less-than-satisfactory reports and 44 per cent lacked an adequate clinicopathological correlation. Histology was taken in only 37 per cent of cases and its absence detracted from the autopsy in 24 per cent of cases. The role of the endoscopy and the disease that led to it were understated in the cause of death, and in 34 per cent of cases the cause of death stated by the autopsy pathologist was judged not to reflect the clinicopathological circumstances (NCEPOD, 2004).

Upper gastrointestinal tract surgery

Irrespective of disease stage, oesophagectomy in patients with oesophageal malignancies remains a dangerous procedure, with a postoperative mortality rate of 4.8–14 per cent (Law et al., 2004; Ra et al., 2008). The risk of death is increased when surgery is performed in a hospital performing fewer than 0.67 cases per year, and patients over the age of 80 years have double the odds of dying due to the surgery (Ra et al., 2008). Patients with a poor preoperative physiological status, as measured using various co-morbidity scores, also have an increased risk of postoperative death (Bartels et al., 1998; Ra et al., 2008). The most common surgical complication is anastamotic leakage, but cardiac rhythm disturbances, sepsis and pulmonary complications are also common (Law et al., 2004). Death may be due to anastamotic leakage, cardiac disease (arrhythmias, myocardial infarction etc.), pulmonary complications, stroke, hepatic failure or progression of malignancy. Fatal pulmonary disease is more common when the patient is older than 70 years, has a proximal tumour and/or has a prolonged operation duration (Law et al., 2004). Tumours located behind the trachea are anatomically unfavourable. There is no difference in the complication rates between thoracoscopic and transthoracic operative routes.

Nasopharyngeal tubes are commonly used in both medicine and surgery, either as a route for feeding or to decompress an obstructed gut. Death associated with the insertion of these devices is rare, but misplacement can result in pneumothorax, haemothorax and pneumonia (Agarwal et al., 2002). In addition, it is notable that nasogastric feeding in patients with advanced dementia reduces their survival rate significantly (Alvarez-Fernandez et al., 2005).

A detailed consideration of the various methods that can be employed in a total gastrectomy is beyond the scope of this chapter. Total gastrectomy is associated with a significant postoperative mortality. Fatal complications occur in approximately 6–14 per cent of patients and include dehiscence of the oesophagojejunal anastamosis with subsequent peritonitis, pneumothorax, hepatic necrosis resulting from ligation of the hepatic artery, and perforation of the jejunal loop by a feeding tube (Budišin et al., 2000). Death is more likely in patients aged over 40 years and in those with significant co-morbidities

(Grossmann *et al.*, 2002; Oňate-Ocaňa *et al.*, 2007). The combination of pancreaticosplenectomy with gastrectomy increases the mortality rate (Lo *et al.*, 2002).

Hepatopancreatobiliary surgery

The risk of postoperative death in patients undergoing surgery on the biliary tract is dependent on the extent of the surgery and whether or not the patient was jaundiced preoperatively (Mishra *et al.*, 2007). In patients undergoing a pancreaticoduodenectomy (Whipple's procedure) the postoperative mortality rate is 0–3.8 per cent in centres routinely performing this procedure, but the risk rises to 17.6 per cent in centres rarely performing the procedure (Birkmeyer *et al.*, 2002). Postoperative renal failure and sepsis are highly predictive of postoperative mortality, and other common complications include wound infection, renal failure, pulmonary complications and gastrointestinal haemorrhage (Mishra *et al.*, 2007).

Surgical advances have meant that it has become possible to resect larger quantities of the liver. In addition to complications unrelated to liver dysfunction, patients may die as a result of portal vein thrombosis (which the pathologist should actively seek at autopsy in these cases), bacterial peritonitis, severe sepsis, renal failure or gastrointestinal haemorrhage. Overall, the postoperative mortality rate is approximately 3.5 per cent, but the risk of death increases markedly in patients who have a low prothrombin time, elevated INR or a high serum bilirubin in the early postoperative period. Most deaths occur more than 14 days after the surgery (Balzan *et al.*, 2005).

Lower gastrointestinal tract surgery

Laparotomy, regardless of the indication for it, carries a significant risk of small bowel obstruction as a result of postoperative intraperitoneal adhesions. Approximately 1 per cent of all patients who undergo a laparotomy will develop a small bowel obstruction due to adhesions within the 12 months following surgery, and 3 per cent will develop a small bowel obstruction in the longer term (Duron *et al.*, 2008). These obstructions will frequently require a second

surgical episode in order to resolve them but this surgery is itself not without risk. Duron *et al.* (2008) have reported that 3 per cent of patients undergoing surgery to relieve small bowel obstruction due to adhesions die in the first 30 days after surgery, either as a result of cardiopulmonary complications or as a result of intestinal necrosis. A further 7 per cent died during long-term follow-up, without recurrence of their small bowel obstruction. The risk factors for early death in these patients include age over 75 years and an ASA score of 3 or worse. These two factors also increase the risk for death in the longer term, as do a non-resected intestinal wall injury, mixed strangulation/volvulus and medical complications. The use of a laparoscopic approach does not reduce the early postoperative mortality rate.

The risk of postoperative death in patients undergoing colorectal surgery is dependent on the nature of the disease that necessitated treatment and whether the surgery was an elective or emergency procedure.

For patients undergoing elective colectomy for ulcerative colitis, the postoperative mortality rate is 2.3 per cent but the risk of death rises when the surgery is performed in a hospital where few such operations are performed, and where the surgery is part of an emergency admission (Kaplan *et al.*, 2008). In patients undergoing emergency colectomy, a protracted interval (more than 6 days) between admission and surgery also increases the risk of death (Kaplan *et al.*, 2008).

Patients undergoing colectomy or colorectal surgery for malignancy have a greater risk of postoperative mortality. Overall, the risk of postoperative death is 3.4 per cent and is increased by age older than 70 years, emergency surgery, loss of more than 10 per cent of body weight, and neurological co-morbidity (Alves *et al.*, 2005). However, the mortality rate for patients undergoing emergency colectomy is much higher at 22.1 per cent and is principally due to medical complications, although age over 70 years, male sex, ASA score above 2, palliative outcome, tumour perforation and splenectomy also increase the risk of death (Iversen *et al.*, 2008).

Operative intervention for patients with colorectal carcinoma and unresectable liver metastases at the time of presentation remains controversial, but may be indicated where complications arise due to the primary tumour, such as severe haemorrhage or bowel obstruction. There is a 2.5 per cent risk of death in the 30 days after surgery, rising to 28 per cent at 3 months, principally due to disease progression (Vilbert *et al.*, 2007). The author has dealt with one such case, in which resection of a proximal colonic tumour was abandoned without anastamosis of the bowel owing to a decline in the cardiorespiratory function of the patient during surgery. The colon had perforated by the time the abdomen was opened and death occurred as a result of faecal peritonitis within 24 hours of surgery. Risk factors for 3-month mortality include age greater than 75 years, symptomatic primary disease, rectal cancer and a serum AST concentration above 50 UI/L (Vilbert *et al.*, 2007).

Obstruction of the large intestine is a common surgical emergency, most commonly due to malignancy, diverticulitis or volvulus. The treatment is commonly surgical, with either a right hemicolectomy or some variant of left-sided resection. Most obstructions are due to disease in the sigmoid colon. Overall, the mortality rate of such interventions is approximately 19 per cent, but one-third of patients undergoing a subtotal colectomy and more than half of patients undergoing a Hartmann's procedure die (Biondo *et al.*, 2004). Patients typically die as a result of sepsis, multiple organ failure, cardiorespiratory disease or gastrointestinal haemorrhage. An ASA score greater than 2, age older than 75 years, preoperative renal failure and proximal colon damage are all significant risk factors for postoperative death (Biondo *et al.*, 2004).

Elective anterior resection has a 30-day postoperative mortality rate of 2.1 per cent, but patients who die are more likely to suffer from an anastomotic leak. Multivariate analysis indicates that increased age, male sex, the presence of distant metastases (Dukes' stage D) and intraoperative adverse events are independent risk factors for death within 30 days or before discharge from hospital (Matthiessen *et al.*, 2006). Patients receiving preoperative radiotherapy are at increased risk of postoperative death compared with patients who do not receive radiotherapy,

but the volume of tissue irradiated does not appear to be a risk factor (Holm *et al.*, 1996).

Orthopaedic surgery

Death as a result of orthopaedic surgery is uncommon but there are several well-recognised potentially fatal complications, including deep venous thrombosis with subsequent pulmonary thromboembolism, hypostatic pneumonia, sepsis, and emboli of fat, bone marrow or bone cement.

In patients undergoing an elective total hip replacement, the 90-day postoperative mortality rate is 0.08–0.55 per cent (Seagroatt *et al.*, 1991; Dearborn, 1998; Parvizi *et al.*, 2007; Ayanardi *et al.*, 2009). Deaths during the surgery are rare. Most deaths associated with total hip arthroplasty are due to cardiovascular complications, and the risk of death rises with male sex, increasing age, increasing body mass index, co-morbidities, and simultaneous bilateral hip replacement (Seagroatt *et al.*, 1991; Parvizi *et al.*, 2001; Ayanardi *et al.*, 2009). The risk of death is greater in those undergoing hip arthroplasty for an acute fracture, and Parvizi *et al.* (2004) report a 30-day mortality rate of 2.8 per cent for such cases. However, 58 per cent of patients suffering life-threatening complications had no risk factors. Most fatal complications arise within 4 days of surgery (Parvizi *et al.*, 2007).

The risk of death following total knee arthroplasty is similar to that of a hip arthroplasty (Gill *et al.*, 2003) and, once again, the risk of life-threatening or fatal complications is greater for simultaneous bilateral procedures (Restrepo and Parvizi, 2007).

Upper limb arthroplasty carries a higher risk of death within 90 days of surgery, with 0.58 per cent of patients dying following shoulder arthroplasty and 0.62 per cent dying following elbow arthroplasty (White *et al.*, 2003; Sanchez-Sotelo *et al.*, 2007). As with lower limb arthroplasty, the risk of death increases with increasing age, and is greater where there are pre-existing medical conditions or where surgery is performed because of a fracture.

The risk of embolism of bone marrow and fat is increased when bone cement is used, because the injection of this material raises the intramedullary pressure, particularly in the fixation of long bone fractures. However, a small number of cases of catastrophic fat embolism have been reported following spinal surgery where polymethylmethacrylate cement and/or pedicle screws have been employed (Temple et al., 2002). Embolic strokes have been reported following the injection of polymethylmethacrylate bone cement during a vertebroplasty, with bone cement emboli present in the middle cerebral artery (Marden and Putman, 2008). Multiple cardiac perforations and fatal pulmonary emboli have also been reported following the use of bone cement for percutaneous vertebroplasty (Monticelli et al., 2004; Lim et al., 2008).

The author has dealt with one case in which the internal iliac artery and vein were torn by a rongeur (an instrument with a sharp edge and scoop-shaped tip that is used to gouge out bone or disc pulp) during a hemidiscectomy for sciatica. The resultant haemorrhage proved fatal.

A careful review of the clinical history, paying particular attention to whether or not anticoagulant prophylaxis was prescribed and administered, is needed. Samples of the lungs and brain should be submitted, unfixed, for frozen section and stained with Oil Red O to exclude fat emboli. Bone marrow emboli can be visualised in the lungs on routine haematoxylin and eosin-stained sections but caution is required in their interpretation. The author has, on numerous occasions, seen bone marrow emboli in post-mortem lungs in cases where there was no history of trauma, cardiopulmonary resuscitation or operative intervention, and death was due to an acute myocardial infarction.

The operative site should be opened and examined under direct vision, and samples collected for bacteriological examination.

Transplantation surgery

Irrespective of the organ(s) transplanted, patients who die following transplantation surgery require a thorough autopsy if the cause of death is to be found. This is true irrespective of the interval between surgery and death. In the early postoperative period, death may be due to acute rejection, sepsis, bleeding or other co-morbidities. In the longer term, sepsis, graft rejection and primary disease recurrence will need to be excluded. Obese patients undergoing liver or renal transplants are at increased risk of postoperative death (Nair et al., 2001). The surgical site must be examined in detail macroscopically, checking the competence and patency of all anastamoses. The transplanted organ should be examined histopathologically with multiple blocks, looking for rejection and disease recurrence. Review of these slides by the pathologists in the centre where the transplant was performed can be invaluable as it permits comparison of the tissue with biopsies taken in life. The pathologist performing the autopsy should remain mindful that transplant recipients are often significantly immunosuppressed and the remaining major organs must be sampled sufficiently extensively to allow the detection of opportunistic infections. This should include the collection of samples for microbiology and virology. The author has seen a case where a liver transplant recipient died of a viral myocarditis, presumably contributed to by the immunosuppression.

Conclusions

The autopsy of patients who die during or after surgery remains a valuable procedure which will, not infrequently, yield findings that were unsuspected in life. However, these autopsies are complex and require a degree of expertise. Pathologists performing these autopsies must familiarise themselves with the patient record prior to starting, and should be aware of the common complications of these surgeries. When the pathologist has doubts over his or her competence to complete the case satisfactorily, it should be declined and the instructing medicolegal authority encouraged to refer it to an appropriate specialist. The value of histology and other investigations cannot be over-emphasised, and pathologists have been repeatedly criticised heavily for not taking such samples in these cases.

References

Abuksis G, Mor M, Segal N *et al.* (2000). Percutaneous endoscopic gastrostomy: high mortality rates in hospitalised patients. *Am J Gastroenterol* **95**:128–32.

Agarwal A, Gaur A, Sahu D, Singh P, Pandey CK (2002). Nasogastric tube knotting over the epiglottis: a cause of respiratory distress. *Anesth Analg* **94**:1659–60.

Aldea GS, Gaudiani JM, Shapira OM *et al.* (1999). Effect of gender on postoperative outcomes and hospital stays after coronary artery bypass grafting. *Ann Thorac Surg* **67**:1097–103.

Alvarez-Fernandez B, Garcia-Ordonez MA, Martinez-Manzanares C, Gomez-Huelgas R (2005). Survival of a cohort of elderly patients with advanced dementia: nasogastric tube feeding as a risk factor for mortality. *Int J Geriatr Psychiatry* **20**:363–70.

Alves A, Panis Y, Mathieu P *et al.* on behalf of the Association Francaise de Chirurgue (2005). Postoperative mortality and morbidity in French patients undergoing colorectal surgery: results of a prospective multicenter study. *Arch Surg* **140**:278–83.

Ayanardi M, Pulido L, Parvizi J, Sharkey PF, Rothman RH (2009). Early mortality after modern total hip arthroplasty. *Clin Orthopaed Rel Res* **467**:213–18.

Balzan S, Belghiti J, Farges O *et al.* (2005). The '50–50 criteria' on postoperative day 5: an accurate predictor of liver failure and death after hepatectomy. *Ann Surg* **242**:824–9.

Bartels H, Stein HJ, Siewert JR (1998). Preoperative risk analysis and postoperative mortality of oesophagectomy for resectable oesophageal cancer. *Br J Surg* **85**:840–4.

Basso C, Burke M, Fornes P *et al.* on behalf of the Association for European Cardiovascular Pathology (2008). Guidelines for autopsy investigation of sudden cardiac death. *Virchows Arch* **452**:11–18.

Biondo S, Parés D, Frago R *et al.* (2004). Large bowel obstruction: predictive factors for postoperative mortality. *Dis Colon Rectum* **47**:1889–97.

Birkmeyer JD, Siewers AE, Finlayson EVA *et al.* (2002). Hospital volume and surgical mortality in the United States. *N Engl J Med* **346**:1128–37.

Brady AR, Fowkes FG, Greenhalgh RM *et al.* (2000). Risk factors for postoperative death following elective surgical repair of abdominal aortic aneurysm: results from the UK small aneurysm trial. *Br J Surg* **87**:742–9.

Budišin N, Majdevac I, Breberina M, Gudurić B (2000). Total gastrectomy and its early postoperative complications in gastric cancer. *Arch Oncol* **8**:91–4.

Calland JF, Adams RB, Benjamin DK *et al.* (2002). Thirty-day postoperative death rate at an academic medical centre. *Ann Surg* **235**:690–8.

Damhuis RAM, Schütte PR (1996). Resection rates and postoperative mortality in 7899 patients with lung cancer. *Eur Resp J* **9**:7–10.

Dearborn JT (1998). Postoperative mortality after total hip arthroplasty: an analysis of deaths after 2736 procedures. *J Bone Joint Surg (Am)* **80**:1291–4.

Duron J-J, du Montcel ST, Berger A *et al.* (2008). Prevalence and risk factors of mortality and morbidity after operation for adhesive postoperative small bowel obstruction. *Am J Surg* **195**:726–34.

Fujita RA, Barnes GB (1996). Morbidity and mortality after thoracoscopic pneumonoplasty. *Ann Thorac Surg* **62**:251–7.

Gill GS, Mills D, Joshi AB (2003). Mortality following primary total knee arthroplasty. *J Bone Joint Surg (Am)* **85**:432–5.

Gomes da Silva R, Glotz de Lima G, Laranjeira A *et al.* (2004). Risk factors, morbidity, and mortality associated with atrial fibrillation in the postoperative period of cardiac surgery. *Arq Brasil Cardiol* **83**:105–10.

Grossmann EM, Longo WE, Virgo KS *et al.* (2002). Morbidity and mortality of gastrectomy for cancer in Department of Veterans Affairs Medical Centers. *Surgery* **131**:484–90.

Hickling MF, Pontefract DE, Gallagher PJ, Livesey SA (2007). Post-mortem examinations after cardiac surgery. *Heart* **93**:761–5.

Holm T, Rutqvist LE, Johansson H, Cedermark B (1996). Postoperative mortality in rectal cancer treated with or without preoperative radiotherapy: causes and risk factors. *Br J Surg* **83**:964–8.

Iversen LH, Bulow S, Christensen IJ *et al.* on behalf of the Danish Colorectal Cancer Group (2008). Postoperative medical complications are the main cause of early death after emergency surgery for colonic cancer. *Br J Surg* **95**:1012–19.

Juvin P, Teissière F, Briom F, Desmonts J-M, Durigon M (2000). Postoperative death and malpractice suits: is autopsy useful? *Anesth Analg* **91**:344–6.

Kaplan GG, McCarthy EP, Ayanian JZ *et al.* (2008). Impact of hospital volume on postoperative morbidity and mortality following a colectomy for ulcerative colitis. *Gastroenterology* **134**:680–7.

Kieffer E, Chiche L, Godet G *et al.* (2008). Type IV thoracoabdominal aneurysm repair: predictors of postoperative mortality, spinal cord injury, and acute intestinal ischaemia. *Ann Vasc Surg* **22**:822–8.

Lausten GS, Engell HC (1984). Postoperative complications in abdominal vascular surgery. *Acta Chir Scand* **150**:457–61.

Law S, Wong K-H, Kwok K-F, Chu K-M, Wong J (2004). Predictive factors for postoperative complications and mortality after esophagectomy for cancer. *Ann Surg* **240**:791–800.

Lee AHS, Gallagher PJ (1998). Post-mortem examination after cardiac surgery. *Histopathology* **33**:399–405.

Lee AHS, Borek BT, Gallagher PJ *et al.* (1997). Prospective study of the value of necropsy examination in early death after cardiac surgery. *Heart* **78**:34–8.

Lim SH, Kim H, Kim HK, Baek MJ (2008). Multiple cardiac perforations and pulmonary embolism caused by cement leakage after percutaneous vertebroplasty. *Eur J Cardiothorac Surg* **33**:510–12.

Lo S-S, Wu C-W, Shen K-H, Hsieh M-C, Lui W-Y (2002). Higher morbidity and mortality after combined total gastrectomy and pancreaticosplenectomy for gastric cancer. *World J Surg* **26**:678–82.

Loft A, Anderson TF, Bronnum-Hansen H, Roepstorff C, Madsen M (1991). Early postoperative mortality following hysterectomy: a Danish population-based study, 1977–81. *Br J Obstet Gynaecol* **98**:147–54.

Lubitz J, Riley G, Newton M (1985). Outcomes of surgery among the Medicare aged: mortality after surgery. *Health Care Financ Rev* **6**:103–15.

Macrae FA, Tan KG, Williams CB (1983). Towards safer colonoscopy: a report on the complications of 5000 diagnostic or therapeutic colonoscopies. *Gut* **24**:376–83.

Marden FA, Putman CM (2008). Cement-embolic stroke associated with vertebroplasty. *Am J Neuroradiol* **29**:1986–8.

Matthiessen P, Hallbook O, Rutegard J, Sjodahl R (2006). Population-based study of risk factors for postoperative death after anterior resection of the rectum. *Br J Surg* **93**:498–503.

Mishra D, Bhat P, Rodrigues G, Rao A (2007). Analysis of preoperative risk factors affecting mortality and morbidity in patients after surgery of biliary tract: a retrospective study. *Internet J Surg* **13**(1).

Monticelli F, Meyer HJ, Tutsch-Bauer E (2004). Fatal pulmonary cement embolism following percutaneous vertebroplasty (PVP). *Forensic Sci Int* **149** (1):35–8.

Murray S, Charbeneau J, Marshall BC, LiPuma JJ (2008). Impact of Burkholderia infection on lung transplantation in cystic fibrosis. *Am J Respir Crit Care Med* **178**:363–71.

Nair S, Cohen DB, Cohen C *et al.* (2001). Postoperative morbidity, mortality, costs and long-term survival in severely obese patients undergoing orthotopic liver transplantation. *Am J Gastroenterol* **96**:842–5.

National Confidential Enquiry into Perioperative Deaths (1992). *1990*. London: NCEPOD.

National Confidential Enquiry into Perioperative Deaths (1997). *1994/95*. London: NCEPOD.

National Confidential Enquiry into Perioperative Deaths (1998). *1996/97*. London: NCEPOD.

National Confidential Enquiry into Perioperative Deaths (2000). *Percutaneous Transluminal Coronary Angioplasty*. London: NCEPOD.

National Confidential Enquiry into Perioperative Deaths (2001). *Changing the Way We Operate*. London: NCEPOD.

National Confidential Enquiry into Patient Outcome and Death (2004). *Scoping Our Practice*. London: NCEPOD.

National Confidential Enquiry into Patient Outcome and Death (2005). *Abdominal Aortic Aneurysm: A Service in Need of Surgery?* London: NCEPOD.

National Confidential Enquiry into Patient Outcome and Death (2006). *The Coronery's Autopsy: Do We Deserve Better?* London: NCEPOD.

National Confidential Enquiry into Patient Outcome and Death (2008). *Death Following a First-time, Isolated Coronary Artery Bypass Graft: The Heart of the Matter.* London: NCEPOD.

Oñate-Ocaña LF, Becker M, Aiello-Crocifoglio V *et al.* (2007). Prediction of morbidity after gastrectomy for gastric adenocarcinoma using logistic regression analysis. *BMC Cancer* **7**(suppl 1):A35.

Parvizi J, Johnson BG, Rowland C, Ereth MH, Lewallen DG (2001). Thirty-day mortality after elective total hip arthroplasty. *J Bone Joint Surg (Am)* **83**:1524–8.

Parvizi J, Ereth MH, Lewallen DG (2004). Thirty-day mortality following hip arthroplasty for acute fracture. *J Bone J Surg (Am)* **86**:1983–8

Parvizi J, Mui A, Purtill JJ *et al.* (2007). Total joint arthroplasty: when do fatal or near-fatal complications occur? *J Bone Joint Surg (Am)* **89**:27–32.

Pietrantoni C, Minai OA, Yu NC *et al.* (2003). Respiratory failure and sepsis are the major causes of ICU admissions and mortality in survivors of lung transplants. *Chest* **123**:504–9.

Plöchl W, Pezawas L, Hiesmayr M *et al.* (1996). Nutritional status, ICU duration and ICU mortality in lung transplant recipients. *Intensive Care Med* **22**:1179–85.

Pompeo E, Mineo TC on behalf of the Pulmonary Emphysema Research Group (2002). Long-term outcome of staged versus one-stage bilateral thoracoscopic reduction pneumoplasty. *Eur J Cardiothorac Surg* **21**:627–33.

Quine MA, Bell GD, McCloy RF *et al.* (1994). Prospective audit of upper gastrointestinal endoscopy in two regions of England: safety, staffing, and sedation methods. *Gut* **36**:462–7.

Ra J, Paulson EC, Kucharczuk J *et al.* (2008). Postoperative mortality after esophagectomy for cancer: development of a preoperative risk prediction model. *Ann Surg Oncol* **15**:1577–84.

Restrepo C, Parvizi J (2007). Safety of simultaneous bilateral total knee arthroplasty: a meta-analysis. *J Bone Joint Surg (Am)* **89**:1220–6.

Sanchez-Sotelo J, Sperling JW, Morrey BF (2007). Ninety-day mortality after total elbow arthroplasty. *J Bone Joint Surg (Am)* **89**:1449–51.

Sanders DS, Carter MJ, D'Silva J *et al.* (2000). Survival analysis in percutaneous endoscopic gastrostomy feeding: a worse outcome in patients with dementia. *Am J Gastroenterol* **95**:1472–5.

Seagroatt V, Goldacre M (1994). Measures of early postoperative mortality: beyond hospital fatality rates. *Br Med J* **309**:361–5.

Seagroatt V, Tan HS, Goldacre M *et al.* (1991). Elective total hip replacement: incidence, emergency readmission rate, and postoperative mortality. *Br Med J* **303**:1431–5.

Sieg A, Hachmoeller-Eisenbach U, Eisenbach T (2001). Prospective evaluation of complications in outpatient GI endoscopy: a survey among German gastroenterologists. *Gastrointest Endosc* **53**:620–7.

Smith BM, Perring P, Engoren M, Sferra JJ (2000). Hospital and long-term outcome after percutaneous endoscopic gastrostomy. *Surg Endosc* **22**:74–80.

Stuart SP, Tiley EH, Boland JP (1993). Feeding gastrostomy: a critical review of its indications and mortality rate. *Southern Med J* **86**(2):169–72.

Suvarna SK (2008). National guidelines for adult autopsy cardiac dissection and diagnosis: are they achievable? A personal view. *Histopathology* **53**:97–112.

Temple JD, Ludwig SC, Marshall WK, Larsen L, Gelb DE (2002). Catastrophic fat embolism following augmentation of pedicle screws with bone cement: a case report. *J Bone Joint Surg (Am)* **84**:639–42.

Thompson AM, Wright DJ, Murray W *et al.* (2004). Analysis of 153 deaths after upper gastrointestinal endoscopy: room for improvement? *Surg Endosc* **18**:22–5.

Toh K-W, Nadesan K, Sie MY, Vijeyasingam R, Tan PSK (2004). Postoperative death in a patient with unrecognized arrhythmogenic right ventricular dysplasia syndrome. *Anesth Analg* **99**:350–2.

Vernhet H, Serfaty JM, Serhal M *et al.* (2004). Abdominal CT angiography before surgery as a predictor of postoperative death in acute aortic dissection. *Am J Radiol* **182**:875–9.

Viiala CH, Zimmerman M, Cullen DJE, Hoffman NE (2003). Complication rates of colonoscopy in an Australian teaching hospital environment. *Intern Med J* **33**:355–9.

Vilbert E, Bretagnol F, Alves A *et al.* (2007). Multivariate analysis of predictive factors for early postoperative death after colorectal surgery in patients with colorectal cancer and synchronous unresectable liver metastases. *Dis Colon Rectum* **50**:1776–82.

Watanabe S, Asamura H, Suzuki K, Tsuchiya R (2004). Recent results of postoperative mortality for surgical resections in lung cancer. *Ann Thorac Surg* **78**:999–1003.

White CB, Sperling JW, Cofield RH, Rowland CM (2003). Ninety-day mortality after shoulder arthroplasty. *J Arthroplasty* **18**:886–8.

Chapter 19

THE RADIOLOGICAL AUTOPSY

Amanda J Jeffery and Vimal Raj

Introduction

During the Royal College of Pathologists' National Pathology Week in 2008, the post-mortem examination was described as the ultimate surgical operation. In the past, radiology played a complementary role to the traditional examination. This has changed in the last few decades and radiology now has the potential to be used as an alternative to an autopsy in selected cases. This progression can be attributed to many factors, examples being advances in technology, new innovations in radiology, increasing

Box 19.1 Recognised uses of radiological investigations in post-mortems

- *Identification.* Useful when a body is not identifiable by other means.
- *Firearm death.* Useful where location and retrieval of projectiles is of forensic importance.
- *Child abuse or non-accidental injury.* Skeletal surveys are crucial for the detection of recent and historical skeletal trauma.
- *Barotrauma or suspected air embolism.* Such entities can be difficult to demonstrate at post-mortem.
- *Traumatic subarachnoid haemorrhage.* Contrast angiography is a recognised method for examination of the integrity of the vertebral arteries.
- *Other complex cases* – where the examination and interpretation is compromised by destruction of the body (e.g. fire damage, decomposition, dismemberment, or fragmentation).

numbers of post-mortem examination relative to the numbers of pathologists undertaking them, and ethico-religious considerations. This changing trend, however, is not so apparent in the UK, where the majority of post-mortems do not make use of this valuable adjunct.

The advantages of post-mortem radiology are already recognised in some special circumstances (Box 19.1). In modern practice, it is forensic and paediatric pathologists who primarily undertake post-mortem radiology (Crane, 2000; Kahana and Hiss, 1999). Around the world a few radiologists have also embraced it as a special interest and collaborate with the forensic pathologists for optimal results.

Development of post-mortem radiology in the UK

Post-mortem radiology owes its conception to the two basic discoveries of the x-ray and magnetic resonance imaging (MRI). The humble x-ray has come on leaps and bounds since its discovery in the late nineteenth century and is used in the majority of radiological procedures. In 1994, it was proposed that computerised tomography (CT) may address a declining number of post-mortems that had resulted from increased clinical commitments of pathologists and ethico-religious considerations (Donchin *et al.*, 1994). In 1997, at the request of the local Jewish population, an MRI service was set up in Manchester in the UK as an alternative to the invasive post-mortem procedure.

In the *British Medical Journal*, radiologists reported achieving a confident cause of death in 87 per cent of cases, but the findings were not correlated with the autopsy findings (Bisset *et al.*, 2002). This work highlighted the potential for the development of non-invasive imaging-based post-mortem examinations (Bisset, 1998). Since then, concerns have been raised as to the validity of these suggestions (Swift, 2002). In May 2008, the Manchester experience was communicated to the general public within a local newspaper article entitled 'Body scans instead of post-mortems' (Britton, 2008). In July of the same year, the topic was raised in the House of Commons and the Lord Chancellor and Secretary of State for Justice, Jack Straw, announced that he was in discussion with others regarding rolling out this service to the rest of the UK (Hansard, 2008). As the British government looks to 'roll out' an autopsy imaging service across the country, questions regarding the accuracy of post-mortem radiology in detecting pathology and cause of death remain unanswered.

The radiological hand

Different modalities of radiology available to pathologists can be viewed as the five fingers of a hand (Fig. 19.1). The fingers correspond to x-ray (post-mortem radiography; PMR), computerised tomography (CT), magnetic resonance imaging (MRI), ultrasound (US), and fluoroscopy/angiography. Each individual modality has its own use and limitations; the latter can be overcome when used in conjunction with each other.

Recent advances in technology, especially in the field of CT and MRI, allow visualisation of anatomy and pathology more accurately with the ability to reconstruct images in three-dimensional planes. After a brief look at the other four modalities, this chapter will focus on the role of CT as it is the workhorse in this field and will be used more frequently in future.

Post-mortem radiography

The role of plain-film radiography, although still valuable, is declining. PMR is readily available and does not need the same extensive training in interpretation as CT. PMR can localise metallic foreign bodies and help in assessing skeletal injuries in multiple traumas and non-accidental injury.

Magnetic resonance imaging

In many ways, MRI can be considered as the 'new kid in town' as far as post-mortem radiology is concerned. In ante-mortem clinical practice, MRI can not only demonstrate soft tissue injury but also predict the timing of injury. MRI can also assess the central nervous system in more detail than can CT. MRI, however, has many limitations that restrict its routine use in all centres. Metallic or other magnetic substances cannot be scanned by MRI and can be a health hazard to the operators; this precludes the scanning of mass casualty patients or patients with suspected firearm injuries. MRI is by no means fast and it can take up to 30 minutes to scan the thorax alone. One further disadvantage is the limited availability of scanner facilities and technical or reporting expertise around the country. As it stands, MRI has great prospects and may significantly contribute in the field of post-mortem imaging in the years to come.

Fluoroscopy

Fluoroscopy holds one strong advantage over other forms of imaging and that is the ability to provide

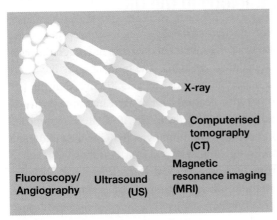

Figure 19.1 The 'radiological hand'.

the operator with real-time images. Even with multiplane images, some foreign bodies can be notoriously difficult to locate. Real-time imaging greatly assists the location and removal of objects that may be of forensic importance or represent hazards to the pathologist or anatomical technologist. This explains its use in mass fatality scenarios such as the London bombings of 2005.

Angiography

Angiography can assist, for example, in cases of basal subarachnoid haemorrhage caused by aneurysm rupture or traumatic tearing of vessels. When the base of the brain is coated with blood clot it can be difficult to identify the source of the bleeding. Contrast angiography can be coupled with fluoroscopy or other imaging modalities such as CT. Post-mortem angiography can be complicated and time-consuming and hence it is not regularly practised.

Ultrasound

Ultrasound scanning is not generally used as a form of post-mortem imaging owing to the clear advantages of the other imaging modalities.

Computerised tomography

Basic structure and the scanning process

Computerised tomography is often referred to as 'computerised axial tomography' (CAT). It was developed in 1972 by Godfrey Hounsfield and Allan Cormack, with a view to producing cross-sectional images of the body. Unlike plain-film radiography, which uses a photographic plate, CT involves the passage of x-ray beams through the body of a subject to be read by a series of circular detectors. The x-ray tube rotates around the body to produce the cross-sectional images. At their advent, CT scanners had a single row of detectors (single-slice/detector CT). In a modern CT scanner there are multiple rows of detectors closely aligned to each other (multiple-detector CT; MDCT). For post-mortem imaging,

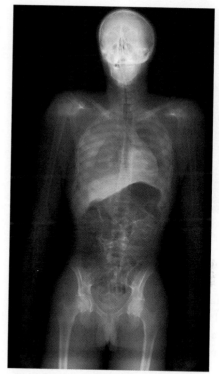

Figure 19.2 Example of a scout image.

although 64-slice MDCT is ideal, 16-slice MDCT may be adequate.

The spatial resolution (sharpness) of the image produced depends on the number of detectors, the rotation speed of the x-ray tube, and electronic post-processing and image reconstruction. The slice thickness acquired can be manipulated by collimation of the detector and/or the x-ray beam.

Several developments in CT technology over recent years have made the scanners more robust and not only quicker in acquiring images but also faster in image reconstruction. As a result, in less than a minute the whole body can be imaged in a nearly perfect 3D acquisition (i.e. the resolution in the z-plane is almost as good as in the x- and y-planes; isotropic imaging). This allows manipulation of the images and review in any desired plane (multi-planar reconstruction; MPR).

In practical terms, anything and everything can be scanned – body bags, charred remains, unidentified tissue material etc. The first image acquired is known as the 'scout image' (Fig. 19.2). This is used to

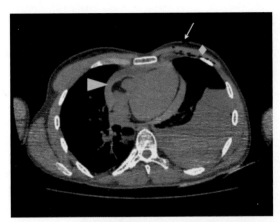

Figure 19.3 Axial image of a victim of a stab wound to the chest, showing the skin wound (arrow), underlying subcutaneous emphysema (diamond) and haemopericardium (arrow head).

define the target area for scanning and is a two-dimensional image akin to standard radiography.

Multiple axial slices can be viewed (as is routine in clinical practice) and the data can be reconstructed to produce 3D images (Figs 19.3 and 19.4). Post-processing manipulation can also allow virtual dissection of the body (Fig. 19.5).

The current status of CT

The field of post-mortem computerised tomography (PMCT) is a relatively new entity that is expanding rapidly, replacing the use of other more traditional forms of radiology as novel applications evolve. The capabilities of PMCT have been championed within the literature – with many suggesting that it has the potential to replace the invasive post-mortem in the future (Dirnhofer *et al.*, 2006; Hoey *et al.*, 2007; Leth, 2007; Rutty, 2007).

A research group in Switzerland coined the term 'Virtopsy®' to represent the concept of the radiological virtual autopsy (Thali *et al.*, 2003a). Within the UK, the Ministry of Justice, Ministry of Defence, Department of Health and the Home Office have worked together to recruit a group of experts to push forward research into the non-invasive or so-called 'near-virtual' autopsy. In our multicultural world, the idea of rapid, non-invasive examination of the dead is undoubtedly an enviable prospect. However, most of the current literature pertains to individual case reports rather than a true assessment of whether the scan would be fit for medicolegal purposes.

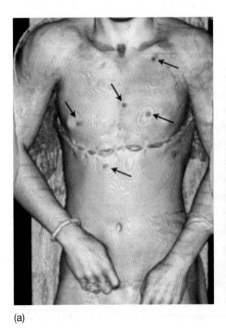

(a)

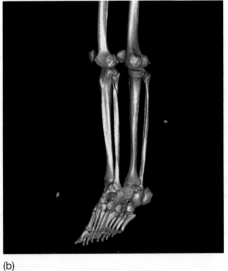

(b)

Figure 19.4 (a) Example of three-dimensional surface reconstruction showing multiple entry wounds of shotgun (arrows). (b) Three-dimensional skeletal reconstruction showing fracture of the left proximal fibula.

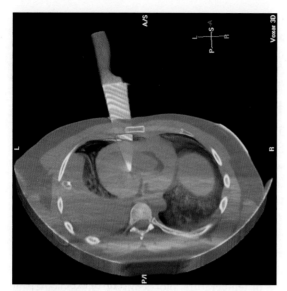

Figure 19.5 Virtual dissection of a three-dimensional reconstruction of stabbing, detailing the exact position of an in-situ weapon.

In May 2005, the Victorian Institute of Forensic Medicine (VIFM), Victoria, Australia, installed a 16-slice CT scanner within their mortuary facility (O'Donnell *et al.*, 2007). The Victoria state government funded this project because of the scanner's potential to enhance the state's counter-terrorism capabilities. Over 15 000 bodies have been scanned and publication of their experience is anticipated. Within Victoria, PMCT has proven to be a valuable adjunct when the next of kin have objected to post-mortem examinations in cases of inspection and report (similar to the Scottish system of view and grant) and when death certificates are scrutinised (O'Donnell and Woodford, 2008).

CT in post-mortem practice

The principal questions asked by HM coroners in relation to the death of an individual are who the individual is and when, where and how that individual came to his or her death. Indeed a large proportion of the pathologists work is concentrated on how they came to their death.

Who is the deceased?

Radiology is a well-established method of human identification. PMCT can identify natural or unnat-ural bone pathology and medical implants/prostheses (Dedouit *et al.*, 2007a). A case report has demonstrated successful identification of an unknown corpse by correlation of multiple features within the lumbar spine (Riepert *et al.*, 1995a). It is easier to compare two conventional x-rays or two CT scans, but only if the ante-mortem records are available. In traditional x-rays, it can be difficult to achieve identical orientation with a post-mortem x-ray. Post-processing manipulation and reorientation of CT-generated images can circumvent this problem (Pfaeffli *et al.*, 2007). Researchers are also developing computer software to assist comparisons between different radiological modalities (Riepert *et al.*, 1995b).

There are, however, a number of areas of the human skeleton that are considered as unique as a fingerprint. The unique morphology and permanence of the frontal sinuses has made them an important tool in the armoury of the forensic anthropologist when attempting to identify skeletal remains. PMCT has been shown to be a potentially useful alternative to plain radiology when ante-mortem scans are available for comparison (Reichs, 1993; Smith *et al.*, 2002). Anthropologists have used CT scanning to obtain important data from archaeological remains to avoid destruction of mummified corpses such as Otzi, the iceman discovered in Tyrol in 1991 (Recheis *et al.*, 1999; Rühli and Böni, 2000).

In cases of marked decomposition, anthropological measurements may be taken from the skeleton of the deceased without time-consuming and potentially damaging defleshing of the bones (Dedouit *et al.*, 2007a). The potential exists, therefore, for anthropological indicators of age and sex to be obtained from non-destructive PMCT (Pasquier *et al.*, 1999; Uysal *et al.*, 2005; Dedouit *et al.*, 2007b, 2008a, 2008b; Robinson *et al.*, 2008).

Reconstructed 3D data from skulls may also be used in the process of facial reconstruction (Quatrehomme, 1997; Wilkinson *et al.*, 2006). Ante-mortem CT scans have already been used to gather information regarding the variable thickness of facial soft tissues in different racial subgroups (Phillips and Smuts, 1996).

Dental evidence

Forensic odontology is an established means of identification. The dentition of the deceased may be
correlated with prior dental records or photographs
of the deceased smiling. This is traditionally
achieved by physical examination of the dentition by
an odontologist and contemporaneous or subsequent comparison with available dental records. In
mass fatality situations, the use of conventional
x-rays to record dentition can be particularly time-
consuming, with radiography becoming a
rate-limiting factor in body processing. It is important to remember that all modes of dental
identification are, of course, fundamentally dependent on the existence of dental records for comparison.
The absence of prior dental records caused significant difficulty in the identification of the victims of
the Asian tsunami on 26 December 2004 (Petju et
al., 2007).

Software packages are available for CT scanning
which are clinically used by maxillofacial surgeons
(Au-Yeung et al., 2001). It has been proposed that
PMCT could attain more detailed dental imaging
within minutes, circumventing the need for the
presence of odontologists within an already over-
populated temporary mortuary facility and
superseding the conventional radiology (Jackowski
et al., 2006a). Others have, however, expressed concerns over the apparent high error rate resulting
from streak artefacts despite the use of an extended
CT scale and the difficulty in differentiating some
dental materials such as ceramics from the native
dentine and enamel (Kirchhoff et al., 2008).

Mass fatality radiology

In mass fatality scenarios, identification of the individuals becomes a prime concern. The standard
approach used in previous incidents – such as the
terrorist bombings in London in July 2005 – has seen
fatalities move through up to three separate radiology stations, standard radiography, fluoroscopy and
dental radiography. Truck-mounted CT scanners
could be mobilised to the area via road, or containers
could be airlifted into place. These CT scanners have
the potential to provide a quick, permanent record of
individual characteristics for future comparison

(Sidler et al., 2007) and may, in the future, provide an
all-encompassing radiology facility acquiring all the
necessary data in one, more time-efficient, station
(Rutty et al., 2007a, 2007b).

Where and when did death occur?

The place of discovery of a body may not necessarily
be the place of death. In the majority of cases this
will be ascertained from witness statements, scene
investigation and circumstantial evidence rather
than invasive pathological evidence.

The case is similar for the estimation of the time
of death. There is a wealth of research regarding the
estimation of time since death when such information is not available – it includes, for example, the
use of temperature, biochemistry, entomology, and
muscle excitability (Anderson, 2004; Henßge and
Madea, 2004; Madea, 2005). These investigations are
largely non-invasive.

As invasive pathological examination has limited
capabilities in determining where and when a person
has died, it would appear that radiological investigations are unlikely to be able to assist further in these
areas.

How did death occur?

Natural deaths

One of the main criticisms faced by forensic PMCT
is the argued inability to detect certain natural
causes of death with any degree of certainty. In particular its ability to diagnose cardiac causes of death
and pulmonary thromboembolism does cause concern. Although calcification of the coronary arteries
can be demonstrated, any pathologist undertaking
post-mortem examinations will be aware that non-
calcified coronary arteries may be significantly
stenosed and become thrombosed while some
severely calcified vessels are remarkably patent. The
appearance of the myocardium in the post-mortem
period may be altered by relative hypostasis and
decomposition. It has been argued that MRI can differentiate between post-mortem clotting and
ante-mortem thrombus, and that areas of myocardial infarction can be visualised (Jackowski et al.,

2005a, 2006b). Electron-beam CT has been shown to provide excellent images of the coronary circulation, but these have been contrast-infused explanted hearts (Prigent and Steingart, 1997; Rah *et al.*, 2001). These ideas are all still in the research phase and at present remain impossible with standard PMCT alone.

While radiology may have the potential to replace a post-mortem examination, one has to consider the additional information gained from the hands-on approach and the supplementary investigations that can be undertaken by pathologists – for example toxicology, histology and microbiology.

In addition to the assessment of pathology within the body, the organs are routinely weighed at the time of post-mortem. The weights may then be compared with standardised tables of weights expected for that particular sex, weight and height. In practice these weights often add little to the interpretation of the findings. The more important are, arguably, the heart and brain, where an excessive weight will alert the pathologist to the potential of underlying cardiac disease and brain swelling, respectively. There is a single paper that has investigated the ability of PMCT and PMMRI to provide accurate assessment of organ weight (Jackowski *et al.*, 2006c). It showed an excellent correlation between both CT and MRI estimations of organ mass with that found at autopsy, with some limitation in decomposed cases where there may be gaseous degradation. The paper, however, concentrated on the liver and spleen alone and did not address the issues of assessing a non-homogeneous organ.

While toxicological samples may be taken by needle aspiration, further consideration is required for microbiological and histological examination. MDCT fluoroscopy-guided needle biopsies have been proposed and preliminary research would suggest that the amount of tissue that can be harvested is sufficient for histopathological assessment (Aghayev *et al.*, 2007). It is important to note, however, that there was no autopsy correlation of this work. Many may consider the needle autopsy approach inadequate, but it may still have value when there could be be a high infection risk to the pathologist and mortuary staff.

Unnatural deaths

CT is used clinically as a screening tool in cases of trauma. It is therefore unsurprising that it can be of value in assessing traumatic injuries in the deceased (Hoey *et al.*, 2007). The case reports which frequent the literature, however, often provide only a cursory overview of the positive achievements of the imaging rather than displaying a critical review of the findings.

Firearm deaths

The use of radiology in the location of projectiles within the body is commonplace in modern practice. It is easy to appreciate the advantages of 3D imaging over multiple 2D traditional x-rays (Figs 19.6 and 19.7).

Bevelling of the skull is used in conjunction with the external wound appearances to differentiate between entrance and exit wounds. CT has been shown to demonstrate this feature (Oehmichen *et al.*, 2004). It is also argued that the track of the projectile can be determined, but this appears to largely

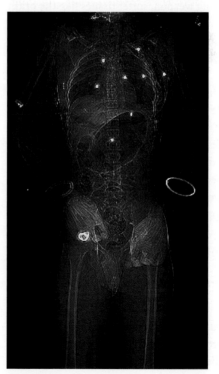

Figure 19.6 Scout image of a shotgun fatality showing multiple pieces of buck shot.

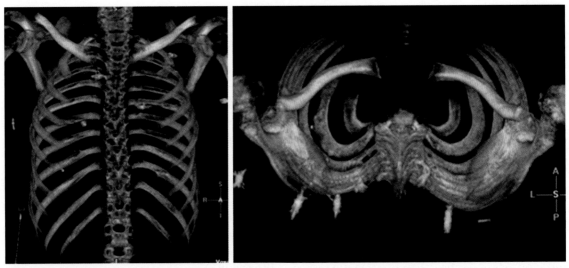

Figure 19.7 Three-dimensional images of the position of the pieces of shot (blue/green colour) in relation to the rib cage.

depend on aligning the entrance and exit wounds and pattern of bone fragmentation rather than demonstrating the tract itself (Oehmichen *et al.*, 2003; Thali *et al.*, 2003b). It is important to remember that following the passage of the projectile or the removal of a penetrating weapon, softer tissues like the brain will collapse, obscuring the track. Bleeding into the defect will also affect the tissue density differentiation that is required to visualise the true path of the injury.

It has been suggested that gunshot residues may be detectable using CT (Stein *et al.*, 2000; Thali *et al.*, 2003c). The authors propose that the presence of detectable residues within the soft tissue of a victim may be used to ascertain the range of shot. It is acknowledged that the assessment would be dependent on the weapon and ammunition used. However, there did not appear to have been consideration of the artefactual introduction of external foreign material into the wound and projectiles from an intermediate target. Modern primers are also lead-free, reducing the universal application of such techniques.

Military trauma

There is increasing use of PMCT in cases of military trauma. Following pressure from families and the refusal of permission for invasive post-mortem procedures, the Israel Defense Forces Medical Corps commenced PMCT scanning. Their preliminary findings showed that PMCT used in conjunction with conventional post-mortem examination revealed more details than either method used in isolation (Farkash *et al.*, 2000).

Problems encountered in CT assessment of military casualties have involved intersecting projectile paths, and paths that involved limbs that may be insufficiently scanned owing to the limitation of the field of view of the scanners. Bodies may have to be manipulated in the post-mortem room to assess the possibility of traversing limbs and re-entering the body – something which may not be appreciable on CT scans (Levy *et al.*, 2006).

Paediatric non-accidental injury

The skeletal survey has been an essential part of the assessment of non-accidental injury in children for some years. It has been shown in animal studies that CT scans may overestimate the number of fractures present depending on the fracture orientation in relation to the orientation of the scanning plane (Cattaneo *et al.*, 2006). However, owing to the high fracture detection rate, the work suggests that a cranial CT scan should be undertaken in children with suspected head injury. One specific area in which CT was shown to have a lower rate of fracture detection than conventional x-ray was the rib-cage, which was believed to be a consequence of the tangential slices viewed in conventional CT reporting. This work highlights the value of combining multiple forms of examination to reap the most accurate results.

Shaken baby syndrome remains an area of great controversy in forensic pathology. Contrast-enhanced PMCT of the bridging veins, the proffered source of the classical subdural haemorrhage, has been put forward as an adjunct to the post-mortem (Stein *et al.*, 2006); however, as this involves needling of the fontanelle prior to direct observation of the contents of the skull, this may not meet with support from many pathologists. It is also important to recognise that variations in the density of subdural haematomas cannot reliably be interpreted as re-bleeding in the setting of a chronic subdural haemorrhage (Sargent *et al.*, 1996). As such, histological examination is required when timing of the bleed is crucial. It has been demonstrated that post-mortem lividity within the posterior cranial fossa may be mistaken for traumatic subarachnoid haemorrhage in infants because increased density in the area of the tentorium is used clinically as an indication (Kibayashi *et al.*, 2005).

Knife injuries

The use of CT in stab injuries has been reported (Nathoo *et al.*, 2000; Thali *et al.*, 2002a). These reports, however, involve ante-mortem CT scans with the use of a contrast medium and one with the knife left *in situ*. In the latter, there is no apparent consideration of the implications had the knife been removed from the wound. The position of the wound track and its effects are understandably easier to ascertain if there is a weapon *in situ* and a functioning circulation. In forensic pathological practice the circulation is certainly absent and the same is often true of the weapon. The wound track collapses, making visualisation of the track difficult if not impossible. Although the scans may be able to show the clinical sequelae of the injury, whether or not they can provide the forensically relevant information that would be obtained through post-mortem examination remains to be proven.

Head injury

The position and morphology of fractures to the skull are regularly assessed by forensic pathologists to differentiate between falls and blunt-force assaults. Multi-planar and 3D imaging can demonstrate these features in a sterile manner for jury members with the adjunct of digital overlays of potential weapons used in cases of assault. Forensic pathologists are also asked for opinions in cases of assault where the victim has survived. In such cases the clinical CT scans may provide important forensic evidence (Bauer *et al.*, 2004).

Forensic examination of head injury usually involves not only a thorough post-mortem examination but also specialist neuropathological examination. At present neither PMCT nor PMMRI can assess findings in the scalp or temporalis muscles as accurately as naked eye observation, and many small lesions such as thin-film subdural haemorrhages and contusions are easily missed in imaging (Yen *et al.*, 2007).

Air embolism

Radiology is an excellent method of confirming air within tissue and the cardiovascular system. Demonstration of an air embolism at post-mortem is not impossible but requires specialist techniques that would not be undertaken if the entity was not given prior consideration. PMCT is an excellent modality for the identification and quantification of air embolism assuming gaseous decomposition is considered (Plattner *et al.*, 2003; Jackowski *et al.*, 2004). In deaths due to decompression sickness, PMCT and PMMRI imaging are more successful in identifying gas bubbles in the meningeal vessels than is post-mortem examination (Ozdoba *et al.*, 2005).

It is important to remember, however, that, if a person dies from an unrelated pathology while diving, so called 'off-gassing' of the tissues on ascent of the body will still occur so the presence of arterial gas does not necessarily indicate arterial gas embolism due to barotrauma (Cole *et al.*, 2006). Taking this pitfall into consideration, the Royal College of Pathologists in Australia recommends the use of CT in the post-mortem examination of diving fatalities (Oliver *et al.*, 1999).

Fatal pressure on the neck

While PMCT is able to show fractures of the hyoid bone, in order to ascertain whether this occurred prior to or after death MRI scanning must be used as CT alone cannot reliably show areas of associated soft tissue haemorrhage (Bolliger *et al.*, 2005). The use of CT and MRI in clinical forensic medicine is attracting great interest where it is suggested that radiological imaging of a surviving victim can prove trauma to the neck in the absence of external findings, thus assisting in prosecution of the assailant (Yen *et al.*, 2005)

Other complex cases

In cases where decomposition or destruction of the body by other means such as fire makes external evidence of injury difficult to identify, PMCT may be invaluable in highlighting areas of internal trauma prior to internal post-mortem examination (Thali *et al.*, 2002b, 2003d). However, in cases of decomposition, more needs to be learnt about the imaging appearances of gaseous decomposition and other changes such as adipocre (Jackowski *et al.*, 2005b).

Foreign body interpretation using CT

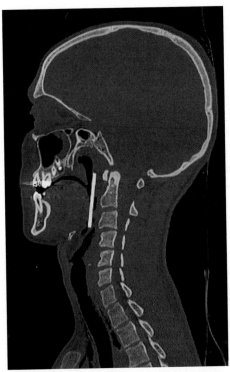

Figure 19.8 Sagittal view showing non-metallic foreign body within the pharynx.

The ability to detect radio-opaque materials such as metals is unquestionable. However, the presence of non-metallic foreign bodies needs further consideration. There are clinical examples of wooden foreign bodies that have been missed on CT (Imokawa *et al.*, 2003). The images we see on CT scan are a representation of the variation in tissue densities within the body (Fig. 19.8). A foreign body within a tissue of a similar density will be difficult to detect. Wooden objects have been shown to produce hypodense areas on CT scans that can be misinterpreted as air but also hyperdense areas if left *in situ* in the longer term (Krimmel *et al.*, 2001). These considerations are of particular importance when dealing with injuries caused by explosions. The explosive device may disperse metal or non-metallic components such as plastics, and body parts may themselves become secondary projectiles (Eshkol and Katz, 2005; Wong *et al.*, 2006).

Some investigators have commented on the varied radiological appearances of ammunition components (Levy *et al.*, 2006). Even with prior radi-

ological investigation, small fragments of projectile may elude even the most thorough of pathologists. If CT were able to identify which of the fragments were likely to be of most forensic importance, this would focus the efforts on the fragments of most value.

Artefacts and interpretative difficulties

In the UK there is a collaboration of forensic radiographers – the International Association of Forensic Radiographers: (www.afr.org.uk) – but at present there is no equivalent body of clinical radiologists trained in diagnostic imaging and specialising in forensic imaging. While post-mortem CT remains a relatively new venture, it is vital that those undertaking the scans share their experiences with others.

The scan process itself has a significant learning curve and has some significant differences from clinical ante-mortem scanning. In the writers' expe-

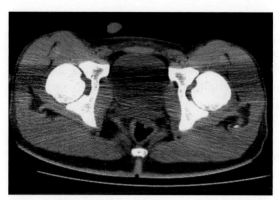

Figure 19.9 The streaking seen here is an example of a beam hardening artefact.

rience, scan protocols (x-ray tube current and voltage) have to be modified for different parts of the body in order to obtain optimal images. Most subjects are scanned in body bags with the subject's arms by the side of the trunk; this is again different from clinical scanning, in which the arms are held above the head when scanning the trunk. The former leads to significant artefacts (beam hardening artefact) and can significantly deteriorate image quality (Fig. 19.9).

There are a number of changes that occur to the body after death. While the knowledge base is still growing, simple post-mortem artefacts may be mistaken for ante-mortem injuries or pathologies. Visceral hypostasis is evident in PMCT particularly within the lungs (Shiotani *et al.*, 2004).

An apparent post-mortem change identified on CT is hyperattenuation of the aortic wall (Shiotani *et al.*, 2002). Although causes such as atherosclerosis and arteritis have been identified in clinical situations, it was noted in 100 per cent of the post-mortem cases in that particular study. The authors suggest that this may be due to the loss of blood pressure and relative condensation of the fibrous components of the vessel wall and blood dilution following peri-arrest resuscitation attempts.

Dilatation of the cardiac chambers has been recognised in PMCTs undertaken following cases of cardiac arrest, but it is unclear whether this is truly post-mortem artefact or the consequence of fluid resuscitation and ensuing cardiac failure (Shiotani *et al.*, 2003).

Air has been reported within the hepatic portal vein on PMCT. Although this may be seen in the presence of intra-abdominal pathology, it may simply represent a post-mortem change or artefact produced by artificial respiration during attempts at cardiopulmonary resuscitation (Yamazaki *et al.*, 2003, 2006; Shiotani *et al.*, 2004).

Many of the unusual findings seen in PMCT involve post-mortem decompositional gas production. As part of our collaborative work in Leicester, it has been noted that air trapping is often present within the vertebral bodies apparently outlining the fine vascular networks present. This observation is supported by the work of others who have used CT scanning to identify air pockets and similar patterns in donor bone grafts which had been confused with lytic pathology when viewed with conventional radiography (Rotman *et al.*, 2007). The authors considered this to be a post-mortem phenomenon arising as a consequence of decomposition.

The future of post-mortem radiology

Owing to significant advances in recent times, post-mortem radiology is going through a very dynamic and perhaps volatile phase of transition. It is vital that this specialist field be well nurtured and supported in this phase. Expectations from the pathologists are high and this will keep increasing owing to various socioeconomic and political factors. Radiological autopsy may provide the answer to these problems. It has been shown to be fast, reliable, easily transportable, reproducible and sensitive to the ethico-religious needs of the public.

Another arena in which post-mortem radiology has the potential to excel is the courtroom. Jurors are rarely shown photographs taken from the post-mortem examination unless it is deemed absolutely necessary, owing to their potentially distressing nature. Radiology can provide sanitised images of extensive traumatic injuries such as skull fractures (Fig. 19.10), avoiding the current dependence on the drawing skills of the pathologist or external graphics companies.

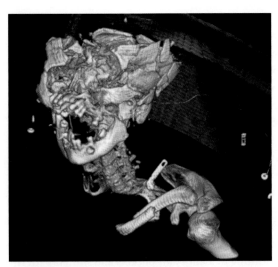

Figure 19.10 CT images can produce sanitised images of gross trauma for court purposes. This individual suffered massive head and facial injuries in a road traffic collision.

We believe the use of CT and MRI in post-mortem assessment will continue to increase in future as more and more evidence becomes available about its sensitivity and specificity in detecting abnormalities. No definitive evidence is currently available to suggest that it will replace the traditional post-mortem examination. As the use of these techniques increases, more centres around the world will be able to provide this service. For optimal results, post-mortem radiology should be performed and reported by a pathologist and radiologist in conjunction. The journey of post-mortem radiology can be summed up as: 'Indistinct past, budding present, but a bold future'.

References

Aghayev E, Thali MJ, Sonnenschein M *et al.* (2007). Post-mortem tissue sampling using computed tomography guidance. *Forensic Sci Int* **166**:199–203.

Anderson GS (2004). Determining time of death using blow fly eggs in the early postmortem interval. *Int J Legal Med* **118**:240–1.

Au-Yeung KM, Ahuja AT, Ching ASC, Metreweli C (2001). DentaScan in oral imaging. *Clin Radiol* **56**:700–13.

Bauer M, Polzin S, Patzelt D (2004). The use of clinical CCT images in the forensic examination of closed head injuries. *J Clin Forensic Med* **11**:65–70.

Bisset RAL (1998). Magnetic resonance imaging may be alternative to necropsy. *Br Med J* **317**:1450.

Bisset RAL, Thomas NB, Turnbull IW, Lee S (2002). Postmortem examinations using magnetic resonance imaging: four-year review of a working service. *Br Med J* **324**:1423–4.

Bolliger S, Thali M, Jackowski C *et al.* (2005). Postmortem non-invasive virtual autopsy: death by hanging in a car. *J Forensic Sci* **50**:455–60.

Britton P (2008). Body scans instead of post-mortems. *Manchester Evening News*, 29 May.

Cattaneo C, Marinelli E, Di Giancamillo A *et al.* (2006). Sensitivity of autopsy and radiological examination in detecting bone fractures in an animal model: implications for the assessment of fatal child physical abuse. *Forensic Sci Int* **164**:131–7.

Cole AJ, Griffiths D, Lavender S, Summers P, Rich K (2006). Relevance of postmortem radiology to the diagnosis of fatal cerebral gas embolism from compressed air diving. *J Clin Pathol* **59**:489–91.

Crane J (2000). Forensic radiology: from Belfast to Bosnia. *Imaging* **12**:284–91.

Dedouit F, Telmon N, Costagliola R *et al.* (2007a). New identification possibilities with postmortem multislice computed tomography. *Int J Legal Med* **121**:507–10.

Dedouit F, Telmon N, Guilbeau-Frugier C *et al.* (2007b). Virtual autopsy and forensic identification. Practical application: a report of one case. *J Forensic Sci* **52**:960–4.

Dedouit F, Bindel S, Gainza D *et al.* (2008a). Application of the Iscan method to two- and three-dimensional imaging of the sternal end of the right fourth rib. *J Forensic Sci* **53**:288–95.

Dedouit F, Guilbeau-Frugier C, Telmon *et al.* (2008b). Virtual autopsy and forensic anthropology of a mummified fetus: a report of one case. *J Forensic Sci* **53**:208–12.

Dirnhofer R, Jackowski C, Vock P, Potter K, Thali MJ (2006). Virtopsy: minimally invasive, imaging-guided virtual autopsy. *Radiographics* **26**:1305–33.

Donchin Y, Rivkind AI, Bar-Ziv J *et al.* (1994). Utility of postmortem computed tomography in trauma victims. *J Trauma Injury Infect Crit Care* **37**:552–5; discussion 555–6.

Eshkol Z, Katz K (2005). Injuries from biologic material of suicide bombers. *Injury* **36**:271–4.

Farkash U, Scope A, Lynn M *et al.* (2000). Preliminary experience with postmortem computed tomography in military penetrating trauma. *J Trauma Injury Infect Crit Care* **48**:303–8; discussion 308–9.

Hansard (2008). House of Commons debate, 15 July, London (www.parliament.uk).

Henßge C, Madea B (2004). Estimation of the time since death in the early post-mortem period. *Forensic Sci Int* **144**:167–75.

Hoey BA, Cipolla J, Grossman MD *et al.* (2007). Postmortem computed tomography, 'CATopsy', predicts cause of death in trauma patients. *J Trauma Injury Infect Crit Care* **63**:979–85; discussion 985–6.

Imokawa H, Takasi T, Natuki S, Daisuke O, Kiyomi Y (2003). Penetrating neck injuries involving wooden foreign bodies: the role of MRI and the misinterpretation of CT images. *Auris Nasus Larynx* **30**(Suppl):S145–7.

Jackowski C, Thali M, Sonnenschein *et al.* (2004). Visualization and quantification of air embolism structure by processing postmortem MSCT data. *J Forensic Sci* **49**:1339–42.

Jackowski C, Schweitzer W, Thali M *et al.* (2005a). Virtopsy: postmortem imaging of the human heart *in situ* using MSCT and MRI. *Forensic Sci Int* **149**:11–23.

Jackowski C, Thali M, Sonnenschein M *et al.* (2005b). Adipocere in postmortem imaging using multislice computed tomography and magnetic resonance imaging. *Am J Forensic Med Pathol* **26**:360–4.

Jackowski C, Aghayev E, Sonnenschein M *et al.* (2006a). Maximum intensity projection of cranial computed tomography data for dental identification. *Int J Legal Med* **120**:165–7.

Jackowski C, Thali M, Aghayev E *et al.* (2006b). Postmortem imaging of blood and its characteristics using MSCT and MRI. *Int J Legal Med* **120**:233–40.

Jackowski C, Thali MJ, Buck U *et al.* (2006c). Noninvasive estimation of organ weights by postmortem magnetic resonance imaging and multislice computed tomography. *Invest Radiol* **41**:572–8.

Kahana T, Hiss J (1999). Forensic radiology. *Br J Radiol* **72**:129–33.

Kibayashi K, Shojo H, Sumida T (2005). Dural hemorrhage of the tentorium on postmortem cranial computed tomographic scans in children. *Forensic Sci Int* **154**:206–9.

Kirchhoff S, Fischer F, Lindemaier G *et al.* (2008). Is post-mortem CT of the dentition adequate for correct forensic identification? Comparison of dental computed tomograpy and visual dental record. *Int J Legal Med* **122**:471–9.

Krimmel M, Cornelius CP, Stojadinovic S, Hoffmann J, Reinert S (2001). Wooden foreign bodies in facial injury: a radiological pitfall. *Int J Oral Maxillofac Surg* **30**:445–7.

Leth P (2007). The use of CT scanning in forensic autopsy. *Forensic Sci Med Pathol* **3**:65–9.

Levy AD, Abbott RM, Mallak CT *et al.* (2006). Virtual autopsy: preliminary experience in high-velocity gunshot wound victims. *Radiology* **240**:522–8.

Madea B (2005). Is there recent progress in the estimation of the postmortem interval by means of thanatochemistry? *Forensic Sci Int* **151**:139–49.

Nathoo N, Boodhoo H, Nadvi SS, Naidoo SR, Gouws E (2000). Transcranial brainstem stab injuries: a retrospective analysisi of 17 patients. *Neurosurgery* **47**:1117–22.

O'Donnell C, Woodford N (2008). Post-mortem radiology: a new sub-speciality? *Clin Radiol* **63**:1189–94.

O'Donnell C, Rotman A, Collett S, Woodford N (2007). Current status of routine post-mortem CT in Melbourne, Australia. *Forensic Sci Med Pathol* **3**:226–32.

Oehmichen M, Gehl HB, Meissner C *et al.* (2003). Forensic pathological aspects of postmortem imaging of gunshot injury to the head: documentation and biometric data. *Acta Neuropathol* **105**:570–80.

Oehmichen M, Meissner C, Konig HG, Gehl HB (2004). Gunshot injuries to the head and brain caused by low-velocity handguns and rifles: a review. *Forensic Sci Int* **146**:111–20.

Oliver J, Lyons TJ, Harle R (1999). The role of computed tomography in the diagnosis of arterial gas embolism in fatal diving accidents in Tasmania. *Australas Radiol* **43**:37–40.

Ozdoba C, Weis J, Plattner T, Dirnhofer R, Yen K (2005). Fatal scuba diving incident with massive gas embolism in cerebral and spinal arteries. *Neuroradiology* **47**:411–16.

Pasquier E, Pernot LDSM, Burdin V *et al.* (1999). Determination of age at death: assessment of an algorithm of age prediction using numerical three-dimensional CT data from pubic bones. *Am J Phys Anthropol* **108**:261–8.

Petju M, Suteerayongprasert A, Thongpud R, Hassiri K (2007). Importance of dental records for victim identification following the Indian Ocean tsunami disaster in Thailand. *Public Health* **121**:251–7.

Pfaeffli M, Vock P, Dirnhofer R *et al.* (2007). Post-mortem radiological CT identification based on classical ante-mortem X-ray examinations. *Forensic Sci Int* **171**:111–17.

Phillips VM, Smuts NA (1996). Facial reconstruction: utilization of computerised tomography to measure facial tissue thickness in a mixed racial population. *Forensic Sci Int* **83**:51–9.

Plattner T, Thali MJ, Yen K *et al.* (2003). Virtopsy: postmortem multislice computed tomography and magnetic resonance imaging in a fatal scuba diving incident. *J Forensic Sci* **48**:1347–55.

Prigent FM, Steingart RM (1997). Clinical value of electron-beam computed tomography in the diagnosis and prognosis of coronary artery disease. *Curr Opin Cardiol* **12**:561–5.

Quatrehomme GC, Subsol S, Delingette G *et al.* (1997). A fully three-dimensional method for facial reconstruction based on deformable models. *J Forensic Sci* **42**:649–52.

Rah BR, Katz RJ, Wasserman AG, Reiner JS (2001). Post-mortem three-dimensional reconstruction of the entire coronary arterial circulation using electron-beam computed tomography. *Circulation* **104**:3168.

Recheis W, Weber GW, Schäfer K *et al.* (1999). Virtual reality and anthropology. *Eur J Radiol* **31**:88–96.

Reichs KJ (1993). Quantified comparison of frontal sinus patterns by means of computed tomography. *Forensic Sci Int* **61**:141–68.

Riepert T, Rittner C, Ulmcke D, Ogbuihi S, Schweden F (1995a). Identification of an unknown corpse by means of computed tomography of the lumbar spine. *J Forensic Sci* **40**:126–7.

Riepert T, Ulmcke D, Jendrysiak U, Rittner C (1995b). Computer-assisted simulation of conventional roentgenograms from three-dimensional computed tomography data: an aid in the identification of unknown corpses (FoXSIS). *Forensic Sci Int* **71**:199–204.

Robinson C, Eisma R, Morgan B *et al.* (2008). Anthropological measurement of lower limb and foot bones using multi-detector computed tomography. *J Forensic Sci* **53**:1289–95.

Rotman A, Hamilton K, O'Donnell C (2007). 'Lytic' lesions in autologous bone grafts: demonstration of medullary air pockets on post mortem computed tomography. *Forensic Sci Med Pathol* **3**:270–4.

Rühli F, Böni T (2000). Radiological aspects and interpretation of post-mortem artefacts in ancient Egyptian mummies from Swiss collections. *Int J Osteoarchaeol* **10**:153–7.

Rutty G (2007). Are autopsies necessary? The role of computed tomography as a possible alternative to invasive autopsies. *Rechtsmedizin* **17**:21–8.

Rutty GN, Robinson C, Jeffery A, Morgan B (2007a). Mobile computed tomography for mass fatality investigations. *Forensic Sci Med Pathol* **3**:138–45.

Rutty GN, Robinson CE, Bouhaidar RM, Jeffery AJM, Morgan BB (2007b). The role of mobile computed tomography in mass fatality incidents. *J Forensic Sci* **52**:1343–9.

Sargent S, Kennedy JG, Kaplan JA (1996). 'Hyperacute' subdural hematoma: CT mimic of recurrent episodes of bleeding in the setting of child abuse. *J Forensic Sci* **41**:314–16.

Shiotani S, Mototsugu K, Noriyoshi O *et al.* (2002). Hyperattenuating aortic wall on postmortem computed tomography. *Radiation Med* **20**:201–6.

Shiotani MK, Ohashi N, Yamazaki K *et al.* (2003). Dilatation of the heart on postmortem computed tomography: comparison with live CT. *Radiation Med* **21**:29–35.

Shiotani S, Kohno M, Ohashi N *et al.* (2004). Non-traumatic postmortem computed tomographic findings of the lung. *Forensic Sci Int* **139**:39–48.

Sidler M, Jackowski C, Dirnhofer R, Vock P, Thali M (2007). Use of multislice computed tomography in disaster victim identification: advantages and limitations. *Forensic Sci Int* **169**:118–28.

Smith DR, Keith GL, Hoffman JM (2002). Identification of human skeletal remains by comparison of bony details of the cranium using computerised tomographic scans. *J Forensic Sci* **47**:937–9.

Stein KM, Bahner ML, Merkel J, Ain S, Mattern R (2000). Detection of gunshot residues in routine CTs. *Int J Legal Med* **114**:15–18.

Stein KM, Ruf K, Ganten MK, Mattern R (2006). Representation of cerebral bridging veins in infants by postmortem computed tomography. *Forensic Sci Int* **163**:93–101.

Swift BSR (2002). Postmortem radiology is useful but no substitute for necropsy. *Br Med J* **325**:549.

Thali MJ, Schwab CM, Tairi K, Dirnhofer R, Vock P (2002a). Forensic radiology with cross-section modalities:

spiral CT evaluation of a knife wound to the aorta. *J Forensic Sci* **47**:1041–5.

Thali MJ, Yen K, Plattner T *et al.* (2002b) Charred body: virtual autopsy with multi-slice computed tomography and magnetic resonance imaging. *J Forensic Sci* **47**:1326–31.

Thali MJ, Yen K, Schweitzer W *et al.* (2003a). Virtopsy, a new imaging horizon in forensic pathology: virtual autopsy by postmortem multislice computed tomography and magnetic resonance imaging: a feasibility study. *J Forensic Sci* **48**:386–403.

Thali MJ, Schweitzer W, Yen K *et al.* (2003b). New horizons in forensic radiology: the 60-second digital autopsy-full-body examination of a gunshot victim by multislice computed tomography. *Am J Forensic Med Pathol* **24**:22–7.

Thali MJ, Yen K, Vock P *et al.* (2003c). Image-guided virtual autopsy findings of gunshot victims performed with multi-slice computed tomography and magnetic resonance imaging and subsequent correlation between radiology and autopsy findings. *Forensic Sci Int* **138**:8–16.

Thali MJ, Yen K, Schweitzer W *et al.* (2003d). Into the decomposed body: forensic digital autopsy using multislice computed tomography. *Forensic Sci Int* **134**:109–14.

Uysal S, Dilek G, Mahmut K, Iåÿil T, Uäÿur K (2005). Estimation of sex by 3D CT measurements of the foramen magnum. *J Forensic Sci* **50**:1310–14.

Wilkinson C, Rynn C, Peters H *et al.* (2006). A blind accuracy assessment of computer-modeled forensic facial reconstruction using computed tomography data from live subjects. *Forensic Sci Med Pathol* **2**:179–87.

Wong J, Marsh D, Abu-Sitta G *et al.* (2006). Biological foreign body implantation in victims of the London July 7th bombings. *J Trauma* **60**:402–4.

Yamazaki K, Shiotani S, Ohashi N, Doi M, Honda K (2003). Hepatic portal venous gas and hyper-dense aortic wall as postmortem computed tomography finding. *Legal Med* **5**:S338–41.

Yamazaki K, Shiotani S, Ohashi N *et al.* (2006). Comparison between computed tomography and autopsy findings in cases of abdominal injury and disease. *Forensic Sci Int* **162**:163–6.

Yen K, Thali MJ, Aghayev E *et al.* (2005). Strangulation signs: initial correlation of MRI, MSCT, and forensic neck findings. *J Magn Reson Imaging* **22**:501–10.

Yen K, Lovblad K-O, Scheurer E *et al.* (2007). Post-mortem forensic neuroimaging: correlation of MSCT and MRI findings with autopsy results. *Forensic Sci Int* **173**:21–35.

Chapter 20

THE DECOMPOSED BODY AND THE UNASCERTAINED AUTOPSY

Julian L Burton

Introduction

It is very easy to feel disheartened when, at the end of the macroscopic examination, no cause of death has been identified. Trainees in particular may feel that they have in some way 'failed'. While it may be that a macroscopically evident cause of death has been missed, or misinterpreted, it must be remembered that not all causes of death are identifiable by naked examination alone. Furthermore the autopsy, while considered by some to be the gold standard for the determination of the cause of death, is not an infallible investigation and is not expected to yield a cause of death in every case.

In the author's practice, which is heavily skewed towards deaths occurring in the community and to the autopsy of decomposed bodies, it is not uncommon for a careful macroscopic examination to fail to yield a cause of death. Overall it has been estimated that when all investigations have been completed the cause of death will remain unascertained in 2–5 per cent of cases (Milroy, 2007). Factors that make it less likely to ascertain a cause of death are summarised in Box 20.1. More experienced autopsy pathologists tend to be more willing to list a cause of death as unascertained, perhaps through greater confidence that they have not missed a macroscopic diagnosis. (Indeed, some pathologists would state a cause of death as 'Unascertainable', but this is not recommended.) With experience one becomes more critical of minor disease changes and less willing to

accept them as a cause of death. If it is not possible to determine a cause of death on the balance of probability, it is better to state the cause of death as being unascertained, rather than attempt to bluff one's way through a spurious diagnosis.

One would expect that all unascertained autopsies are performed on the instruction of a coroner (or other medicolegal authority). In England and Wales, a hospital (consent) autopsy can be performed only when a cause of death can be stated on a medical certificate of the cause of death. Although a diagnosis of 'unascertained' is frustrating for the pathologist and for the relatives, the autopsy still has utility for the coroner, who will want to know whether death is due to a natural or an unnatural cause. In these cases, the

Box 20.1 Factors making it more likely that the cause of death will remain unascertained after autopsy

- Increasing experience of the pathologist
- Deceased age <35 years
- Decomposition
- Death occurring in the community rather than in hospital
- Poor autopsy technique
- Failure to retain samples for histopathological examination
- Failure to retain samples for toxicological examination
- Failure to retain samples for microbiological investigation
- Failure to retain samples for genetic testing

pathologist can assist the coroner both in the autopsy report and in the inevitable inquest with a statement as follows:

> A detailed autopsy examination, including external examination, dissection and macroscopic (naked eye) inspection of the internal organs, histopathological examinations of the internal organs, toxicological and microbiological examinations, has not revealed a cause of death. The cause of death is therefore considered to be unascertained. It is notable that there were no findings to suggest that death was due to the actions or inactions of a third party. It is likely, therefore, that death was due to an unascertained natural cause. It is recognised that the autopsy will not yield a cause of death in 2–5 per cent of autopsies, and that it is more likely that the cause of death will remain unascertained when the deceased was less than 35 years of age or significantly decomposed.

The autopsy should, of course, be performed to a high standard and should comply with the latest guidelines set out by the Royal College of Pathologists. While some cases will remain truly unascertained, a cause of death can be identified in many other cases where the macroscopic examination fails to find a cause. This chapter provides an approach to the autopsy of decomposed bodies before considering occult causes of death by organ system. Toxicological examinations are considered in detail in Chapter 15.

The decomposed body

Many autopsying pathologists are reluctant to perform autopsies on decomposed bodies – perhaps unsurprisingly given the unpleasant sights and smells associated with the examination. There is a tendency to perform the examination as quickly as possible, but this results in a cursory substandard autopsy, for which pathologists have rightly been criticised (NCEPOD, 2006). The pathologist who accepts the autopsy of a decomposed body should perform the examination to the same high standard that they would employ for the non-decomposed. In the author's experience, the autopsies of decom-

posed bodies will reveal a macroscopic cause of death in more than 50 per cent of cases, rising to 80–90 per cent after histological and toxicological examinations have been undertaken.

In some cases the identification of the deceased is unknown or uncertain. The degree of decomposition may be such that facial features are unrecognisable. In cases where the identity of the deceased is suspected but not certain, it is advisable to obtain any and all available medical records prior to commencing the examination. Operative interventions may prove useful in confirming the identification of the deceased.

The autopsy follows the same sequence as in other cases, with a review of the available history, a detailed external examination, sample collection, evisceration, internal dissection, further sampling and further investigations. These are discussed in detail in the earlier chapters of this book, and only those elements particular to the decomposed body will be considered here.

External examination

The external examination of a decomposed body must be thorough. Both the front and the back of the body must be examined in every case. In addition to looking for identifying features, evidence of trauma, disease and medical intervention, the pathologist should document the external extent of decomposition. The speed at which putrefactive decomposition progresses depends on a variety of factors, including the ambient temperature of the environment in which the body lay, the humidity (and any water immersion), and the extent of any animal or insect predation. The presence or absence of maggot infestation should be recorded. In a temperate climate, putrefactive decomposition progresses through a relatively defined sequence (Table 20.1). This can only be taken as a guide. The author has examined bodies where the deceased was seen alive less than 24 hours prior to the autopsy examination but in which there was marked bloating of the abdomen and scrotum, with extensive venous marbling and blister formation.

In addition to putrefactive decomposition, bodies

Table 20.1 Progression of putrefactive decomposition in a temperate climate

Days since death	Changes observed
0–1	Dependent post-mortem hypostasis Rigor mortis develops
1–2	Green discolouration of the anterior abdominal wall, beginning in the right iliac fossa, due to bacterial action converting haemoglobin into sulphaemoglobin
2–3	Bloating of the abdomen begins
3–4	Venous marbling begins due to bacterial decomposition of blood
5–6	Abdominal bloating established Skin slippage and blister formation
14	Marked bloating of the abdomen and scrotum
21	General softening of the tissues Eyes bulge
28	Generalised blackening of the skin Skin liquefaction

may undergo mummification if the environment is dry, or adipocere formation if the environment was wet. More than one form of decompositional change can be present in the same body and they should be recorded. Mummification retards the speed of putrefactive decomposition.

Paradoxically, decompositional changes can make the identification of the body easier. When skin slippage develops, the epidermal layers can be easily wiped away using a soft cloth. Any underlying tattoos will appear more vivid and can be photographed. Because the epidermis contains melanin, the skin of Afro-Caribbean and Indo-Pakistani individuals will appear white when this has been done.

Conversely, decomposition may mask signs of injury and previous operative intervention. The body, and especially the neck, should be examined carefully for bruising. Penetrating injuries may more readily attract maggot activity than the surrounding skin. The presence of purged fluid at the nose and mouth, a common finding, should not be confused with trauma and does not indicate gastrointestinal haemorrhage or haemoptysis. Scars may be rendered all but invisible on the putrefied and/or mummified body.

The autopsy report should include an estimation of the date of death based on the clinical history and the external examination findings. It is prudent not to attempt to be overly precise when stating the date of death, and of course not to state a date of death that precedes the time at which the deceased was last seen alive.

Evisceration

Decomposed bodies are eviscerated in the same way as all others. However, once putrefactive decomposition with bloating has developed, any assessment of the presence or absence of air in the pleural cavities will be spurious. In such cases, the presence of gas in the pleural cavities does not indicate that the deceased had a pneumothorax.

Initial specimen collection

It is the author's practice to always collect samples for toxicological analysis when eviscerating a decomposed body, it being easier to discard them if not needed than to attempt to obtain samples if the internal dissection fails to reveal a cause of death. When decomposition is not advanced, it is usually possible to obtain samples of blood, urine and vitreous humour, as described in Chapter 15. As decomposition progresses it becomes more difficult to obtain blood and vitreous humour. In that case, fluid from the abdominal or chest cavities, appropriately labelled as such, can be retained, as can samples of the psoas muscle and bile. In cases of suspected carbon monoxide poisoning, for example due to a faulty central heating boiler, psoas muscle can be submitted for an assessment of carboxymyoglobin. The toxicologist should be advised of the state of decomposition.

Internal examination

As putrefactive decomposition progresses, the internal organs become progressively lighter, and this must be remembered when comparing the weights of the organs with standardised tables. The author addresses this by including the following statement in the autopsy report:

All the internal organs were affected by decompositional changes, rendering many of them autolysed. The internal organs become lighter as decomposition progresses. It should be noted, therefore, that the organ weights recorded at autopsy may not reflect the weights of the internal organs at the time of death.

Organs that are naturally rich in fibrous tissue or muscle are the most resistant to decompositional changes. Disease processes that result in the deposition of calcium or fibrous tissue are also resistant to decompositional changes, so diseases such as coronary artery atherosclerosis, myocardial fibrosis and cirrhosis can usually be identified.

Care must be taken not to confuse the changes of decomposition with pathological processes. For example, as decomposition progresses the brain develops a greenish-grey hue and then liquefies. In such cases it is not possible to make any detailed comment about the brain, although one can usually comment on whether or not there was any intracranial haemorrhage. (The author has seen cases in which the brain was completely destroyed by maggot activity.)

The heart becomes soft, brown and flabby. The presence of a ruptured myocardial infarct with resultant haemopericardium can usually be easily identified.

The lungs blacken, solidify and become filled with decompositional fluids, some of which may have been purged from the stomach. This should not be confused with pneumonia or pulmonary oedema. The author's practice when there is purging at the nose and mouth is to state that decompositional changes precluded an assessment of the presence or absence of pulmonary oedema and congestion.

The mucosa of the gut rapidly decomposes. While it may be possible to identify a gastrointestinal haemorrhage, it is not uncommon for the cause of this to remain unidentifiable. The action of gas-forming bacteria will result in a 'Swiss-cheese' appearance of the liver, while the spleen becomes liquefied and blackened – an appearance that should not be confused with the diffluence seen in patients dying of septicaemia. The pancreas and the endocrine organs autolyse rapidly and in a decomposed body may be unidentifiable. The kidneys become softened and the cortico-medullary junction rapidly becomes blurred and then unidentifiable. The bladder and internal genital organs, particularly the uterus and prostate, typically resist the decompositional process and remain identifiable until decomposition is very advanced.

Further investigations

All the internal organs should be sampled for histopathological examination. Sometimes this may yield only amorphous eosinophilic tissue, but in many cases sufficient histological detail remains to confirm or exclude pathology. Immunohistochemistry can also be successfully performed on tissue removed from a decomposed body (Lowe, 1997). Tissue can be stored for genetic studies if required. In the author's experience, the widespread bacterial and fungal growth present within a decomposed body renders microbiological examination of little value in the autopsy of decomposed bodies.

The unascertained autopsy

In the majority of autopsies the macroscopic examination of the body will yield the cause of death, and most often this will be present within the heart. However, a number of potentially fatal pathological processes are not readily detectable by naked-eye examination, and deaths due to these will initially be considered to have an unascertained cause.

This section of the chapter considers how to approach these cases. The intention is not to present a detailed discussion of pathophysiology but rather to provide a practical approach. In all such cases the first step is to remain calm and not to panic. The pathologist should then review the clinical history and organ dissection again, placing special emphasis on the heart. If no macroscopic pathology that could account for death can be found, the following sections can be considered.

Sudden cardiac death when the heart is macroscopically normal

In many cases where the cause of death is initially unascertained by macroscopic examination, the cause of death will lie within the heart. It has been estimated that in England there are 11 per 100 000 sudden unexpected deaths due to cardiac or unascertained causes each year (Bowker *et al.*, 2003). Coronary artery atherosclerosis is by far the most common cardiac cause of death (Fabre and Sheppard, 2006). When present to a degree that can cause death, atherosclerosis is visible on naked-eye examination; but it can be very focal, so significant stenoses may be missed if the examination of the arteries is not sufficiently thorough.

It is imperative that the heart be correctly and adequately examined. In some cases the available clinical history will provide clues to the pathologist that the cardiac examination will fall outside his or her competence. When this occurs, the autopsy should be referred to a pathologist with a special interest in cardiac pathology. Where this is not practicable, the heart should be retained, fixed and referred to a cardiac pathologist (Suvarna, 2008). In such cases it is the author's practice to perform the autopsy but to limit the cardiac dissection to an examination of the coronary arteries. The posterior walls of the ventricles are then incised to aid fixation and the heart is retained and fixed in formalin prior to submission to a cardiac pathologist.

Sudden arrhythmic death syndrome

In recent years the concept of SADS has emerged to encompass those deaths believed to be of cardiac origin in which no cause of death can be found despite extensive post-mortem investigation. Also known as sudden adult death syndrome, SADS has its corollaries in sudden unexpected death in infancy (SUDI) and sudden unexpected death in epilepsy (SUDEP), in that it is a diagnosis of exclusion. Behr *et al.* (2007) recently reported that these deaths are typically seen in young adult males, with a mean age of 32 years, although deaths have been ascribed to SADS in individuals as young as 7 years and as old as 64 years. In 18 per cent of cases there was a pre-existing family history of premature death (Behr *et al.*, 2007). It is estimated that the annual incidence of SADS is 0.10–0.16 per 100 000 (Behr *et al.*, 2007). This may mean that a country the size of England could expect to have 500 SADS deaths per year.

Examining the heart

The examination of the heart should be systematic and thorough. National guidelines for this dissection have been proposed and the author favours those set out by Suvarna (2008). All abnormalities should be recorded and, ideally, photographed.

Prior to its evisceration the heart should be examined *in situ* to assess its gross architecture and vascular connections for the presence of congenital anomalies – having first opened and examined the pericardial sac. This done, the pulmonary artery is opened and the distal pulmonary artery is probed with a finger to exclude the presence of a saddle pulmonary thrombo-embolus. On no account should the probing finger be directed proximally towards the pulmonary valve (Suvarna, 2008). The heart can now be severed from its vascular attachments and examined in more detail.

The coronary arteries should next be examined, slicing them transversely at 2–3 mm intervals looking for the presence of atherosclerosis, anatomical variations, myocardial bridging, dissection, haemorrhage and thrombus (Biggs *et al.*, 2009). The most severely diseased portions of each major coronary artery are retained for histopathological evaluation. Heavily calcified coronary arteries may be dissected free, fixed and decalcified prior to slicing. Alternatively the pathologist may elect to attempt to cut the vessels using scissors. If facilities are available, post-mortem coronary artery angiography can be performed (Suvarna, 2008).

The myocardium is examined after the coronary arteries. Two or three transverse parallel slices are made through the left and right ventricles, approximately 10 mm apart, starting at the apex and aiming towards the base but avoiding the valves. The remainder of the heart is then opened by following the direction of blood flow, taking time to inspect the cardiac valves carefully before making any incision into them (Suvarna, 2008). The heart should be weighed and its weight compared with reference tables for the deceased's height and weight.

If no cause of death is identified, a more detailed examination of the heart is warranted. This will include dissection of the cardiac conduction system (Chapter 11) and extensive sampling of the heart for

Table 20.2 Sampling the heart for histopathological evaluation in SADS and cardiomyopathies[a]

Block number	Tissue sample
1	Left main stem and left anterior descending coronary artery
2	Right coronary and posterior interventricular coronary arteries
3	Circumflex and obtuse marginal arteries
4	Sino-atrial node
5	Sino-atrial node
6	Atrio-ventricular node
7	Atrio-ventricular node
8	Atrio-ventricular node
9	Atrio-ventricular node
10	Atrio-ventricular node
11	Bundle of His, bundle branches
12	Bundle of His, bundle branches
13	Basal interventricular septum
14	Right and left atium
15	Apical interventricular septum
16	Right ventricular outflow tract
17	Anterior left ventricular myocardium
18	Lateral left ventricular myocardium
19	Apical left ventricular myocardium
20	Posterior left ventricular myocardium
21	Jumbo block of both ventricles
22	Jumbo block of both ventricles
23	Jumbo block of both ventricles

[a] Each block should be labelled to indicate site of origin within the heart. If present, a pacemaker should be retained and submitted to the local ECG department for testing (Suvarna, 2008). However, pacemaker malfunction is a rare cause of death (Suvarna et al., 1999; Suvarna 2008).

histopathological examination (Table 20.2). It must be remembered that diseases such as myocarditis and cardiomyopathy can be reliably excluded as a cause of death only if the heart has been appropriately and widely sampled. A single block of myocardium from the left and right ventricles is not sufficient for this purpose. When sampling the macroscopically abnormal heart, a single block of tissue may suffice. In general the author's practice is to retain, as a minimum, blocks of the coronary arteries, the right ventricle (one or two samples), the interventricular septum,

and the anterior, lateral and posterior walls of the left ventricle (a total of six to eight blocks). As a minimum the myocardium should be stained with haematoxylin and eosin, a Perl's stain and a connective tissue stain, remembering that other stains may be needed to exclude other diseases such as amyloidosis and storage disorders. A number of further samples other than the heart should be retained (Table 20.3).

Channelopathies

In recent years there has been an increasing appreciation and understanding of the fact that genetically based abnormalities in the transport of ions into and out of cardiac myocytes may cause disease and death. Collectively, these conditions are referred to as the 'channelopathies' and include Brugada syndrome, long QT syndrome, Lev–Lenègre syndrome, short QT syndrome and familial atrial fibrillation (Glatter et al., 2006; Brugada et al., 2007).

Some understanding of these unusual conditions is essential for pathologists engaged in autopsy practice. The deceased is typically a young adult and the macroscopic and microscopic examination will be unrewarding. Toxicological and microbiological investigations are used to exclude other causes of death. Ultimately the diagnosis may depend on a knowledge of the deceased's family history, analysis of electrocardiograms (ECGs) taken in life, the absence of positive findings at autopsy, and molecular cytogenetic testing performed on splenic tissue retained at autopsy (Brugada, 2000; Glatter et al., 2006; Suvarna, 2008).

The long QT syndrome is caused by dysfunction of sodium ion channels which result from gain-of-function mutations in the SCN5A sodium channel gene. Such mutations result in prolonged ingress of sodium ions into the myocytes, extending the time taken for them to return to resting action potential. The clinical result is, as the name suggests, a prolongation of the QT interval on the ECG and an increased risk of sudden death, particularly while at rest or in sleep as a result of a fatal polymorphic ventricular tachycardia (Brugada, 2000).

Long QT syndrome may be congenital or acquired. Numerous genetic mutations have been linked to the congenital form of long QT syndrome

Table 20.3 Other tissue samples that should be taken when investigating a potential sudden arrhythmogenic syndrome death

Investigation	Tissue samples required	Comments
Histopathology	Sample all other major organs and any macroscopic lesions	In addition, consider retaining the brain for detailed examination
Microbiology	Blood Samples of both lungs Liver Urine	Collect samples for bacteriological culture and virology (Chapter 16)
Toxicology	Blood Urine Vitreous humour Gastric contents	Plain and preserved samples
Electron microscopy	Myocardium	Fix in cold gluteraldehyde
Genetic studies	2 cm^3 sample of spleen	Submit rapidly to local molecular cytogenetics laboratory for DNA extraction

From Suvarna (2008).

(Roden and Viswanathan, 2005; Goldenberg and Moss, 2008). A detailed discussion of these genetic mutations is beyond the scope of this book and the advice of a clinical geneticist may be invaluable in such cases. Acquired long QT syndrome may be associated with the use of a wide variety of cardiac and non-cardiac medications including sotalol, quinidine, dofetilide, terfenadine, cisapride, haloperidol, methadone, erythromycin, amiodarone, sertindole and terodiline (Roden and Viswanathan, 2005). Acquired long QT syndrome may also develop in patients suffering from a myocardial infarction, cardiac failure, hypokalaemia, hypomagnesaemia, subarachnoid haemorrhage or starvation (Roden and Viswanathan, 2005). Prolongation of the QT interval is also seen in chronic alcoholics with liver or pancreatic disease, with a concomitant increased risk of sudden death (Milroy, 2007).

Brugada syndrome is an autosomal dominant inherited disorder that has variable penetrance. Several dozen SCN5A mutations have been associated with the syndrome which, in contrast to long QT syndrome, result in a loss of function of the sodium ion channel. Patients are typically male and in the fourth or fifth decade of life at the time of diagnosis and have ST elevation in ECG leads V1–V3. Sudden cardiac death occurs either as a result of ventricular fibrillation or polymorphic ventricular tachycardia (Brugada et al., 2007). It has been suggested that

patients with Brugada syndrome who have QRS prolongation are at increased risk of sudden cardiac death (Takagi et al., 2007).

Catecholaminergic polymorphic ventricular tachycardia is a potentially fatal cardiac arrhythmia that is precipitated by stress, emotion or physical exertion. The disease has both autosomal dominant and recessive varients and typically first becomes manifest in childhood or adolescence (Milroy, 2007).

A degree of circumspection and careful consideration is needed, in the author's opinion, before stating that a death was caused by a channelopathy. Other possible causes of death must be carefully excluded, and it should be remembered that, while these syndromes can cause death, they rarely do so.

Myocarditis

Myocarditis may cause death and it is typical for the heart to appear macroscopically normal or to display only subtle so-called 'tiger-striping' change – pale yellow linear stripes in the myocardium (Fabre and Sheppard, 2006). The disease not uncommonly goes undiagnosed in life. Kytö et al. (2005) found that, of all cases of fatal myocarditis identified at autopsy in Finland between 1970 and 1998, the diagnosis was not considered in life in two-thirds of cases.

Lymphocytic myocarditis, which is commonly of viral origin, is characterised histologically by the presence of a myocardial lymphocytic infiltrate which surrounds and destroys individual cardiac myocytes and is associated with interstitial oedema. Granulomatous myocarditis, known to some as cardiac sarcoidosis, is characterised by the presence of well-formed non-caseating 'naked' granulomas within the myocardium without associated eosinophils. Toxic myocarditis, characterised by an influx of macrophages and eosinophils, may also on occasion be seen, associated with either drug therapy or thyrotoxicosis (Fabre and Sheppard, 2006). Giant cell myocarditis, in which the myocardium is infiltrated by multinucleate giant cells, macrophages, eosinophils and lymphocytes, is rare and of uncertain aetiology – although fatal cases associated with non-steroidal anti-inflammatory drug use have been reported (Adachi *et al.*, 2001). *Toxoplasma gondii* infection in patients with human immunodeficiency virus infection has been reported to rarely cause a fulminant myocarditis (Eza and Lucas, 2006).

Myocarditis may be only focally present, so wide histological sampling of the atria and ventricles is needed to diagnose or exclude these diseases. In the author's experience, sampling of the heart, lungs, liver and blood for virological studies can also be useful in determining the aetiology of lymphocytic myocarditis, and this must be considered at the time of the macroscopic examination. Myocarditis causes death by producing arrhythmogenic foci within the myocardium and by causing cardiac failure (Weber *et al.*, 2008).

Immunohistochemistry may play a valuable role in the diagnosis of chronic myocarditis. Normal myocardium contains low numbers of CD45RO immunoreactive T-cells. Provided that the clinical history is appropriate, the presence of 15 or more CD45RO immunoreactive lymphocytes or macrophages per square millimetre of myocardium is indicative of a diagnosis of chronic myocarditis (Feeley *et al.*, 2000). Lower counts are not specific and may be present in patients dying from a wide variety of non-cardiac diseases (Feeley *et al.*, 2000).

Intrinsic cardiomyopathies

While some cardiomyopathies will result in a mac-roscopically abnormal heart, they can also be present in hearts that appear macroscopically normal and give rise to sudden unexpected death. The intrinsic cardiomyopathies include hypertrophic cardiomyopathy, arrhythmogenic right ventricular cardiomyopathy (dysplasia), and idiopathic diffuse left ventricular cardiac fibrosis.

All the intrinsic cardiomyopathies are uncommon. In life, they are often discovered coincidentally and the first manifestation of the disease may be sudden death. Consequently these diseases may be missed by the autopsy pathologist if not specifically sought.

Hypertrophic (obstructive) cardiomyopathy (HCM) is an autosomal dominant disease caused by mutations in the genes coding for the structural components of the thick and thin filaments that constitute the cardiac sarcomere. It affects 1 in 500 of young adults but may affect individuals of any age from infancy to old age (Hughes, 2004). Marcoscopically HCM is typically associated with cardiac hypertrophy due to an asymmetrical hypertrophy of the left ventricular and in particular the septal myocardium. Symmetrical hypertrophy may also occur, so symmetrical hypertrophy does not exclude the disease (Phadke *et al.*, 2001). As sub-aortic outflow obstruction develops, endocardial fibrosis occurs beneath the anterior leaflet of the mitral valve and chordae – the mitral impact lesion (Hughes, 2004). Fabre and Sheppard (2006) observed that in their series the heart was macroscopically normal in approximately one-sixth of cases. In 10 per cent of cases the heart becomes dilated (Hughes, 2004). Microscopically there is regional myocyte disarray arranged around foci of interstitial collagen. Wide sampling is needed to detect these (see Table 20.2), and the blocks should be taken perpendicular to the long axis of the heart to increase the opportunity of identifying the disarray (Hughes, 2004).

Arrhythmogenic right ventricular cardiomyopathy (formally known as arrhythmogenic right ventricular dysplasia) has both autosomal dominant and recessive inheritance and an incidence of 1 per 2500–5000. The disease is caused by mutations in genes coding for phakoglobulin, desmoglein, desmocollin and desmoplakin, affecting mechanical cell junctions and causing intercalated disc remodelling. The disease is usually most prominent in the right ventricle but the septal and left ventricular myocardium is not uncommonly affected (Thiene *et al.*, 2007). While thinning of the right ventricular wall may be macroscopically apparent, the heart may appear macroscopically normal (Fabre and Sheppard, 2006). The disease is diagnosed histologically when there is infiltration of fatty and fibrous connective tissue throughout the full thickness of the right ventricular myocardium (Thiene *et al.*, 2007). Patients with the disease may be treated by the implantation of a cardioverter defibrillator. However, fatal ventricular fibrillation may be the first manifestation of the disease (Dalal *et al.*, 2005; Thiene *et al.*, 2007).

Idiopathic diffuse left ventricular cardiac fibrosis may cause sudden death, and approximately half of patients will have a macroscopically normal heart without scarring or thinning (Fabre and Sheppard, 2006). The disease is characterised by the presence of increased fibrosis in the left ventricular myocardium in the absence of ischaemic heart disease or systemic hypertension. Other diseases that can produce cardiac fibrosis – including hypereosinophilia, scleroderma, sarcoidosis, viral myocarditis, radiation and drug effects – must be excluded (Lakhan and Harle, 2008). The aetiology is unknown, but Hookana *et al.* (2008) have reported a case in which a lamin A/C gene mutation was associated with left ventricular fibrosis and fatal cardiac arrest.

Non-atheromatous disease of the coronary arteries

Fatal non-atheromatous disease of the coronary arteries has been reported. These include the anomalous origin and course of coronary arteries and myocardial bridging. In the cases reported by Fabre and Sheppard (2006), the bridged segment was 20–40 mm in length and 2–5 mm deep. Other diseases include vasculitis and coronary artery spasm with associated focal contraction band necrosis or infarction (Fabre and Sheppard, 2006). Fineschi *et al.* (1999) reported a case of late Kawasaki disease in which a 20-year-old man collapsed and died and was found to have calcified thin-walled aneurysms of the coronary arteries.

Diseases affecting the conducting system

Sometimes the fatal disease is localised to the cardiac conducting system, but this is rare. Evans and Suvarna (2005) report a fatal cystic atrioventricular tumour in which a young adult male collapsed and died suddenly, with no macroscopic cardiac pathology.

Pneumonia

Pneumonia is a common cause of death. Bronchopneumonia is typically seen in the very young and in the elderly and lobar pneumonia more commonly affects adults aged 20–65 years of age. The macroscopic diagnosis of pneumonia at autopsy is not always easy and is certainly not always reliable (Burton and Underwood, 2007). False-positive and -negative diagnoses are possible. The author has seen neoplastic changes and adult respiratory distress syndrome confused with pneumonia, and has examined many cases where the diagnosis of pneumonia could only be made histologically.

Experienced autopsy pathologists are more likely to make a correct macroscopic diagnosis of the presence or absence of pneumonia than trainees. Roulson *et al.* (2005) reported that the diagnosis of pneumonia could be confirmed microscopically in only 23 per cent of cases, and macroscopic diagnosis was overturned by histology in 31 per cent of cases (Burton and Underwood, 2007). Sampling of the lungs for histopathological and microbiological examination may yield a cause of death. The author has seen cases where no pneumonia was present histologically but where organisms typically associated with pneumonia were present on bacterial culture of the lungs (which should be sterile). The discrepancy is probably due to sampling error.

It should be remembered that a fatal pneumonitis or secondary bacterial pneumonia may complicate influenza infection. In cases where there is a history of influenza-like symptoms in the days preceding death, or where other family members have influenza-like symptoms, it is the author's practice to submit nasal and tracheal swabs for virological analysis.

Table 20.4 Distinguishing diabetic ketoacidosis from alcoholic ketoacidosis and hyperosmolar hyperglycaemic non-ketotic syndrome (HHNS)

	Diabetic ketoacidosis	Alcoholic ketoacidosis	HHNS
Blood β-hydroxybutyrate concentration	+++	+++	N
Vitreous glucose concentration	N / +++	+	N / +++
Urine glucose concentration	+++	0	+++

0, negative; +, low; N, normal; +++, elevated.

Diabetes mellitus

While it is well recognised that diabetes mellitus contributes to the development of atherosclerosis and can cause significant renal disease, it must also be remembered that, like epileptics, diabetics are prone to sudden and unexplained death. These deaths fall into three categories: those due to diabetic ketoacidosis, those due to hyperosmolar hyperglycaemic non-ketotic syndrome (HHNS), and those due to the 'dead in bed' syndrome. In addition, the possibility of a deliberate or accidental suicidal or homicidal insulin overdose must not be overlooked. Deaths in each of the categories will typically yield no significant positive findings on macroscopic examination of the body.

Diabetic ketoacidosis and HHNS

Diabetic ketoacidosis is typically seen in patients with insulin-dependent diabetes mellitus. While HHNS is seen in patients with insulin-dependent diabetes it more commonly occurs in patients with non-insulin-dependent diabetes mellitus.

In insulin-dependent diabetes there is an absence of circulating insulin, which is treated by the therapeutic administration of either animal or human insulin. In the insulin-dependent diabetic who omits their insulin therapy, the blood glucose concentration rises as insulin is required for glucose to enter cells. Consequently, although the blood glucose concentration is normal or elevated glucose cannot be used as a metabolic fuel. When this is the case the liver converts fatty acids to ketones, which can be used as an energy source by the brain. When the concentration of ketones within the blood rises the patient develops a metabolic acidosis, and this can be fatal.

Patients with non-insulin-dependent diabetes are more prone to HHNS. Circulating levels of insulin are typically high but there is insulin resistance in the target tissues. As the blood sugar concentration rises there is increased renal excretion of glucose, and the resulting glycosuria causes an osmotic diuresis. This diuresis causes dehydration, which may be fatal.

Macroscopic examination of the body is typically unremarkable, although the liver may show fatty change. All of the major organs should be sampled for histopathological examination to exclude other causes of death. Analysis of the blood glucose concentration is of no value at post-mortem. The diagnosis will depend on toxicological examination of the vitreous humour, blood and urine (Table 20.4). Vitreous glucose concentration can be used as a marker of hyperglycaemia if normal or elevated at autopsy. The vitreous glucose concentration normally declines rapidly after death, so a low value cannot be taken to indicate ante-mortem hypoglycaemia. When hypoglycaemia is suspected, blood samples should be taken for insulin assay.

'Dead in bed' syndrome

In some insulin-dependent diabetics, a thorough macroscopic examination accompanied by toxicological, microbiological and extensive histological investigation will fail to find a cause of death. Typically the deceased is an adolescent or young adult taking human insulin, who was well during the day and evening before death and who is found dead in bed the next morning. As a consequence, these deaths have been given the unfortunately frivolous-sounding name of 'dead in bed' syndrome. Some authors have estimated that the syndrome accounts for 5–6 per cent of deaths in insulin-dependent diabetics (Koltin and Daneman, 2008). There may be no history of ante-mortem hypoglycaemia or poor diabetic control.

Much has been written about the possible cause(s) of 'dead in bed syndrome'. It is known that insulin-induced hypoglycaemia results in prolongation of the QT interval (Heller, 2002). It is currently believed that death occurs as a result of a ventricular dysrhythmia due to prolongation of the QT interval, which is caused by either hypoglycaemia or a cardiac autonomic neuropathy (Heller, 2002; Suys *et al.*, 2006; Start *et al.*, 2007; Koltin and Daneman, 2008; Tu *et al.*, 2008).

Alcoholism and ketoacidosis

Alcohol has a wide range of toxic effects on the human body. As well as predisposing to gastritis and peptic ulcer disease, which may result in fatal gastrointestinal haemorrhage, excess alcohol consumption may cause fatty liver, cirrhosis, pancreatitis and alcoholic cardiomyopathy. These are generally readily identifiable macroscopically if the history of alcoholism is known and, in the case of cardiomyopathy, if histology is taken to exclude other causes. Fatty liver does not itself cause death, but in the context of alcoholism it should prompt the pathologist to consider the possibility of a fatal ketoacidosis.

Acute alcohol intoxication can be fatal but it is difficult to know at what level alcohol becomes toxic. In England and Wales the maximum blood alcohol concentration that is permitted while driving is 80 mg/100 mL. Tolerance develops with time, and on occasion individuals driving with a blood alcohol concentration of 2000 mg/100 mL have been reported. In practice, a blood alcohol level of approximately 350–380 mg/100 mL is probably sufficient to cause death (Milroy, 2007). Binge drinking can be associated with the development of supraventricular and ventricular tachycardias, which can be fatal (Milroy, 2007).

Acute alcohol intoxication increases the risk of inhalation of gastric contents. However, the autopsy pathologist should be extremely cautious in ascribing death to this. It is common for gastric contents to shift into the lungs passively after death and they are frequently found within the trachea. Passive post-mortem shift may result in gastric contents being present in the alveoli. As a result, death should be ascribed to inhalation of gastric contents only if they are present in the distal lung parenchyma and are associated with an inflammatory reaction (Milroy, 2007).

The individual dying from alcoholic ketoacidosis typically has a history of chronic excess alcohol consumption. There may be a history of binge drinking. The individual typically has a poor diet and has sourced most of their calorific intake from alcohol and so has low glycogen stores in the liver. After a period of abstinence these glycogen stores are rapidly depleted and the liver begins to metabolise fatty acids to ketones. Typically then there is a history of heavy alcohol use, a period of abstinence followed by nausea and vomiting, lethargy, dehydration, confusion and ultimately coma and death. Macroscopic examination of the body often yields few or no positive findings though the liver usually shows profound fatty change. The diagnosis is made on the basis of toxicological examination of vitreous humour, blood and urine (see Table 20.4).

The chronic alcoholic who suddenly stops drinking can be expected to suffer withdrawal symptoms within 6–8 hours. These may include seizures and delirium tremens, which can in rare cases be fatal (Milroy, 2007).

Sudden unexpected death in epilepsy

Patients with epilepsy may die from their epilepsy (status epilepticus, accidents sustained during a seizure, treatment-related deaths), from the underlying disease which causes the epilepsy, or from an unrelated cause. The neuropathological autopsy is discussed in detail in Chapter 12, but it is worth noting here that in a proportion of sudden deaths in epileptics no cause will be found at autopsy. These have come to be known as sudden unexpected deaths in epilepsy (SUDEP; Box 20.2). The mechanism of death is unknown but it has been suggested that it may be due to neurological pulmonary oedema or a cardiac arrhythmia.

The diagnosis of SUDEP is, ultimately, one of exclusion. A complete autopsy should be performed. Samples of all the major organs must be examined histopathologically and blood should be submitted for toxicological examination and microbiological culture. Urine, gastric contents and vitreous humour are also sent for toxicological examination. Hair

Box 20.2 Features of a sudden unexpected death in epilepsy

- The patient is known to have epilepsy (recurrent unprovoked seizures)
- Death was unexpected and occurred rapidly (but most are unwitnessed)
- The deceased was in a reasonable state of health
- Autopsy examination fails to reveal a cause of death
- Death was not due to status epilepticus

may be sent for anti-epileptic toxicology analysis to demonstrate compliance. It is the author's practice and recommended best practice to routinely retain the brain and refer it for examination by a neuropathologist in these cases, and to strongly consider retention of the heart for a detailed examination. These deaths typically occur in young adults and sudden cardiac death must be excluded as discussed earlier in this chapter. In true SUDEP, these investigations reveal no positive findings, although the brain may yield findings consistent with epilepsy and/or a cause of the deceased's epilepsy. Toxicological examination should include a request for assays of the deceased's anti-epileptic medication and may demonstrate non-compliance (Royal College of Pathologists, 2006).

Epilepsy increases the risk of drowning, for example in the bath, and the author has seen such cases. When drowning has occurred, a diagnosis of SUDEP is not appropriate (Royal College of Pathologists, 2006) and a more acceptable cause of death would be:

1a – Drowning
1b – Idiopathic primary generalised epilepsy

Anaphylaxis

The investigation of deaths that may be due to anaphylaxis is discussed in detail in Chapter 17. It is worth reiterating here that there may be few signs to see at autopsy and the key to reaching the diagnosis is a high index of suspicion and the collection of appropriate samples for immunological analysis.

The unascertained autopsy where the cause of death is unnatural

When no cause of death is identified by a careful and thorough macroscopic examination, the pathologist must remain mindful of the fact that the cause of death may be unnatural. If the cause is to be identified, a high index of suspicion is needed, principally because many of the potential unnatural causes will require specific tests to be requested and performed, typically as part of the toxicological examination.

The body should be carefully reviewed for the presence of injuries and other marks, and the clinical history reviewed. Examination of photographs taken at the scene where the body was found may prove invaluable.

Commotio cordis

Sudden application of blunt force trauma to the anterior chest wall at the correct point in the cardiac cycle can trigger a fatal ventricular fibrillation cardiac arrest. This is analogous to the administration of a precordial thump to a patient in cardiac arrest, in which the mechanical energy is converted into the equivalent of an approximately 20 J shock which affects the cardiac rhythm. This is known as 'commotio cordis' (Maron et al., 2002). Animal experimentation has shown that a blow to the chest wall precisely within 10–30 milliseconds before the peak of the T wave consistently results in ventricular fibrillation (Madias et al., 2007). The diagnosis is made on the basis of a history of immediate collapse following a blow to the chest by a non-collapsible projectile, for example a cricket ball, baseball or hockey puck. The autopsy reveals no positive findings, and detailed cardiac examination, neuropathology, histology, microbiology and toxicological investigations are negative.

Unascertained unnatural respiratory causes of death

The airway effectively can be considered to extend, in the unanaesthetised individual, from the atmosphere to the cellular mitochondria. Abnormalities in any part of this pathway may result in death, leaving few or no abnormalities to be detected on macroscopic examination of the body.

On occasion, death will result because the deceased entered an environment where the atmosphere was irrespirable (i.e. contained no oxygen). Such an environment may be found in grain silos or rusty ship cargo holds with insufficient ventilation. Germinating grain or rusting iron may deplete or displace the oxygen content of the air.

The author has seen several cases where death was due to the deliberate inhalation of an irrespirable atmosphere, typically helium. In such cases the deceased may have constructed an elaborate device to allow inhalation of the gas. If the pathologist receives no information regarding the presence of this equipment and the associated helium gas canisters, determination of the true cause of death may be impossible. Helium is a light inert gas and not all toxicology departments are able to test samples for its presence although it is technically possible to do so (Auwaerter *et al.*, 2007). Determination of the cause of death in such cases may rest purely on the circumstantial evidence of the scene of death. It is notable that a number of publications are readily available to the public on the Internet describing helium inhalation as a method of suicide.

Other individuals may die because, while the atmosphere contains oxygen, it also contains toxic gases. Most commonly this will be carbon monoxide formed as a by-product of incomplete combustion. Haemoglobin has a much higher affinity for carbon monoxide than for oxygen. The pathologist may suspect that death is due to carbon monoxide poisoning either because of the circumstances in which a body has been found or because of a characteristic 'cherry pink' discolouration of the body and tissues. In the author's experience, this cherry pink discolouration is most vividly seen in the musculature during the evisceration, rather than in the skin, giving the muscles a vibrant 'fresh' appearance. This discolouration can be seen in patients with a low carboxyhaemoglobin concentration and cannot therefore be regarded as being pathognomonic.

In bodies recovered from fires, death may be due to the inhalation of other toxic products of combustion, including hydrogen cyanide, rather than carboxyhaemoglobin.

Plastic bag asphyxia may be suicidal or acciden-

tal, as in the case of the individual who accidentally or deliberately places a plastic bag over their head (Saint-Martin *et al.*, 2009). This too has been described in popular literature as a means of suicide. It is not necessary for the bag to be secured around the neck. If the person finding the body removes the bag and the pathologist is not made aware of the fact that a bag was present, it will be impossible to determine the true cause of death. Plastic bag asphyxiation may also be homicidal.

Homicidal occlusion of the nose and mouth, as seen in smothering, may also leave no signs on the body, particularly if the deceased does not struggle against the assailant. So-called cardinal signs of asphyxia, such as conjunctival petechial haemorrhages, circumoral pallor and 'hyperfluidity of the blood', are so non-specific as to be meaningless.

It is notable at this point that a search for petechial haemorrhages in the conjunctivae and mouth should be made in every autopsy, but care is needed in their interpretation. While they may be present in smothering and positional asphyxia (see below), they are also seen in a small proportion of deaths due to hanging and in approximately one-fifth of acute cardiac deaths. The presence of petechiae therefore cannot be taken to indicate that death was due to asphyxia. However, if petechiae are found, this should prompt a careful examination of the neck for signs of trauma, and the neck veins should be decompressed before dissecting the muscles of the anterior and posterior compartments of the neck in layers to look for bruising.

Cyanide poisoning may also cause an asphyxial death: it inhibits cellular respiration. Although cyanide has an odour of burnt almonds, many individuals are anosmic to this. Cyanide poisoning may result in a characteristic 'brick red' discolouration of the skin and tissues, and is identifiable on toxicological examination.

Positional asphyxia occurs when an individual becomes trapped in a position so that he or she is unable to expand the chest and therefore cannot breathe. There may be few or no findings at autopsy, and indeed other possible causes of death must be excluded macroscopically, histopathologically and with the aid of microbiology and toxicology. A detailed knowledge of the position in which the body was found, ideally obtained by visiting the scene or reviewing the photographs of the scene of death, is essential if this diagnosis is to be made. 'Found collapsed at bottom of stairs, ? positional asphyxia' is not sufficient information on which to make this diagnosis. The body must have been in a position that would prevent gas exchange, and there should be a reason why the deceased was unable to move out of that position (Belviso *et al.*, 2003).

Hypothermia

Hypothermia may leave few or no positive findings at autopsy, so a detailed account of the circumstances in which the body was found is essential (Ogata *et al.*, 2007). What was the temperature of the environment? Was the death witnessed? Was the body dressed? Where was the body found?

As the core temperature falls, uncontrollable shivering begins in an attempt to raise body temperature. Shivering gradually stops and the individual becomes confused. This may be associated with paradoxical undressing, and so the body may be found naked or partially clothed. In a state of confusion, the hypothermic individual may stumble about the environment sustaining injuries which mimic an assault, or may crawl into small enclosed spaces – the 'hide and die' syndrome. Ultimately coma and death ensue. The elderly and middle-aged individuals who have consumed alcohol outdoors appear to be at particular risk (Taylor *et al.*, 2001).

The body should be examined by the pathologist as soon as possible and, if practicable, before it has been refrigerated in the mortuary. Hypothermia may result in reddish discolouration of the skin over the bony prominences. However, such changes will also be seen in many bodies where death was due to a demonstrable natural cause and where the body has spent a weekend in mortuary refrigeration. A complete and thorough autopsy examination should be made. Intramuscular haemorrhages have been reported in individuals dying from hypothermia and it has been suggested that these are caused by uncontrollable shivering (Ogata *et al.*, 2007). Histopathological examination of the pancreas may reveal vacuolation of the acinar cells, which assists in the diagnosis of hypothermia (Preuss *et al.*, 2007). Toxicological analysis of the urine may reveal elevated catecholamine levels.

The author has made a diagnosis of hypothermia based on the history alone in one case, where a climber was trapped by bad weather in the company of friends and was embalmed before repatriation and autopsy examination some weeks after death occurred. In that case, the macroscopic, histopathological and toxicological examinations were negative.

Drugs and poisons

By far the most common cause of death in autopsies where there are no significant pathological macroscopic findings in the author's practice is death as a result of an illicit or prescribed drug. The collection of samples for appropriate toxicological investigation in such circumstances is discussed in Chapter 15. Plain and preserved samples of blood, urine and vitreous humour, and a sample of gastric contents, should be submitted for analysis.

Drugs commonly implicated in the cause of death include aspirin, paracetamol, opiates, benzodiazepines, methadone, cocaine, amphetamines and barbiturates, and the author's practice is to ask for an analysis for all of these, plus alcohol. The toxicologist should be informed of the prescription medications available to the deceased as these may not form part of a routine toxicological screen. Even when there is a clear history of substance misuse, samples should be retained for histopathological analysis: sometimes the toxicological findings are negative.

Conclusion: formulating the cause of death

As we have seen in this chapter, there are numerous causes of death that are not apparent on macroscopic examination and that come to light only when further investigations are undertaken. Even when extensive histological, toxicological and microbiological investigations have been performed with (as appropriate) detailed cardiac and neuropathological studies, the cause of death will remain unascertained in a small proportion of cases.

When no cause of death can be identified, the pathologist is faced with the dilemma of what to state as the cause. For those with epilepsy, SUDEP is an acceptable cause of death. Sudden arrhythmogenic death syndrome is slowly gaining acceptance (Milroy, 2007). In general, the author's practice is to state that these deaths are 'unascertained'. The discussion section of the autopsy report can then be used to explain the investigations that have been performed. To assist the investigating medicolegal authority, the pathologist should note whether there was anything at autopsy to suggest that death was due to an unnatural cause, or whether it is likely, on the balance of probability, that death was due to an unknown but natural cause.

References

Adachi Y, Yasumizu R, Hashimoto F *et al.* (2001). An autopsy case of giant cell myocarditis probably due to a non-steroidal anti-inflammatory drug. *Pathol Int* **51**:113–17.

Auwaerter V, Perdekamp M, Kempf J *et al.* (2007). Toxicological analysis after asphyxial suicide with helium and a plastic bag. *Forensic Sci Int* **170**:139–41.

Behr ER, Casey A, Sheppard M *et al.* (2007). Sudden arrhythmic death syndrome: a national survey of sudden unexplained cardiac death. *Heart* **93**:601–5.

Belviso M, De Donno A, Vitale L, Introna F (2003). Positional asphyxia: reflection on two cases. *Am J Forensic Med Pathol* **24**:292–7.

Biggs MJP, Swift B, Sheppard MN (2009). Myocardial bridging: is it really a cause of sudden cardiac death. In: Tsokos M (ed.) *Forensic Pathology Reviews*, Vol. 5. Totowa, NJ: Humana Press.

Bowker TJ, Wood DA, Davies MJ *et al.* (2003). Sudden, unexpected cardiac or unexplained death in England: a national survey. *Q J Med* **96**:269–79.

Brugada R (2000). Use of intravenous antiarrhythmics to identify concealed Brugada syndrome. *Curr Control Trials Cardiovasc Med* **1**:45–7.

Brugada J, Brugada R, Brugada P (2007). Channelopathies: a new category of diseases causing sudden death. *Herz* **32**:185–91.

Burton JL, Underwood J (2007). Clinical, educational, and epidemiological value of autopsy. *Lancet* **369**:1471–80.

Dalal D, Nasir K, Bomma C *et al.* (2005). Arrhythmogenic right ventricular dysplasia: a United States experience. *Circulation* **112**:3823–32.

Evans CA, Suvarna SK (2005). Cystic atrioventricular node tumour: not a mesothelioma. *J Clin Pathol* **58**:1232.

Eza DE, Lucas SB (2006). Fulminant toxoplasmosis causing fatal pneumonitis and myocarditis. *HIV Med* **7**:415–20.

Fabre A, Sheppard MN (2006). Sudden adult death syndrome and other non-ischaemic causes of sudden cardiac death. *Heart* **92**:316–20.

Feeley KM, Harris J, Suvarna SK (2000). Necropsy diagnosis of myocarditis: a retrospective study using CD45RD immunohistochemistry. *J Clin Pathol* **53**:147–9.

Fineschi V, Reattelli LP, Baroldi G (1999). Coronary artery aneurysms in a young adult: a case of sudden death. A late sequelae of Kawasaki disease? *Int J Legal Med* **112**:120–3.

Glatter KA, Chiamvimonvat N, He Y, Chevalier P, Turillazi E (2006). Postmortem analysis for inherited ion channelopathies. In: Rutty GN (ed.) *Essentials of Autopsy Practice: Current Methods and Modern Trends*. London: Springer.

Goldenberg I, Moss AJ (2008). Long QT syndrome. *J Am Coll Cardiol* **51**:2291–300.

Heller SR (2002). Abnormalities of the electrocardiogram during hypoglycaemia: the cause of the dead in bed syndrome? *Int J Clin Pract Suppl* **129**:27–32.

Hookana E, Juntilla MJ, Sarkioja T *et al.* (2008). Cardiac arrest and left ventricular fibrosis in a Finnish family with the lamin A/C mutation. *J Cardiovasc Electrophysiol* **19**:743–7.

Hughes SE (2004). The pathology of hypertrophic cardiomyopathy. *Histopathology* **44**:412–27.

Koltin D, Daneman D (2008). Dead-in-bed syndrome: a diabetes nightmare. *Pediatric Diabetes* **9**:504–7.

Kytö V, Saukko P, Lignitz E *et al.* (2005). Diagnosis and presentation of fatal myocarditis. *Hum Pathol* **36**:1003–7.

Lakhan SE, Harle L (2008). Cardiac fibrosis in the elderly, normotensive athlete: case report and review of the literature. *Diagn Pathol* 3:12.

Lowe J (1997). The obscure autopsy and neuroleptic malignant syndrome. *Med Sci Law* 37:79–81.

Madias C, Maron BJ, Alsheikh-Ali AA, Estes NAM, Link MS (2007). Commotio cordis. *Indian Pacing Electrophysiol J* 7:235–45.

Maron BJ, Gohman TE, Kyle SB, Estes NAM, Link MS (2002). Clinical profile and spectrum of commotio cordis. *JAMA* 287:1142–6.

Milroy CM (2007). The autopsy in cases of unascertained sudden death. *Curr Diagn Pathol* 13:401–9.

National Confidential Enquiry into Patient Outcome and Death (2006). *The Coroner's Autopsy: Do We Deserve Better?* London: NCEPOD.

Ogata M, Ago K, Ago M *et al.* (2007). A fatal case of hypothermia associated with hemorrhages of the pectoralis minor, intercostal, and iliopsoas muscles. *Am J Forensic Med Pathol* 28:348–52.

Phadke RD, Vaideeswar P, Mittal B, Deshpande J (2001). Hypertrophic cardiomyopathy: an autopsy analysis of 14 cases. *J Postgrad Med* 47:165–70.

Preuss J, Lignitz E, Dettmeyer R, Madea B (2007). Pancreatic changes in cases of death due to hypothermia. *Forensic Sci Int* 166:194–8.

Roden DM, Viswanathan PC (2005). Genetics of acquired long QT syndrome. *J Clin Invest* 115:2025–32.

Roulson J, Benbow EW, Hasleton PS (2005). Discrepancies between clinical and autopsy diagnosis and the value of post mortem histology; a meta-analysis and review. *Histopathology* 47:551–9.

Royal College of Pathologists (2006). *Guidelines on Autopsy Practice. Scenario 6: Deaths Associated with Epilepsy.* Available online at: www.rcpath.org/resources/pdf/AutopsyScenario6Jan05.pdf.

Saint-Martin P, Prat S, Bouyssy M, O'Byrne P (2009). Plastic bag asphyxia: a case report. *J Forensic Legal Med* 16:40–3.

Start RD, Barber C, Kaschula ROC, Robinson RTCE (2007). The 'dead in bed syndrome': a cause of sudden death in type 1 diabetes mellitus. *Histopathology* 51:843–5.

Suvarna SK (2008). National guidelines for adult autopsy cardiac dissection and diagnosis: are they achievable? A personal view. *Histopathology* 53:97–112.

Suvarna SK, Start RD, Tayler OI (1999). A prospective audit of pacemaker function, implant lifetime, and cause of death in the patient. *J Clin Pathol* 52:677–80.

Suys B, Heuten S, De Wolfe D *et al.* (2006). Glycemia and corrected QT interval prolongation in young type 1 diabetic patients. *Diabetes Care* 29:427–9.

Takagi M, Yokoyama Y, Aonuma K, Aihara N, Hiraoka M (2007). Clinical characteristics and risk stratification in symptomatic and asymptomatic patients with Brugada syndrome: multicenter study in Japan. *Cardiovasc Electrophysiol* 18:1244–51.

Taylor AJ, McGwin G, Davis GG *et al.* (2001). Hypothermia deaths in Jefferson County, Alabama. *Injury Prev* 7:141–5.

Thiene G, Corrado D, Basso C (2007). Arrhythmogenic right ventricular cardiomyopathy/dysplasia. *Orphanet J Rare Dis* 2:45.

Tu E, Twigg SM, Semsarian C (2008). Sudden death in type 1 diabetes: the mystery of the 'dead in bed' syndrome. *Int J Cardiol* 138:91–3.

Weber MA, Ashworth MT, Risdon RA *et al.* (2008). Clinicopathological features of paediatric deaths due to myocarditis: an autopsy series. *Arch Dis Child* 93:594–8.

Chapter 21

RECONSTRUCTION OF THE BODY

Steven Donlon and Guy N Rutty

Show me the manner in which a nation or community cares for its dead and I will measure, with mathematical exactness, the tender sympathies of its people, their respect for the laws of the land and their loyalty to high ideals.

William Gladstone (1871)

Introduction

Reconstruction of the body after autopsy is a very important and often overlooked part of the overall investigation, and would normally be entrusted to the anatomical pathology technologist (APT) – though most forensic pathologists would be reasonably well versed in this procedure.

Before performing an autopsy one should consider how the body is going to be reconstructed afterwards and what the final cosmetic appearance will look like. This will be determined by the incisions that one makes and the parts of the body inspected or removed. Consented autopsies (hospital autopsies) often have restrictions attached, and for this reason both the pathologist and the technologist should be aware of any restrictions that have been included, by carefully studying all sections of the consent form. One must also be aware that it is not uncommon in today's climate for coroners to attach restrictions and exclude or indeed include or indicate a specific organ or procedure in consultation with next of kin and on direction and advice from the pathologist.

A satisfactory reconstruction can be achieved only if the autopsy procedure itself has been performed to the highest standard and the pathologist understands how a body is reconstructed after the autopsy. One should aim to produce the most aesthetically pleasing end result possible. The aim is not, however, to 'improve' on the ante-mortem appearance. If, for example, a patient has undergone a bilateral orchidectomy the scrotum should not be reconstructed to simulate the presence of testes. Treatment of the body with respect and dignity are the most important factors. One must remember that the body may be viewed for the first time by the relatives for the purpose of formal identification after the autopsy. Reconstruction therefore plays a key role in the presentation of the dead to the relatives. Poor reconstruction or rough handling of the cadaver can lead to unnecessary distress and potential complaints.

One must always remember that in some areas of the world the pathologist will have no option but to be able to reconstruct a body to a satisfactory standard. Having said this, the APT is specifically trained in the art of reconstruction and therefore is usually the person who will perform these procedures – although in some areas of the world this may be assigned to staff within a funeral home. The technologist should always ask the pathologist for permission to reconstruct the body prior to any such undertaking.

General preparation

At the end of the evisceration, the body cavity will usually have residual body fluids, tissues and even bowel contents within it. All of these must be removed to prevent leakage. In the UK, with the introduction of legislation by the Human Tissue Authority (HTA), 'tissue' includes blood products – so residual blood and cellular material should remain with the body. This has created a dilemma for the technologist delegated to the reconstruction, as blood-stained fluid such as ascites and pleural fluid have in the past been removed and disposed of. Clarification was sought from the HTA on this specific subject. The HTA stated that 'residual tissue is any tissue taken for a specific purpose'. As this residual fluid is not for a specific purpose, it can be disposed of as waste products; however, the body should be as complete as possible.

Fluids are removed with the use of a ladle and jug and can be disposed of into a sluice, which is connected to a designated mortuary drainage system. Some autopsy tables may have integrated suction incorporated in the design for this purpose. Any tissue is removed by hand or other appropriate method and returned to the body in an environmentally friendly unlettered plastic bag with the other body tissues. All organs must be returned to the body unless prior consent for retention has been obtained. No foreign objects (e.g. universal containers, blood tubes, syringes, needles, gloves, aprons etc.) are to be placed inside the body: they should be disposed of separately through appropriate designated clinical waste routes. If the body contained sharp objects, such as inferior vena cava filters, glass or needles, these should be disposed of into a sharps bin.

Once the body cavities are dry, the pelvic cavity and the posterior pleural cavities are lined with sufficient wadding or cotton wool to soak up any remaining body fluids or fluids that might continue to leak following the reconstruction (Fig. 21.1). This ensures that no fluid leaks from the body after reconstruction. Cotton wadding is also placed into the neck to reconstruct its normal contour. Most establishments use cotton wool as the wadding although alternative materials have been used in the

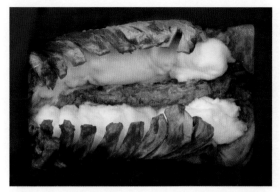

Figure 21.1 The body cavities are packed with wadding.

past, for example towelling, clothing or even sawdust or newspaper. The use of such alternative materials is now deemed inappropriate, as is the use of descriptive items such as incontinence pads, clinical waste bags or black refuse bags, as a negative inference could be drawn from their use. Clear or opaque bags should be used to contain the returned organs. Some mortuaries use specific absorbent crystals (e.g. embalming crystals) that soak up excess fluid.

The organs should not be placed free into the body cavities, but be returned in an environmentally friendly plastic bag (as mentioned above). This bag is sealed and placed into the cavity on top of the wadding. This is another step that tries to prevent leakage from the body.

Suturing

General principles

Traditionally, suturing was performed using single good-quality mattress twine attached to a long cutting needle, straight or serpentine depending on personal preference. This type of twine has in general (owing to negative inferences associated with its use) now been replaced by suture twine supplied for this specific purpose. The choice of suture is important. Lesser quality materials, for example string or polythene twine, may cause knotting and/or suture breakdown.

A knot is placed at the end of the suture to locate and secure the start. Suturing then proceeds using a technique known as under-stitching, whereby the

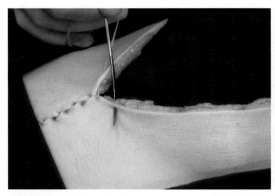

Figure 21.2 Under-stitching.

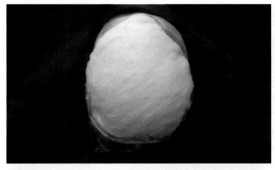

Figure 21.3 The cranial cavity is packed with wadding.

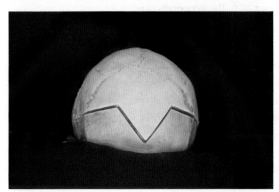

Figure 21.4 A triangular notch cut in the frontal bone prevents the skull-cap slipping.

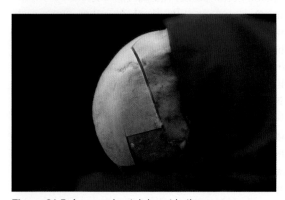

Figure 21.5 A second notch is cut in the squamous temporal bone to stop the skull-cap slipping.

skin is sewn from below (Fig. 21.2). This method is chosen out of preference to other stitching styles as it produces a flatter cosmetic result and much of the suturing is hidden from view at the end of the procedure. The stitches should be tight and placed approximately 1 cm apart. Each suture is placed approximately 5 mm from the incision edge to ensure that as much of the suture as possible is hidden from view. Suture depths greater than 5 mm are not appropriate in the average body as they may draw fat up into the suture line, giving a poor cosmetic result. Care must also be taken not to catch cotton wool in the sutures, for example when closing the neck.

The head

The stripped dura and the brain are placed into the plastic bag with the other body tissues. Any bones (e.g. the orbital plates or middle ears), if not sampled for histology, are placed back into their anatomical sites. Sufficient wadding is placed into the cranial cavity to soak up any fluid (Fig. 21.3). While it is often assumed that this has to fill the entire cranial cavity to prevent the skull-cap from moving, there are in fact better ways to achieve this (see below). A lesser amount of packing is therefore permissible. In children the brain should be placed back inside the cranial cavity whenever possible to retain a natural feel (parents will commonly want to hold the baby after post-mortem examination); although this is technically difficult, care should be taken to maintain a realistic weight to body size ratio.

The skull-cap can now be replaced. When the skull was opened one should have considered how to stop any movement of the skull after reconstruction. This can be achieved by placing a triangular or square notch in the midline of the frontal bone incision (Fig. 21.4). The point of the triangle should point towards the nose to avoid glove puncture injuries while removing the brain. A second notch is placed in either or both of the squamous temporal

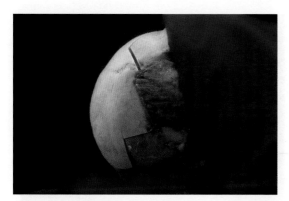

Figure 21.6 The temporalis is replaced.

bones (Fig. 21.5). Finally, the posterior skull incision should be angled at approximately 150 degrees to the incision in the squamous temporal bones. Thus the skull-cap can be appropriately relocated and have minimal movement. A poor reconstruction will produce an unsightly bony ridge to the forehead owing to movement of the skull-cap.

The temporalis muscles, which were originally dissected off the skull, are relocated. This hides the incision in the cranial vault at the sides and prevents lateral movement of the skull (Fig. 21.6). To further stabilise the skull one could suture the muscles to the periosteum at the sides. An alternative method is to tie both muscles together with a length of suture that goes over the vertex of the skull. Metal fixing clips are a further alternative technique.

The scalp is then brought back into its original position. From time to time, during the removal of the scalp, the skin may stretch. Thus when the two halves are brought back together the edges may overlap. Careful suturing by a skilled technologist can overcome this problem to ensure a tight fit. An alternative technique is to remove a thin strip of scalp, placing it into the organ bag. This will allow a tight scalp closure to be achieved.

The scalp incision is closed working from ear to ear using the under-stitching method described above. During this procedure the hair is wetted and a comb or brush is used to stop the hair becoming entangled in the twine as one sews. Having reached the other ear the suture is tied off, burying the knot in the process.

The eye and orbit

If the only procedure that has been performed to the eye is the removal of the vitreous humour, an equal quantity of sterile water or preservative (such as saline) is injected into the posterior chamber using the same syringe, needle and hole until the globe is re-inflated. Care should be taken not to over-inflate the eye.

In cases where the eye has been removed and retained, the orbit must be reconstructed. The back of the orbit is first packed with dry cotton wool. Damp cotton wool is then added on top of this to mimic an eye globe. This gives a superior cosmetic result. A clear eye shield is placed over the cotton wool and the lids closed. Particular care should be taken to avoid damaging the eyelashes or the skin of the face. If necessary, the upper eyelid can be glued to the eyeshield. There is no need to draw a 'pupil' on the wadding if the eyelids are properly closed.

The neck

Although some argue that a Y-shaped incision results in poor neck reconstruction and hampers viewing of the body, this is not the authors' experience. A careful incision as posterolateral as possible will not show when reconstructed and the deceased is lying in the funeral home or funeral casket, clothed, on a pillow with bedding appropriately placed. The 'standard' midline incision, which should be avoided, can easily result in a poor cosmetic result if the upper end is sited too high on the neck.

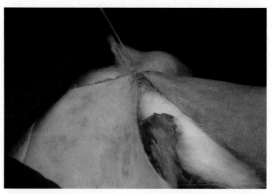

Figure 21.7 The neck is sutured, beginning with an 'anchor suture'.

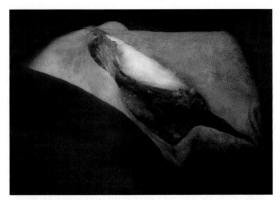

Figure 21.8 Wadding is added to the neck to reconstruct a life-like contour.

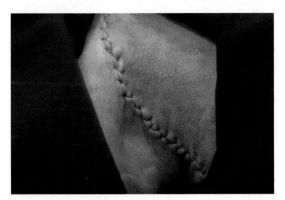

Figure 21.9 The neck is sutured closed.

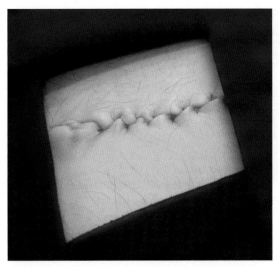

Figure 21.10 The body is closed using neat sutures.

Thorax and abdomen

Having closed the neck incisions and returned the bag containing the organs and tissues to the body cavities, the thorax and abdomen can be closed. Wadding placed on top of the bag assists in stopping leakage and is helpful in reconstructing the original shape of the chest. The sternal rib-shield is placed on top of the bag and wadding such that the cut ends of the ribs meet. The suturing proceeds where one left off from the start of the neck reconstruction. One-centimetre, under-sewn sutures are continued to the suprapubic region, where the suture is tied off and buried (Fig. 21.10).

The limbs

Sometimes it is necessary to open the limbs during an autopsy, when seeking the presence of subcutaneous and muscular injuries, deep vein thromboses or fractures. Incisions into the limbs should be placed on their extensor surfaces where possible. At the end of the examination, the incision is packed with cotton wadding. The incision can then be closed using the under-sewn suturing method described above. If long bones are removed, further specialist reconstruction techniques are required, as considered below. Where the shoulders and buttocks have been examined, care must be taken during reconstruction not to cause distortion of the local anatomy. This is a particular

The three points of the neck and chest skin incisions must first be joined with a securing stitch, before sewing several centimetres down the midline chest incision (Fig. 21.7). The neck suture can then begin behind either ear. As with the head, suturing is performed using the under-stitching method. The suturing is continued downwards from the ear until the midline is reached.

After replacing any false teeth the mouth and neck are packed with wadding (Fig. 21.8). To minimise any potential leakage the wadding should reach the line of the incision. The suture is then continued upwards to the other ear, packing the neck as one proceeds. During the sewing process the neck is shaped so that it resembles the living neck as far as possible. If excessive packing is used, the body will look bloated. When the ear is reached the suture is tied off, burying the knot in the process (Fig. 21.9).

problem with the buttocks. A stabilising, locating stitch similar to that used for the neck can be used to join the midline back incision to those running down the buttocks and legs. Once this is performed, suturing can start at the most distal lower limb site and work back up each side to the natal cleft area. Where tattoos have been incised, care should be taken to try to ensure that the suture line brings the tattoo back to as near to its original state as possible.

Long bones and spinal column

Sometimes a long bone (e.g. femur) may have to be removed for examination and retained at autopsy. In the past, an equal-sized length of broomstick covered by wadding was placed into the space left by the long bone to enable shape reconstruction and to soak up any excess fluid. However, this would be unacceptable with modern regulations. Whenever possible the original bone should be replaced. Custom-made prosthetic units are available but expensive. The limb should be packed to avoid leakage, then sutured closed as above.

If the spinal cord has been removed, the space is lined by wadding and the vertebral column replaced. In cases where the spinal cord has been removed using a posterior approach, wadding is placed over the vertebral column to minimise leakage, and the incision is closed using the under-stitching technique.

Washing down

After the body has been reconstructed it must be cleaned of any residual bodily fluids that have been spilt during the autopsy. Hot water should be avoided as this may remove the skin – although most mortuaries will have the hot water thermostatically controlled to avoid scalding and alleviate this problem. Mild detergents/disinfectants may be added to a bowl of warm water to assist the washing process. The body and tray are thoroughly washed using a clean sponge, making sure that all traces of blood, tissue, bowel contents and fat have been removed. The back of the body and the hair must be washed. The body and tray are then rinsed with warm water. The body and tray are next dried using clean dry sponges, clean dry cotton towels or dispos-

able paper towels. Further drying can be done using clean dry towels or disposable-type paper towel roll. Once again the back and the hair must be dried.

With a head block placed under the neck, the hair can now be combed. Wherever possible, this is done to recreate the original ante-mortem style. Although this may require the assistance of a specialist, for example an embalmer or embalmer's assistant, competent APTs should be able to achieve this without assistance.

Finally, the body should be dressed in a shroud and a clean white sheet, or placed in a plastic body sheet or zip-type body bag. On no account should a body be left uncovered; dignity and respect must be maintained at all times. All of the identification labels must be clearly accessible and visible. A waterproof write-on wristband may be placed on the body at this point, before returning the body to the storage area. At least two bands should be placed on each body, preferably at different locations (e.g. the wrist and ankle or both wrists). Toe tags should be avoided as they tend to fall off. The use of modern electronic tagging systems, although available for cadavers, have as yet not been generally accepted owing to unproven concern over the public response to the use of such devices.

Special circumstances

Danger of infection with category 3 pathogens

Regardless of whether or not there is a potential or known risk of infection with a category 3 pathogen (see Chapters 6 and 7), the same level of care should be given during the reconstruction of the body. The only difference is that at the end of the procedure bodies suspected or known to harbour such pathogens are placed into sealed body bags that should bear a clearly visible 'biohazard' label. Funeral directors should be alerted to the risk posed, with the provision of a non-specific infection control notification sheet that states the route of transmission (e.g. aerosol, blood), and the category of infection. On no account should the specific infection be divulged, so as to preserve patient confidentiality. The custodian of the body, whether it is a National Health Service or public mortuary, has a duty of care to any third party handling the remains.

Chemical risk, category 4 pathogens, or radiation contamination

There are certain circumstances in which, assuming an examination has occurred in the first place, the body would not be reconstructed. Category 4 pathogens and some instances of chemical and radiological contaminated bodies fall into this category. These bodies would simply be placed in a purpose-designed body bag and disposed of following advice from the local Health Protection Agency.

Decomposition

If the body has decomposed, the level of reconstruction will be determined by the state of the body. Sutures may need to be wider apart and placed deeper into the tissue (or other suturing techniques used) to enable the body cavities to be sealed without the tissue tearing. The body is then placed into sealed tubular plastic sheeting or an equivalent body bag.

Wounds and incisions

If there are any wounds or surgical incisions to the body, these are closed with suturing, but only if a second autopsy examination is not to be performed. Small lacerations and incised wounds can be closed with tissue glue. In the case of homicide, these wounds should be closed only after the opportunity for a second examination of the injuries has occurred, and only then after consultation with, and approval by, the lead pathologist.

Pelvic dissection

In cases where the genital tract has been removed *en bloc*, the pelvic bone wedge is replaced to reconstruct the pelvic ring. A series of strong deep sutures starting at the most posterior aspect and working anteriorly will reconstruct this area.

Fetal and paediatric reconstruction

After a paediatric autopsy the basic principles are the same as for an adult, with the goal being to produce a high standard of cosmetic reconstruction. The choice of suture material may be different in view of the size of the body. The use of thick, black suture material should be avoided at all costs. It should be remembered that family members often pick up children after the autopsy, so careful reconstruction and dressing of the body is critical.

After a fetal autopsy, the fragility of the skin occasionally makes suturing an unsuitable method of reconstruction. The body should be lightly dried with absorbent paper towels and loosely packed with cotton wool (or other suitable wadding). The soft tissues and skin are then reunited using a fast-acting tissue adhesive. Care should be taken to avoid using excess glue as this produces an exothermic reaction.

Further reading

Gau GS, Napier K, Bhundia J (1991). Use of tissue adhesive to repair fetal bodies after dissection. *J Clin Pathol* **44**:759–60.

Gresham GA, Turner AF (1979). Reconstruction of the body after post-mortem examination. In: *Post-mortem Procedures: An Illustrated Textbook*, pp. 131–2. London: Wolfe Medical.

Hoggarth P, Poole B (2001). A pathologist's guide to embalming. In: Rutty GN (ed.) *Essentials in Autopsy Practice*, Vol. 1. London: Springer-Verlag, pp. 23–42.

Online:
Care and Respect in Death: Good Practice Guidance for NHS Mortuary Staff, 2005 (www.dh.gov.uk)

HTA Code of Practice. 3. Post-mortem Examinations (www.hta.gov.uk)

Modernising Pathology: Good Practice Guidance, 2004 (www.dh.gov.uk)

Chapter 22

AUTOPSIES AND CLINICAL AUDIT

James Underwood

Introduction

Clinical audit is the systematic analysis of the quality of patient care with the aim of identifying possible improvements. The use of autopsy data in clinical audit is obvious in the consideration of cases in which the outcome has been fatal; autopsy findings can be compared with the clinical diagnosis and the certified cause of death. However, the role of the autopsy in monitoring the incidence and consequences of previously undiagnosed non-fatal conditions, discovered only at autopsy, should not be ignored.

Effective audit demands a high autopsy rate and high standards of autopsy performance and reporting (Underwood *et al.*, 1989), but the autopsy rate continues to fall. This decline has early origins. Thomas Sydenham (1624–1689) scorned 'Some physicians [who] pompously and speciously prosecute the promotion of medicine by search into the bowels of the dead' (cited by McPhee and Bottles, 1985). While dramatic medical advances were resulting from autopsy observations in Germany by Rokitansky (1804–1878), John Bennett in 1844 in Britain opined that 'It is daily becoming more and more apparent that the results of post-mortem examination have ceased to furnish us with facts sufficiently novel and important enough to advance the study of pathology.'

This opinion is now entrenched in the minds of many senior clinicians, as is evident from surveys of their attitudes to requesting and attending autopsies (Chane *et al.*, 1990). Numerous studies, however, continue to reveal significant discrepancies between clinical diagnoses, including certified causes of death, and the actual conditions or causes of death as determined by autopsy (Roulson *et al.*, 2005; Burton and Underwood, 2007). It is essential, therefore, for autopsy data to be a major component of clinical audit.

For simplicity and to acknowledge the different legal processes in various countries, the discussion in this chapter will make no distinction between medicolegal (e.g. coroners') and clinical (hospital) autopsies in their potential to contribute information for clinical audit. Even deaths outside hospital and falling within medicolegal jurisdiction have the potential to yield information for clinical audit, particularly if the deceased individual recently attended a general practitioner or a hospital outpatient clinic.

Verification of clinical diagnoses

Among the first and largest studies of the accuracy of clinical diagnoses is that of Cabot (1912). In 3000 autopsies, he discovered that 77 per cent of cases of spinal tuberculosis, 61 per cent of cases of cirrhosis and 26 per cent of cases of lobar pneumonia had been missed clinically. Cabot acknowledged that these discrepancies were probably attributable to limited diagnostic methods rather than to errors of clinical interpretation or judgement. According to Wells (1923), 33 per cent of tumours discovered at autopsies in two Chicago hospitals had not been diagnosed in life.

Of course, since these early studies there have been considerable advances in clinical practice and some of the conditions common previously (e.g. spinal tuberculosis) are now relatively rare. Nevertheless, in every subsequent study of clinical versus autopsy diagnoses a significant incidence of discrepancies has been found. For example, Gruver and Freis (1957) found that bacterial pneumonia, meningitis, endocarditis and tumours accounted for approximately half of the 6 per cent of diagnostic discrepancies discovered in a series of 1106 autopsies performed during 1947–1953 at the V.A. Hospital, Washington, DC. Another review (McPhee and Bottles, 1985) cited published rates of missed major diagnoses of clinical relevance as high as 40 per cent and exceeding 10 per cent in most surveys. A particularly thorough survey of 33 separate publications from 1980 to 1986 and involving 30 983 autopsies (Nemetz et al., 1987) reveals a wide range of discrepancy rates, from as low as 0.3 per cent for previously undiagnosed endometrial carcinoma up to 55.5 per cent for previously undiagnosed prostatic carcinoma (occult and, therefore, clinically probably insignificant in just over half).

Not all errors or discrepancies carry equal weight: some are relatively inconsequential (such as occult prostatic carcinoma), but others have considerable impact and might have influenced patient survival if recognised during life (such as pulmonary tuberculosis or infective endocarditis). Goldman et al. (1983) asserted that 12 per cent of autopsies in 1970 revealed conditions that, if they had been diagnosed and treated correctly during life, might have resulted in survival of the patient. Cameron et al. (1980), reporting their experience in Edinburgh, found that the main diagnosis had been missed in 15 per cent of autopsied cases and that in 5 per cent the patient might have benefited if the correct diagnosis had been made in life. However, neither the length of stay in hospital nor the confidence with which the diagnosis was held correlated with clinical diagnostic accuracy (Cameron and McGoogan, 1981).

In one of the most recent and thorough (c.90 per cent autopsy rate) published studies of diagnostic error rates revealed by autopsy, the frequency of major discrepancies declined from 30 to 14 per cent over a 20 year period, although the frequency of minor errors doubled to 42 per cent (Sonderegger-Iseli et al., 2000). The improved rate of major errors resulted mainly from a significant increase in clinical diagnostic specificity for cardiovascular diseases. It is inconceivable that the improvement in clinical diagnostic accuracy was not, to some extent, due to feedback from post-mortem examinations, but this intervention has not been tested experimentally.

With advances in medical imaging, microbiology, clinical biochemistry etc. it was inevitable that diagnostic discrepancies discovered at autopsy might be attributed increasingly to errors of clinical judgement, though not necessarily, of course, due to culpable negligence. Because an autopsy may reveal that a fatal outcome might have been averted if the correct diagnosis had been made in life, clinicians may be tempted to 'bury their mistakes' in the increasingly litigious environment of modern medical practice. This reluctance, even resistance, to autopsies must be overcome.

Undeniably, there is an irreducible lower limit of unavoidable diagnostic errors attributable to the vagaries of disease eluding even the most competent diagnostician.

Death certification and the autopsy

The causes of most deaths in most countries are certified without confirmation by autopsy. Because there are frequent discrepancies between the clinically presumed and the actual cause of death, even in hospital cases that have been subjected to thorough investigation during life, the reliability of death certification data for epidemiological purposes must be questioned. Accurate morbidity and mortality data are essential for monitoring a nation's health, for earlier detection of environmental hazards, and for planning the allocation of limited resources for healthcare.

In the USA, discrepancy rates between certified and actual (as determined by autopsy) causes of death range from 25 to 56 per cent (Kircher et al., 1985). In Trieste, where a remarkably high autopsy rate of about 90 per cent has been achieved lately, previously undiagnosed cancer was discovered in 27 per cent of cases (Gobbato et al., 1982). Discrepancy rates of up to 30 per cent have been reported in the UK. The apparent higher incidence of deaths attributed to ischaemic heart disease in Scotland, compared with England and Wales, could be explained partly by the lower frequency of confirmation of this cause of death by autopsy under the medicolegal procedures of the Procurator Fiscal system.

The financial consequences of using the actual cause of death, rather than the certified cause, are most evident with the system of diagnosis-related-group (DRG) reimbursement. Any increased DRG reimbursement would have to be offset against the increased cost of performing autopsies at a rate high enough to yield a sufficient number of altered diagnoses attracting a higher DRG-based income. Several studies have shown that it is at least theoretically possible to increase DRG reimbursement if autopsy data are used (Kircher, 1990).

Auditing perioperative deaths

During the twentieth century, medicine became more dangerous and surgery became safer, owing to advances in anaesthesia, antisepsis and surgical techniques; perioperative deaths remain, however, a serious problem. The possibility of litigation may arise in some perioperative deaths but is not relevant here and the threat should not inhibit clinical audit.

In the UK, the Confidential Enquiry into Perioperative Deaths (CEPOD – later to become the National Confidential Enquiry into Patient Outcome and Death, NCEPOD) was begun in 1982. It was coordinated by the Associations of Anaesthetists and of Surgeons and funded by two medical charities. The reviews concentrated on three National Health Service regions and the participation rate was 95 per cent. The day after publication of the first CEPOD report in 1987, the British government promised that funds would be provided to support the NCEPOD review of all perioperative deaths in England; the process was soon extended to include Wales and Northern Ireland and hospitals in the independent (private) sector.

The NCEPOD 1989 report (Camplin et al., 1990) records a participation rate by consultant anaesthetists and surgeons of 99.8 per cent, indicating a high degree of willingness to review such cases. It is of interest that three of the six recommendations concerned the care of children: surgeons and anaesthetists should not undertake occasional paediatric practice; consultants with paediatric responsibilities must maintain their professional competence; and no trainee should anaesthetise or operate on any child without their consultant's advice and approval. With regard to pathologists' involvement, 76 per cent (224) of all perioperative deaths were reported to a coroner, but in only 58 per cent was an autopsy directed. Of those cases not referred to a coroner or not accepted as falling within medicolegal jurisdiction, the autopsy rate with relatives' consent was just over 50 per cent.

The NCEPOD 1990 report (Camplin et al., 1992) concluded that, in respect of autopsies, 'The infrequency of this useful investigation revealed in this Enquiry is to be deplored' and that 'communications between pathologists (both hospital and coroners') and clinicians is so poor that useful lessons can often not be learnt'. The report recommended that the quality of information in post-mortem records should be improved and that efforts should be made to increase the number of examinations.

Of the 2558 deaths surveyed in the 1990 NCEPOD report, 32 per cent were accepted for coroners' autopsy in addition to only 7 per cent subjected to 'hospital' autopsy with a relative's consent. Even allowing for the other commitments of surgeons, it is remarkable that, in this series of perioperative deaths, consultants personally requested relatives' consent in only 20 out of 417 cases. Just as lamentable, however, is the finding that in less than half of the autopsied cases was the surgical team informed of the date and time of the post-mortem examination.

Auditing medical treatment

Concomitant with auditing clinical diagnosis by autopsy is the opportunity to assess the effects – desirable and adverse – of treatment. It is remarkable how often deaths of cancer patients are attributed, without autopsy confirmation, to their disease rather than to treatment or some natural intervention. Most pathologists with sufficient experience of autopsies will be familiar with occasional cases in which no evidence of residual or recurrent tumour is found at autopsy and yet the death certificate has recorded death as being due to 'carcinomatosis'. Surely when some of medicine's most toxic drugs have been administered it is desirable to monitor their clinical appropriateness and iatrogenic consequences by autopsies in the event of a fatal outcome.

Auditing diagnostic imaging

Most patients who have died in hospital will have had some form of diagnostic imaging, most commonly an x-ray examination, but increasingly an ultrasound scan, a multi-detector computerised tomography (MDCT) scan, or a magnetic resonance imaging (MRI) procedure. While radiologists have considerable expertise in interpreting these images, radiology, like histopathology, is a fallible process and errors of interpretation are not unknown.

Autopsies provide radiologists and pathologists unrivalled opportunities to correlate the morbid images obtained during life with the corresponding morbid anatomy revealed after death. When examining the organs in such cases, it is helpful if the pathologist slices the relevant organs in the same plane (e.g. sagittal, coronal) as that of the diagnostic image; in this way the features can be matched more precisely.

Sampling and selection of cases for audit

The utility of the autopsy for audit is likely to be greatest in those cases in which there is no perceived prior necessity for the examination. If autopsies are done only on those cases in which there is genuine doubt about the clinical diagnosis, the findings will certainly be informative but less contributory to audit. If autopsies are done routinely in the majority of deaths (which is rarely possible), the sample examined is likely to include a sufficiently high proportion of cases in which there was no perceived prior necessity for the examination.

The report of the Joint Working Party of the Royal Colleges in the UK (1991) recommended that, for effective audit, a sample of at least 10 per cent of general hospital deaths in which there is no perceived prior necessity for autopsy should be examined. It is, however, recognised that there are difficulties in implementing this recommendation. Possibilities include sampling every tenth consecutive death or those cases whose registration numbers end with a particular digit, having first excluded those cases in which an autopsy is deemed necessary; if relatives refuse consent, then the next case would be selected. These procedures would have to be operated with considerable discretion; patients, and their relatives, would be understandably alarmed if they realised that they were destined by lottery for audit by autopsy.

The use of autopsy data in auditing the reliability of ante-mortem clinical diagnoses and causes of death is commonly flawed because of case selection bias (autopsies tend to be requested only in those cases in which there is clinical uncertainty) and variations in autopsy practice (such as inconsistent sampling for histology) even in the same institution. Therefore, Saracci (1991) set out the criteria for determining the validity of autopsy data for use in clinical audit, particularly if comparisons are to be made between institutions or on the basis of trends over time. These criteria are:

- estimating the error rate in the autopsy itself (gross findings should be verified by histology);
- specifying standard conditions and protocols for autopsies;
- ensuring unbiased sampling of deaths for autopsy.

It is recommended also that measures of agreement between clinical and autopsy diagnoses should be expressed in terms of sensitivity and specificity.

Recording autopsy data for audit

Systematic audit requires standard methods for recording and evaluating data. Recording diagnoses is relatively straightforward, particularly if the conditions are assigned SNOP and SNOMED numerical codes.

Discrepancies can be monitored continuously by a computerised system using a relatively simple database in which each diagnosis is entered as a numerical code (Reid *et al.*, 1987). The ante-mortem/post-mortem diagnostic correlation can be classified as agreements, over-diagnoses and under-diagnoses and issued as bar charts to requesting clinicians.

Discrepancies between pre-mortem and post-mortem diagnoses could be quantified by just counting, but this simple method is potentially misleading because autopsies inevitably reveal more morbid changes that were clinically evident, not all of which could be regarded as significant. The relative significance of discrepancies depends on at least three factors.

- *The disease categories of the clinical and autopsy diagnoses.* For example, a discrepant primary site for a malignant neoplasm is likely to be less significant than the discovery of tuberculosis in a case in which death was attributed to carcinomatosis.
- *The treatability of the autopsy diagnosis.* For example, discovery at autopsy of a lung carcinoma in a cardiorespiratory cripple is likely to be relatively insignificant because the patient would not have tolerated investigation or treatment.
- *The quality and quantity of lost life expectancy* (quality-adjusted life years; QALYS). This explains the commendably high level of clinical interest in neonatal and paediatric autopsies.

Table 22.1 Scheme for classifying discrepancies between ante-mortem and post-mortem diagnoses

Category	Discrepancy
Major	Class I: Principal diagnosis definitely affecting clinical outcome
	Class II: Principal diagnosis possibly affecting clinical outcome
Minor	Class III: Secondary diagnosis either symptomatic but not treated or likely to have affected prognosis
	Class IV: Secondary diagnosis that could not have been made clinically
	Class V: None

Adapted from Battle et al. *(1987) and Anderson* et al. *(1990).*

A protocol for classifying diagnostic discrepancies according to their clinical importance is often useful, such as that suggested by Battle *et al.* (1987) and modified by Anderson *et al.* (1990) (Table 22.1). Friederici and Sebastian (1984) proposed a 'concordance score' as a means of quantifying discrepancies based on ranking and categorising diagnoses according to the clinical impact.

Diagnostic errors also need classification according to cause (Table 22.2). Even major diagnostic discrepancies are rarely due to culpable clinical error; the error may be attributable entirely to mimicry of the signs and symptoms of another disease rather than to medical negligence.

Closing the 'audit loop'

The 'audit loop' feeds information from autopsies back into clinical practice with the aim of effecting improvements. This is a gradual and welcome outcome of clinicians witnessing autopsy findings or reading promptly issued autopsy reports on their cases.

Table 22.2 Categorisation of diagnostic errors according to cause.

Category	Cause	Definition
1	Imperfect knowledge	Error due to limitations of contemporary medical knowledge, skills or techniques
2	Innate fallibility	Error due to unpredictable effect of variables in the disease, the patient or the clinical environment
3	Practitioner error	Error due to limited knowledge or skills of the clinician or to inaccurate technical data
4	Negligence	Error due to negligent or wilful disregard of accepted clinical standards

Adapted from Anderson et al. *(1990) and Gorovitz and MacIntyre (1976; cited by Anderson* et al.*).*

Regular mortality meetings, which are now commonplace in some specialties such as neonatology, should involve the active participation of pathologists. Such meetings may result in changes of clinical policy as a result of auditing fatalities. The success of these meetings relies on a spirit of genuine partnership between pathologists and clinicians to achieve improvements in patient care. Clinicians must be receptive of the information from autopsies and willing to concede that serious diagnostic or treatment errors can be made. Concomitantly, pathologists must avoid assuming an adversarial role in morbidity meetings, having taken advantage of the opportunity to perform a meticulous autopsy at relative leisure on a patient who, for example, died after an acute medical or surgical emergency at 4 o'clock in the morning.

The Joint Working Party of the Royal Colleges (1991) recommended systematic monitoring of the discrepancy rates between ante-mortem and post-mortem diagnoses, making the information available to consultants individually or more widely with their consent.

Pathologists can go only part way to closing the 'audit loop'. Completion relies on clinicians changing their practice as a result of autopsy findings, but many pathologists believe that autopsies are ineffective in influencing clinicians' behaviour. Nevertheless, with this motive, clinical audit was a major feature of the UK health service reforms following implementation of the National Health Service and Community Care Act 1990. A study in Peterborough Health Authority surveyed the attitudes of clinicians to autopsy findings in individual cases (Harris and Blundell, 1991). In 44 per cent of cases the autopsy was regarded as 'very valuable', and deemed to be 'of no value' in only 2 per cent. The clinicians stated in 14 per cent of cases that the autopsy results would affect future clinical practice, but others continue to find that evidence for this remains unsubstantiated (Guly, 2005).

Auditing the autopsy

The autopsy itself should not be exempt from audit. The examination is difficult to audit because it is destructive; the organs cannot be reconstituted, the dissection repeated, and the findings reinterpreted. In individual cases it can be attempted by having the thoroughness of the examination, the findings and the interpretations checked by a colleague; this should be mandatory for autopsies done by trainees. There are, however, no published systematic studies of inter-observer agreement on the interpretation of gross autopsy findings.

The performance and reporting of autopsies could be audited by comparison with agreed standards such as requirements to:

- record the measurements of all salient localised lesions, the volumes of all effusions, and the weights of all major organs;
- sample organs for histology according to a protocol;
- issue the report within, for example, 1 week.

Anderson and Hill (1989) surveyed pathology departments in medical schools in the USA and found that the average interval between the autospy and the issue of the report was 55 days, with delays of up to 5 months in some departments. They also found much variation in the format of reports, often resulting in difficulties in ascertaining the important findings.

Histology of autopsy findings can be done to audit the reliability of naked-eye interpretations of morbid changes. The extent to which this is helpful and cost-effective was audited in 160 cases by Reid (1987). He concluded that routine unselected post-mortem histology was not cost-effective, although two unsuspected myocardial infarcts were revealed by histology in 52 hearts deemed grossly to have been normal or near normal.

In a study of the value of post-mortem histology in auditing interpretation of the gross autopsy findings, Zaitoun and Fernandez (1998) concluded that it contributed significantly to the final diagnosis in about 10 per cent of cases and revealed new findings, though not necessarily of clinical significance, in 23 per cent of cases. Using bronchopneumonia as an example, Hunt et al. (1995) revealed a considerable discrepancy rate between the gross diagnosis at autopsy and its confirmation on histology; independent review of the lung histology confirmed bronchopneumonia in only 69.2 per cent of cases in which it had been diagnosed macroscopically and noted in the provisional report. Furthermore, in approximately 20 per cent of all cases in their survey discrepancies between the gross and histological diagnosis had not been resolved in the final report. This illustrates the importance of basing the final autopsy report on a combination of the gross and histological findings if the information is to be used, as it should be, in clinical audit.

Recent problems associated with undisclosed or insufficiently authorised tissue retention have challenged the routine post-mortem sampling for histology and, therefore, the extent to which the gross findings can be audited (Burton and Underwood, 2003; Mcguone and Kay, 2004). However, most relatives readily grant consent for tissue sampling at post-mortem provided that the purposes are sensitively explained. Indeed, prohibiting post-mortem histology may render the overall examination so uninformative that it would be unethical and wasteful to perform it.

Perhaps the easiest aspect of the autopsy to audit is the report – its accuracy, thoroughness and timeliness. The NCEPOD 1990 survey recruited a panel of 10 pathologists to assess anonymised post-mortem information content and clarity. In 8 per cent of reports, major clinical problems had not been addressed; for example, in one case gangrene of the right leg was described by the surgeon but was not mentioned in the autopsy report! Organ weights and volumes of effusions were not recorded in 26 per cent of reports; these are admittedly of little utility in many cases, but they do impart the verisimilitude of objectivity to an otherwise subjective narrative. In 22 per cent of cases the reports failed to reach the clinical team, and when they did the delay exceeded 60 days in almost 8 per cent of cases. The NCEPOD (2006) report focused on the coroner's autopsy, concluding that about 25 per cent of reports were 'poor' or 'unacceptable'. In the most recent findings of the Confidential Enquiry into Maternal and Child Health, Millward-Sadler (2007) stated that about 25 per cent of autopsy reports in maternal deaths were 'poor' or 'appalling'.

In another study, analysis of autopsy reports led to the detection of some significant insufficiencies, but a second audit conducted 2 years after feeding back the results to the pathologists yielded an improvement (Williams *et al.*, 1997).

Rushton (1991) published the results of an audit of perinatal autopsy reports, concluding that 55 per cent failed to achieve an arbitrary set minimum standard. These findings reinforce general concerns about autopsy standards. A high autopsy rate, common in perinatal deaths, does not necessarily equate with a high standard in individual cases. Indeed, any sustained increase in autopsy rates must not be to the detriment of the standard to which they are performed or reported.

Conclusion

Autopsies should be a major feature of clinical audit. In addition to autopsies on those cases in which there is doubt about the cause of death etc., genuine audit must include a sufficiently large sample of cases in which there appear to be no clinical uncertainties. To be effective in improving clinical practice, information from individual autopsies must be made available promptly to the deceased patients' clinicians; aggregated autopsy data should be subjected to regular review by clinicians and by pathologists. Anderson *et al.* (1989) have proposed that institutional funding for audit should be based on achieving target autopsy rates.

It is regrettable, but understandable, that the clinical imperative of diagnostic biopsies has resulted in marginalisation of autopsies unless, apparently, there are pecuniary inducements. More should be done to promote public and professional awareness of the utility of the clinical autopsy in advancing medical knowledge and improving clinical practice. Despite substantial progress in ante-mortem diagnostic methods during the last century, William Osler's (1849–1919) opinion of autopsies should still be commended to today's clinicians:

> *To investigate the causes of death, to examine carefully the condition of organs, after such changes have gone on in them as to render existence impossible and to apply knowledge to the prevention and treatment of disease, is one of the highest objects of the physician.*

The autopsy should be implicit in clinical audit, not relegated to just an option.

References

Anderson NH, Shanks JH, McCluggage GWG, Toner PG (1989). Necropsies in clinical audit. *J Clin Pathol* **42**:897–901.

Anderson RE, Hill RB (1989). The current status of the autopsy in academic medical centers in the United States. *Am J Clin Pathol* **92**:531–7.

Anderson RE, Hill RB, Gorstein F (1990). A model for the autopsy-based quality assessment of medical diagnostics. *Hum Pathol* **21**:174–81.

Battle RM, Pathak D, Humble CG *et al.* (1987). Factors influencing discrepancies between premortem and postmortem diagnoses. *JAMA* **258**:339–44.

Burton JL, Underwood JCE (2003). Necropsy practice after the 'organ retention scandal': requests, performance and tissue retention. *J Clin Pathol* **56**:537–41.

Burton JL, Underwood JCE (2007). Clinical, educational, and epidemiological value of autopsy. *Lancet* **369**:1471–80.

Cabot RC (1912). Diagnostic pitfalls identified during a study of 3000 autopsies. *JAMA* **59**:2295–8.

Cameron HM, McGoogan E (1981). A prospective study of 1152 hospital autopsies: analysis of inaccuracies in clinical diagnosis and their significance. *J Pathol* **133**:285–300.

Cameron HM, McGoogan E, Watson H (1980). Necropsy: a yardstick for clinical diagnosis. *Br Med J* **281**:985–8.

Camplin EA, Devlin HB, Lunn JN (1990). *Report of the National Confidential Enquiry into Perioperative Deaths, 1989.* Available at www.ncepod.org.uk/1989.htm.

Camplin EA, Devlin HB, Hoile RW, Lunn JN (1992). *Report of the National Confidential Enquiry into Perioperative Deaths, 1990.* Available at www.ncepod.org.uk/1990.htm.

Chane J, Rhys-Maitland R, Hon P *et al.* (1990). Who asks permission for an autopsy? *J R Coll Phys (Lond)* **24**:185–8.

Friederici HH, Sebastian M (1984). The concordance score: correlation of clinical and autopsy findings. *Arch Pathol Lab Med* **108**:515–17.

Gobbato F, Vecchiet F, Barbierato D, Melato M, Manconi R (1982). Inaccuracy of death certificate diagnoses in malignancy: an analysis of 1405 autopsied cases. *Hum Pathol* **13**:1036–8.

Goldman L, Saylon R, Robbins S *et al.* (1983). The value of the autopsy in three medical eras. *N Engl J Med* **308**:1000–5.

Gruver RH, Freis ED (1957). A study of diagnostic errors. *Ann Intern Med* **47**:108–20.

Guly H (2005). More autopsies will improve patient care: has the case been made? *Qual Safety Health Care* **14**:397.

Harris MD, Blundell JW (1991). Audit of necropsies in a British district general hospital. *J Clin Pathol* **11**:862–5.

Hunt CR, Benbow EW, Knox WF, McMahon RF, McWilliam LJ (1995). Can histopathologists diagnose bronchopneumonia? *J Clin Pathol* **48**:120–3.

Kircher T (1990). The autopsy and vital statistics. *Hum Pathol* **21**:166–73.

Kircher T, Nelson J, Burdo H (1985). The autopsy as a measure of accuracy of the death certificate. *N Engl J Med* **313**:1263–9.

Mcguone D, Kay EW (2004). The impact of the organ retention controversy on the practice of hospital necropsy: a four-year audit. *J Clin Pathol* **57**:448.

McPhee SJ, Bottles K (1985). Autopsy: moribund art or vital science? *Am J Med* **78**:107–13.

Millward-Sadler H (2007). Pathology. In: Lewis G (ed.) *Saving Mothers' Lives: Reviewing Maternal Deaths to Make Motherhood Safer, 2003–5.* London. Confidential Enquiry into Maternal and Child Health.

National Confidential Enquiry into Patient Outcomes and Death (2006). *The Coroner's Autopsy: Do We Deserve Better?* London: NCEPOD.

Nemetz PN, Ludwig J, Kurland LT (1987). Assessing the autopsy. *Am J Pathol* **128**:362–9.

Reid WA (1987). Cost effectiveness of routine postmortem histology. *J Clin Pathol* **40**:459–61.

Reid WA, Harkin PJ, Jack AS (1987). Continual audit of clinical diagnostic accuracy by computer: a study of 592 autopsy cases. *J Pathol* **153**:99–107.

Roulson J, Benbow EW, Hasleton PS (2005). Discrepancies between clinical and autopsy diagnosis and the value of post mortem histology: a meta-analysis and review. *Histopathology* **47**:551–9.

Rushton DI (1991). West Midlands perinatal mortality survey, 1987: an audit of 300 perinatal autopsies. *Br J Obstet Gynaecol* **98**:624–7.

Saracci R (1991). Is necropsy a valid monitor of clinical diagnosis performance? *Br Med J* **303**:898–900.

Sonderegger-Iseli K, Burger S, Muntwyler J, Salomon F (2000). Diagnostic errors in three medical eras: a necropsy study. *Lancet* **355**:2026–31.

Underwood JCE, Cotton DWK, Stephenson TJ (1989). Audit and necropsy. *Lancet* **i**:442.

Wells HG (1923). Relation of clinical to necropsy diagnosis in cancer and value of existing cancer statistics. *JAMA* **80**:737–40.

Williams JO, Goddard MJ, Gresham GA, Wyatt BA (1997). Audit of necropsy reporting in East Anglia. *J Clin Pathol* **50**:691–4.

Zaitoun AM, Fernandez C (1998). The value of histological examination in the audit of hospital autopsies: a quantitative approach. *Pathology* **30**:100–4.

Chapter 23

REPORTS, DOCUMENTATION AND STATEMENTS

Guy N Rutty

Introduction

Having completed an autopsy examination the pathologist can generate a number of different reports, documentation or statements that differ in their structure, purpose and readership. For the hospital permission autopsy, which has no medicolegal context, the pathologist will produce a report that will be sent to the clinician requesting the examination. In the case of a coroner's autopsy, which is a medicolegal examination no matter whether it is a so-called 'routine' or 'forensic' case, the pathologist may have to produce a report or a statement or both. This chapter outlines the variety of types of documentation that can be used by the pathologist to inform the reader of the findings of the examination.

Autopsy reports and statements should be produced promptly and should be available as soon as possible. Delays in producing autopsy reports render them of less use to clinicians, cause administrative difficulties for medicolegal authorities, can delay funerals and cause undue distress for relatives. The failure to produce a timely autopsy statement for Crown Court could lead to the case being dismissed.

Data storage, transmission and disclosure

Prior to discussion of the different types of document that can be generated, a short discussion con-

cerning data storage, transmission and disclosure is required.

Data storage

Autopsy paperwork contains personal data that should be protected similarly to other forms of medical information. The pathologist can store the report, for example for a coroner, in a secure manner but cannot release the report to any other person without the permission of the coroner. Thus the pathologist must ensure that any paperwork, file or electronic records arising from the autopsy are stored securely and for a period of time appropriate to the case, which in cases of homicide will be indefinitely.

Transmission

Reports and statements can be sent to legitimate interested parties by mail, fax or email, or by using other electronic media. However, the document must be delivered securely. When sending out documents by post then the use of a signature delivery system and a faxable receipt to confirm arrival is advised. With email, faxes and other electronic media the document should be encrypted and password-protected.

Disclosure

With a medicolegal autopsy, all records of all forms including any documentation, photographs, x-rays etc. as well as the location of any retained biological material must be kept together within the autopsy file. This is important as the pathologist must be able to inform or disclose to another interested party what documentation or samples exist. This can be facilitated by use of the Criminal Justice System's disclosure documentation. This documentation of unused material forms Appendix A of the paperwork for criminal justice cases (see page 337 for an example).

Cause of death

The first document that a pathologist will issue is a statement of the cause of death, even if no cause has been identified at the autopsy and further examinations are pending. Strictly speaking this applies only to medicolegal examinations, as permission autopsies by their very nature should already have a cause of death. However, a correctly worded cause of death may have an educational benefit for clinicians who do not always complete death certificates appropriately (Anderson, 1984; Ashworth, 1991). Further, the Office for National Statistics (ONS) may contact clinicians following an autopsy to obtain further information.

The cause of death should be stated in the standard ONS format. It may also be useful to state whether or not death was due to natural causes, although this is typically the remit of the medicolegal authority authorising the autopsy, not the pathologist (although he or she can assist in this function). Alternatively the pathologist may state whether or not, in his or her opinion, the death was contributed to by the actions of a third party. An example of the layout is shown below:

CAUSE OF DEATH
1a   Pulmonary thromboembolism
1b   Deep vein thrombosis
1c   Immobility due to osteoarthritis
Death was due to natural causes. There were no features to suggest that death was due to the action or inaction of a third party.

This should be put in writing and signed and dated by the pathologist. This can be done, for example, by writing the result onto a coroner's officer's form or by using a department pro forma. The original should be sent to the authorising person and a copy kept with the autopsy file. If sent by fax or email then the document must be encrypted and password-protected.

Where a cause of death cannot be issued at the end of the physical examination a cause of death should still be issued but it should indicate that further investigations are continuing. The following is acceptable:

CAUSE OF DEATH
1a   Unascertained – awaiting further tests
1b
1c

On occasion a cause of death can be issued but the pathologist wishes to undertake further laboratory examinations. In England and Wales under current coroner's law this is not permissible if a natural cause of death can be issued. However, under these circumstances it is possible to issue a provisional cause of death indicating that further examinations are to be undertaken, which will allow the pathologist to proceed with these:

CAUSE OF DEATH
1a   Ischaemic heart disease – pending toxicology and
     histological examinations
1b
1c

In addition to the cause of death, a number of other facts should be stated to assist with the timely release of the body.

- The presence or absence of a cardiac pacemaker, radioactive implants or other medical devices remaining in the body at the end of the autopsy should be recorded.
- It should be stated whether or not, in the opinion of the pathologist, the body should be released for humane disposal.

STATEMENT OF WITNESS

(CJ Act 1967, s.9; MC Act 1980, ss.5A (3) (a) and 5B, Criminal Procedure Rules 2005, Rule 27.1)

STATEMENT OF: Dr *y*
DATE OF BIRTH: Over 21 years

This statement consisting of 1 page signed by me is true to the best of my knowledge and belief and I make it knowing that, if it is tendered in evidence, I shall be liable to prosecution if I have wilfully stated in it anything which I know to be false or do not believe to be true.

Signature ....   **Date: 09 February 2010**

Name of Deceased

Reference number

BODY RELEASE STATEMENT

At the request of *x*, HM Coroner for *z*, Dr *y*, registered medical practitioner, *qualifications and place of work*, undertook an autopsy examination on ******** at ******** mortuary, on ******** 2010. I confirm that I understand that there is no pathological reason for the further retention of the body. Samples of tissue and biological fluids have been retained at the autopsy examination as declared upon the organ retention sheet. No whole organs have been retained.

The provisional cause of death following the autopsy examination is:
1a   ********
1b
1c

I will endeavour to produce a full report within ******** weeks. Should this not be possible I will issue a further statement to indicate the reason for the delay and the likely date of submission of a full report.

I confirm that I understand my duty to the Court and that I have complied with that duty.
The information given within this report represents my understanding of the views, opinions and circumstances of this case based on the information that I have received to date, either in writing (all forms) or by oral communication. I recognise that in part this may reproduce or rely upon witness statements, oral communications or hearsay evidence of second parties and that the information given to me by others may or may not be factually correct at the time of my consideration.
I reserve the right to reconsider any aspect of this report should a significant typographical or grammatical error, or factual inconsistency, be identified that could be misinterpreted by a reader.
I also reserve the right to reconsider any aspect of this report should further factual information arise that contradicts the information provided at the time of the postmortem examination, upon which I have based my interpretations.

Name of pathologist
Position
GMC Reg No.

Signed ....   Date ....

Figure 23.1 Example of a body release statement.

- It should be stated whether the pathologist has retained biological material, photographs or radiological imaging.
- There should be an estimate of the time needed to complete the ancillary investigations.

The pathologist may opt to issue a statement that provides this information in one document. Variations of this format can also include the initial findings and interpretations of the autopsy. This type of document is particularly useful in cases where there may be Crown Court proceedings related to the death and where delays in laboratory examinations may mean that the final autopsy report cannot be provided within the normal time frame required by the court for the production of prosecution documentation. An example of such a statement is shown in Fig. 23.1.

Free-from-infection certificate

Bodies that are to be repatriated to their countries of origin will require the pathologist to provide a free-from-infection certificate. This can be in the form of a letter or statement. It is advisable to state on this whether or not any biological tests have been carried out – for example HIV or hepatitis status. If these have not been undertaken then the pathologist cannot state with certainty that the body is free from infection, and the wording of any documentation should reflect this.

Tissue retention form

Since the introduction of the Human Tissue Act 2004 and the amendments to the Coroner's Rules 2008, it has become a requirement that the pathologist declares whether or not any biological material has been retained after the autopsy. Pathologists will have a variety of paper- or computer-based systems for recording what has been retained, where it has been retained, for how long it is to be retained and what the final outcome of the material was – returned to the body, returned to the relatives, retained for research and teaching, or humanely destroyed. The initial tissue retention form should be forwarded to, for example, the coroner's office with a copy kept within the autopsy file. An example is shown in Fig. 23.2.

Autopsy reports and statements

An excellent autopsy may be marred by the presentation of a poor report/statement. Conversely, an excellent report/statement may be generated from a substandard autopsy. It is essential to ensure that the report/statement is complete, concise, clear and factually correct. On this last matter, one is reminded of the wording at the start of a criminal justice statement:

> STATEMENT OF WITNESS
> (CJ Act 1967, s.9; MC Act 1980, ss.5A (3) (a) and 5B; Criminal Procedure Rules 2005, Rule 27.1)
> Statement of: Dr [...]
> Date of birth: Over 21 years
> This statement consisting of 1 page signed by me is true to the best of my knowledge and belief, and I make it knowing that, if it is tendered in evidence, I shall be liable to prosecution if I have wilfully stated in it anything that I know to be false or do not believe to be true.

Similarly to the cause of death, the documentation may be issued based on the macroscopic findings with subsequent supplementary documentation to follow the completion of additional laboratory investigations. This is of benefit as it provides information while the case is fresh in the clinician's mind. The disadvantage is that it may encourage pathologists to, for example, put post-mortem histology aside, resulting in unacceptable delays. However, it is possible, with sufficient effort, to optimise the reporting process so that the macroscopic and microscopic reports are produced together within a few days (Adickes and Sims, 1996). The present author prefers to issue a single complete final report/statement encompassing both the autopsy and laboratory investigations. By use of, for example, a provisional body release statement as illustrated above, this enables essential information to be provided at an early stage with the full report to follow within the time estimated on this provisional documentation.

NAME: _____

PLACE OF EXAMINATION: _____

DATE OF AUTOPSY: _____

PATHOLOGIST: _____

CORONER: _____

TISSUE	SAMPLED (✓)	NUMBER OF PIECES	WHOLE ORGAN (✓)
BRAIN			
SPINAL CORD			
MENINGES			
EYES			
HEART			
VESSEL			
RIGHT LUNG			
LEFT LUNG			
LARYNX			
TRACHEA			
TONGUE			
OESOPHAGUS			
STOMACH			
SMALL INTESTINE			
APPENDIX			
LARGE INTESTINE			
LIVER			
PANCREAS			
GALL BLADDER			
RIGHT KIDNEY			
LEFT KIDNEY			
BLADDER			
PROSTATE			
TESTIS			
UTERUS			
OVARY			
PITUITARY			
THYROID			
ADRENAL			
THYMUS			
SPLEEN			
LYMPH NODE			
TONSIL			
SKIN			
DIAPHRAGM			
MUSCLE			
PERIPHERAL NERVE			
BONE (SPECIFY)			
OTHER (SPECIFY)			

SAMPLES	SAMPLED (✓)
BLOOD	
URINE	
STOMACH	
VITREOUS	
CSF	
BILE	
FAECES	
HAIR	
NAILS	
GUTHRIE CARD	
EFFUSIONS	
ASCITES	

TAKEN	YES (✓)
X-RAY	
CT SCAN	
PHOTOGRAPHS	

PLEASE COMMENT HERE FOR SAMPLES OTHER THAN HISTOLOGY & TOXICOLOGY ON NATURE OF EXAMINATION, E.G. MICROBIOLOGY AND WHERE SAMPLE ARE SENT:

<u>BRAIN</u>

<u>HEART</u> _____

<u>MICROBIOLOGY/VIROLOGY</u>

<u>ADDITIONAL DETAILS:</u> _____

_____

_____

_____

_____

_____

_____

_____

_____

_____

TOXICOLOGY SAMPLES ARE SENT TO THE **XXXX**, UNLESS OTHERWISE STATED

HISTOLOGY SAMPLES ARE SENT TO THE **XXXX**, UNLESS OTHERWISE STATED

PATHOLOGIST

SIGNED: _____

PRINTED: _____

DATED: _____

CORONER

SIGNED: _____

PRINTED: _____

DATED: _____

Figure 23.2 Example of a tissue retention form.

The format

The findings of the autopsy can be provided as a report or a statement or both. Although similar, these two formats are differently defined by the *Oxford English Dictionary*:

- Report – verb: give a spoken or written account of something; noun: an account given of a matter after investigation or consideration.
- Statement – noun: a definite or clear expression of something in speech or writing; a formal account of facts or events, especially one given to the police or in court.

Each format should contain the same basic account of the autopsy finding. The difference lies in the additional wording added to the beginning of a statement. The first addition is illustrated above. The second difference is the inclusion of the following paragraphs at the start of the report. This outlines the pathologist's duty to the court and necessity to compile the index of material for the purposes of disclosure:

> I am an expert in **Forensic Pathology** and I have been requested to provide a statement.
>
> I understand that I owe an overriding duty to the Court to provide independent assistance, to the Court, by way of unbiased opinion in relation to the matters within my expertise and that such advice must be uninfluenced by the exigencies of the case. I have complied with, and will continue to comply with, my duty to the Court.
>
> I confirm that I have read guidance contained in a booklet known as Disclosure: Expert's Evidence and Unused Material which details my role and documents my responsibilities, in relation to revelation as an expert witness. I have followed the guidance and recognise the continuing nature of my responsibilities of revelation. In accordance with my duties of revelation, as documented in the guidance booklet:
>
> (a)   I confirm that I have complied with my duties to record, retain and reveal material in accordance with the Criminal Procedure and Investigations Act 1996, as amended.
>
> (b)   I have compiled an index of all material. I will ensure that the index is updated if I am provided with or generate additional material.
>
> (c)   In the event my opinion changes on any material issue, I will inform the investigating officer, as soon as reasonably practicable, and give reasons.

The final difference is that reports tend to be signed only at the end of the document whereas statements are signed, dated and may be required to be witnessed on every page. The author, however, recommends that all pages should be signed and dated no matter which format is used.

Some departments favour a printed pro forma while others use free text. The use of complete sentences is regarded as essential by some pathologists while others use phrases such as 'Larynx – no significant abnormality'. Some use lists of organs, structures and component parts within anatomical regions or systems while others prefer paragraphs of descriptive text. These issues are best left to the individual. The choice of present or past tense is also a matter of personal preference.

Probity

The autopsy report must, as stressed throughout this chapter, be factually correct and honest. To knowingly falsify any aspect of an autopsy report or misrepresent another's opinion could lead ultimately to a professional investigation, for example by the General Medical Council, or even prosecution for perjury. Of note, unlike so-called 'forensic cases' undertaken in England and Wales, the vast majority of autopsies have no form of independent second examination, audit or checking (Rutty, 2006). The use of an internal so-called 'critical checking system' for autopsy reports is one way to establish audit within a department. The final report can be checked by a second pathologist within the department; and assuming that the procedures that were apparently undertaken, the findings, and the interpretation of any additional laboratory examinations appear 'reasonable', then the report can be issued.

One should always keep good records of the autopsy findings. The practice of undertaking several examinations and then dictating them all from memory either in the mortuary or back in one's office is discouraged as it will at best lead to omissions or at worst fictitious additions. The over-reliance on computer-generated templates is also discouraged as these have the tendency to provide information to the reader that may be factually incorrect – for example, 'Endocrine – pituitary, normal' when the pituitary was not in fact examined. It is better to be honest and state 'Endocrine – pituitary, not examined'.

For those providing criminal justice appendix paperwork, then in addition to appendix A discussed above there is a requirement to produce appendices B and C. Appendix B can be incorporated into the body of the statement or provided separately. Appendix C deals with probity. A police criminal records check may also be required for those who are classified as 'expert' witnesses. (See pages 338 and 339 for examples of these appendices.)

The language used

The language of the autopsy report/statement should be that of the mother tongue of the country of practice, which for the UK is English. Reports should be written such that medical and non-medical professionals as well as lay people can read and understand the findings. After all, the family of the deceased, as an interested party, can have sight of the findings and should be able to understand them (Kees *et al.*, 2008). Medical terminology can be used, although where necessary lay language explanations should be given also to ensure comprehension of the report by the reader. An example would be:

> The coronary arteries showed severe atherosclerosis (a hardening and furring up of the blood vessels that supply blood to the heart).

The spelling and grammar of the report should be as correct as possible. The use of a proofreader is encouraged, although this may represent an additional expense to a department.

Component parts

All autopsy reports/statements should be structured and allow the reader to understand the processes and findings of the examination. The inclusion or omission of any single component is a personal choice, although the present author would encourage that all the following should be included.

The introduction

There should be a unique identifying code to distinguish this from other cases. This should indicate under whose authority the examination was undertaken and who undertook it. The introduction should then contain basic details related to the case as exampled below. Statements should contain the two additional paragraphs of writing as described above. The cause of death in standard ONS format can be included at this stage as well as at the end of the report.

> POST-MORTEM REFERENCE NO. [...]
>
> On the authority of [authority], I [name], a licensed and registered medical practitioner [professional position and qualifications], have been requested to undertake an independent post-mortem examination of:
>
> Name: [...]
>
> Age: [...]   Date of birth: [...]
>
> Address: [...]
>
> Scene of incident: [...]
>
> Date and time of death: [...]
>
> Place, date and time of post mortem: [mortuary name] on [date] starting at [... pm] and finishing at [... pm]
>
> Body identified by: [...]
>
> CAUSE OF DEATH:
>
> 1a   [etc.]

Professional statement

For those writing statements, the inclusion at this stage of a professional summary is required. This should be a brief synopsis of one's professional qualifications and experience within the field, to allow those utilising the statement to decide whether or not you are an expert within the field.

Attendees at autopsy

For those writing statements it is important to disclose who was present during the examination, their name, professional designation and rank as well as the role they undertook. This information should be recorded on the contemporaneous notes of all autopsy examinations even if only a pathologist and techologist were involved. If a mortuary technician undertook the evisceration this should be recorded and disclosed, or the role of a pathology trainee in the examination and writing of the report should be disclosed. An example of how this may be recorded is:

> ATTENDEES AT AUTOPSY
> Pathologist
> STR in Pathology
> Senior Investigating Officer
> Senior Scene of Crime Officer
> Scene of Crime Officer
> Mortuary Technician

Clinical history

The next stage is the inclusion of a brief clinical history. Often this is provided by another person – for example a coroner's officer's report or a police officer attending the mortuary. It should be remembered that this is so-called 'hearsay' evidence and may in fact be factually incorrect. It can be prudent to draw this to the attention of the reader as one can be questioned at a later date, for example at an inquest or Crown Court, as to where this history arose. An example of wording that can be used at the beginning of this section is as follows:

> Clinical History
> The information contained in the section entitled 'Clinical History' is my interpretation of the information that was given to me by the Coroner's Officer's sudden death report prior to the autopsy examination. This information may or may not be factually correct and may alter during the coroner's investigation subsequent to the end of the autopsy examination.

The history recorded within the report/statement should be sufficient to identify the time course of the terminal condition or incident that led to the deceased's death, any significant previous history and relevant medication. However, a balance should be struck between adequate and excessive detail within this section. For example:

> **Clinical History**
>
> This 88-year-old woman was admitted to [...] on 1 January 2010 with a sudden onset of left-sided chest pain. She had restricted mobility due to osteoarthritis, for which she was prescribed ibuprofen. On examination she was found to have a swollen, tender, left calf. Chest x-ray was normal. The ECG showed features consistent with pulmonary thromboembolism. Before treatment could be commenced she suffered a cardio-respiratory arrest. Resuscitation attempts were unsuccessful and she died at 1600 hours on the day of admission.

This history would not be enhanced by the inclusion of unnecessary details such as the obstetric history or childhood illnesses. Disclosure of this information, as with any medical information related to the deceased, must always be justifiable as such information may not be known to the relatives and may breach doctor–patient confidentiality, which does not end on the death of an individual. The list of negatives traditionally included in clinical histories, such as 'no rheumatic fever, no TB' etc., can be omitted from the autopsy report. Care should also be taken not to divulge any clinical history into the public domain that may not have been known by surviving relatives – for example sexual proclivities, HIV status or previous criminal convictions.

A list of any documentation, statements or images that have been provided to the pathologist to assist with the writing of the report/statement should be included at this point. This could include witness statements, clinical photographs or collision investigators' reports. Again this is all part of the principle of disclosure so that the reader knows the source of any information provided to the pathologist that may have been used in the production of the report/statement.

Scene of death

If the pathologist has visited the scene of death or has received photographs or seen a video recording – as may occur in a road traffic accident death – then a brief description of information that has a bearing on the death should be included here. The address, date and time of attendance (arrival and departure) should be stated.

Identification of the deceased

A clear statement of the means of how the deceased was identified to the pathologist should be made. Whether this is a separate component or simply contained in the opening details is a personal preference. For example:

> IDENTIFICATION
>
> The body was identified to me as that of [...] of [...], by [...], at the [mortuary name] on [date] at [time].

The external examination

The account of the external examination details the findings related to general physical observations, identifying features, marks of recent and past medical treatment, natural disease or injury, as well as clothing, jewellery and modifications as detailed in Chapter 8. Rather than present these findings in paragraph format, it can be helpful – particularly when the findings are complex – to present them under subheadings as illustrated below. This provides useful structure, and makes it easier to relate these findings in court. The disclosure of the existence of diagrams from the autopsy examination can be made at this stage. These can be included within the appendices of the report/statement.

> EXTERNAL EXAMINATION
>
> The body was that of a white adult [male or female] in keeping with the stated age of [...]. The hair was [colour] and measured approximately [length in cm] at randomly measured sites. There were no glasses or contact lenses present. The eyes were [colour]. The pupils were midpoint and central. There was no evidence of facial petechiae, cyanosis or congestion. The earlobes were [description].

> Natural teeth were present to the mouth. There was a normal distribution of [male or female] adult body hair. The fingernails measured [length in mm] beyond the tips of the fingers.
>
> The deceased was dressed in the following articles: [...]
>
> The following jewellery was present: [...]
>
> The following tattoos were present: [...]
>
> The following marks were attributed to medical intervention: [...]
>
> The following old marks and injuries were present: [...]
>
> The following fresh marks and changes were present: [...]
>
> Rigor was present throughout; non-blanching post-mortem hypostasis was established in a posterior distribution.
>
> Height: [cm and imperial equivalent]
>
> Weight: [kg and imperial equivalent]
>
> Body diagrams drawn at the time of the autopsy examination are included under Appendix A.

The internal examination

The external examination should be followed by a *systematic* description of the findings in all of the major organ systems. The order is, once again, a matter of personal preference, as is whether to use paragraphs or bullet points. Examples of using the two formats for the cardiovascular system are shown below.

> CARDIOVASCULAR SYSTEM
>
> The heart weighs 350 g and has a normal architecture. The tricuspid, pulmonary, mitral and aortic valves are normal. There is patchy calcified atheroma of the major coronary arteries. The most severe stenoses are as follows: right coronary artery 50%, left anterior descending coronary artery 50%, circumflex artery 80%. No thrombotic occlusions are identified. The left coronary artery is dominant. The myocardium is not hypertrophied, fibrosed or infarcted. The pericardial sac is normal. Mild, uncomplicated atheroma of the aorta is present. The large arteries of the neck and pelvis are unremarkable. The venae cavae are normal. Thrombus is identified in the deep veins of the left calf.

or

> CARDIOVASCULAR SYSTEM
>
> Pericardial sac: Normal
>
> Heart: Weighed at 350 g
>
> Right atrium: Normal
>
> Left atrium: Normal
>
> Right ventricle: Normal
>
> Left ventricle: Normal
>
> Endocardium: Normal
>
> Papillary muscles: Normal
>
> Chordae tendineae: Normal
>
> Valves: Normal
>
> Coronary arteries: A balanced circuit. There was patchy calcified atheroma of the major coronary arteries. The most severe stenoses were as follows: right coronary artery 50%, left anterior descending coronary artery 50%, circumflex artery 80%. No thrombotic occlusions were identified
>
> Aorta: Mild, uncomplicated atheroma
>
> Venous system: Thrombus is identified in the deep veins of the left calf

The use of bold text as illustrated in the second example can allow the reader to skim through a report and pick out the abnormalities present with ease.

Although dismissed as ritual rather than necessity by some authors (Barker, 2000), the weights of all the major organs should be included in the report. The absence of such weights has been used as a quality measure in auditing (Williams *et al.*, 1997). Furthermore, organ weights quoted in the context of normal ranges for the deceased's gender and height or weight can be helpful in explaining the severity of a condition to clinicians and relatives (Start, 2000). This is of particular importance for cardiac weights.

Retained material

Although a biological retention form should be completed at the end of the autopsy as discussed above, a section should be included in the report/statement that indicates what material has been stored following the examination and where it has gone. It should also indicate under whose authority this was undertaken.

> SPECIMENS RETAINED
>
> With the consent of HM Coroner and following discussion with the Senior Investigating Officer, the following were retained:
>
> Histology: [no.] pieces of tissue approximately the size of a postage stamp were placed in plastic cassettes and taken to [place] where they were processed in wax and [no.] glass slides were cut. To date the glass slides and wax blocks remain in the [place]. No whole organs were retained
>
> Toxicology: [sample types] were sent to [place]
>
> Clinical notes: [retained/not retained/photocopies made] by [person]
>
> Photographs: taken by [person or authority]
>
> X-rays: [undertaken/not undertaken] and stored at [place]

Exhibits

In cases where the police are involved, 'exhibits' may be retained during the autopsy examination. A list of the exhibits indicating the unique exhibit number, the description as well as to whom they were handed should be included. If an exhibit is stored in the mortuary or taken to a departmental laboratory, an indication of which exhibit, who took it and to where should also be included here.

This is all part of the process known as 'continuity of evidence' and 'chain of custody'. This is a process where items can be tracked at all stages of their handling, examination and storage and is used for example to show that they have not been tampered with at any stage. Such a system should be employed in normal autopsy practice if only to ensure that the whereabouts of tissue samples is known and logged at all stages (RCPath, 2008). Here is an example:

> EXHIBITS
>
> The following exhibits were handed over to the Scene of Crime Officers at the mortuary:
>
> GR1 – histology samples
>
> GR2 – preserved femoral blood sample
>
> Following the examination, exhibit GR1 was taken by [...] on [date] to [...], where it was processed through the laboratory. GR2 was retained in the mortuary after the examination and taken by [...] on [date] to [...], where it was processed through the laboratory.

Laboratory examinations

The positive findings of any ancillary laboratory examinations should be summarised here. Examples of such investigations include toxicology:

TOXICOLOGY
Forensic toxicological samples were sent to [...]. A copy of the witness statement (Ref: FTOX ...) concerning this examination is in Appendix B. The investigations found [...].

and histology:

HISTOLOGY
Lung: [...]
Heart: [...]
The examination of the remaining organs of the body yielded no additional information that could have caused or contributed to death.

and neuropathology.

In criminal investigations the existence of any laboratory result, *even if it is negative*, arising from a sample derived from the deceased must be disclosed to exist either within the report or on the unused material disclosure form.

Second examination

Bodies may be subject to at least one further examination. If this occurs the pathologist can record this as well as any difference of opinion resulting from the two examinations within the report/statement.

SECOND AUTOPSY
A second independent autopsy was undertaken on the body of the deceased by [...]. It has not been drawn to my attention to date of any differences of opinion between the two autopsy examinations.

Comments and clinicopathological correlation

The report/statement should end with a section outlining the pathologist's conclusions related to the four questions of all autopsy examinations: who the person was, and when, where and how he or she came to die. Although this detail is found within the substance of the report/statement, a brief summary of the major pathological findings in order of their significance should be provided. This can be presented in several formats. The first is a list of the main findings in order of significance:

SUMMARY OF PATHOLOGICAL FINDINGS
1. Pulmonary thromboembolism
2. Pulmonary infarct
3. Deep vein thrombosis
4. Cholelithiasis
5. Uterine fibroids
6. Uncomplicated diverticular disease
7. Resuscitation artefact – rib fractures

The second format is a clinico-pathological correlation:

CLINICOPATHOLOGICAL CORRELATION
Death was due to pulmonary thromboembolism secondary to deep vein thrombosis in the left calf. The clinical history of left-sided chest pain is consistent with the presence of a small pulmonary infarct in the left lower lobe. This indicates that there was at least one episode of thromboembolism prior to the large fatal embolism. The deceased's restricted mobility due to osteoarthritis is likely to have precipitated the deep vein thrombosis.

The combined use of both a summary and a clinico-pathological correlation is recommended. The presence or absence of a clinicopathological correlation has been used as a quality control measure when auditing autopsy reports (NCEPOD, 2006).

The third format is a series of points drawing out the most significant parts of the autopsy findings. This can include expressions of opinion as to how pathologies may have arisen:

COMMENTS
1. The body was that of a white adult [male or female] in keeping with the stated age of [...].
2. The external examination identified [no.] marks which were attributed to medical intervention. These have neither caused nor contributed to death.

3. The external examination identified [no.] single or groups of old injuries which have neither caused nor contributed to death.

4. The external examination identified [no.] single or groups of fresh injuries. These have arisen [opinion as to causation and relevance to cause of death].

5. The internal examination identified the following pathologies: [...].

6. At the time of the deceased's death, he/she [was or was not] under the influence of [drugs or alcohol].

7. I am thus of the opinion that death arose [opinion as to how the deceased came to die].

this case based on the information that I have received to date, either in writing (all forms) or by oral communication. I recognise that in part this may reproduce or rely on witness statements, oral communications or hearsay evidence of second parties and that the information given to me by others may or may not be factually correct at the time of my consideration.

I reserve the right to reconsider any aspect of this report should a significant typographical or grammatical error, or factual inconsistency, be identified that could be misinterpreted by a reader. I also reserve the right to reconsider any aspect of this report should further factual information arise that contradicts the information provided at the time of the post-mortem examination, on which I have based my interpretations.

Coding of the various diagnoses should be undertaken using a system such as SNOMED. It can also be considered to add a disclaimer at the end of the report/statement prior to stating the final cause of death and the signature such as illustrated below. This allows the pathologist to review and revise any aspect should an error have occurred at any stage or new evidence arise in the future in relation to the death.

I confirm that I understand my duty is to the Court and that I have complied with that duty.

The information given within this report represents my understanding of the views, opinions and circumstances of

The report/statement is thus concluded with an indication of the author of the report, with his or her professional designation and GMC number. If a system such as a critical check has been undertaken then an indication of such should be included at this stage. Any documentation such as body diagrams or toxicology reports that the pathologist wishes to produce to support the findings within the report/statement can be included as appendices.

References

Adickes ED, Sims KL (1996). Enhancing autopsy performance and reporting: a system for a 5-day completion time. *Arch Pathol Lab Med* **120**:249–53.

Anderson RE (1984). The autopsy as an instrument of quality assessment: classification of pre-mortem and post-mortem diagnostic discrepancies. *Arch Pathol Lab Med* **108**:490–3.

Ashworth TG (1991). Inadequacy of death certification: proposal for change. *J Clin Pathol* **44**:265–8.

Barker THW (2000). Necropsy organ weights are largely useless. *J Clin Pathol* **53**:243.

Kees E, Brownlee C, Ruff M *et al.* (2008). How well do we communicate autopsy findings to next of kin? *Arch Pathol Lab Med* **132**:66–71.

National Confidential Enquiry into Patient Outcome and Death (2006). *The Coroner's Autopsy: Do We Deserve Better?* London: NCEPOD.

Royal College of Pathologists (2008). *Guidelines for Handling Medicolegal Specimens and Preserving the Chain of Evidence.* London: RCPath.

Rutty GN (2006). Who audits the autopsy? *Forensic Sci Med Pathol* **2**(2):71–2.

Start RD (2000). [Letter]. *J Clin Pathol* **53**:243–6.

Williams JO, Goddard MJ, Gresham GA, Wyatt BA (1997). Audit of necropsy reporting in East Anglia. *J Clin Pathol* **50**:691–4.

APPENDIX FORMS USED IN CRIMINAL JUSTICE CASES

1. Appendix A

EXPERT'S INDEX OF UNUSED MATERIAL

A listing of all the unused material held in relation to this case by:

Name of Expert:

EXPERT'S USE				CPS USE	
No	**Description of material**	**Location**		**Insert C, I or CND**	**Comment**
1					
2					
3					
4					
5					
6					
7					
8					
9					
10					
Completed by: Signed: Date				Reviewing Lawyer: Date: Signature:	

2. Appendix B

DECLARATION

I am an expert in *Forensic Pathology* and I have been requested to provide a statement. I confirm that I have read guidance contained in a booklet known as *Disclosure: Expert's evidence and unused material* which details my role and documents my responsibilities, in relation to revelation as an expert witness. I have followed the guidance and recognise the continuing nature of my responsibilities of revelation. In accordance with my duties of revelation, as documented in the guidance booklist.

a   I confirm that I have complied with my duties to record, retain and reveal material in accordance with the Criminal Procedure and Investigations Act 1996, as amended;

b   I have compiled an Index of all material; I will ensure that the Index is updated in the event I am provided with or generate additional material;

c   in the event my opinion changes on any material issue, I will inform the investigating officer, as soon as reasonably practicable and give reasons.

Signed

Dated

3. Appendix C

Expert Witnesses
Self-Certificate
Revelation of Information
(Criminal Procedure and Investigations Act 1996)

Name of Expert Witness: Date of birth: over 21

Business Address:

Defendant (if known):

I have been instructed to provide expert evidence in relation to the prosecution of the above-named, or an investigation into the following criminal offence.

I confirm that I have read the booklet known as *Disclosure: Expert's evidence and unused material* that has been given to me with this form, and that I am aware of my responsibilities as an expert witness to reveal to the Prosecution Team any information that might undermine any evidence.

1 Have you ever been convicted of, cautioned for, or received a penalty notice for any
   criminal offence (other than minor traffic offences)?   **YES   NO**
2 Are there any proceedings pending against you in any criminal or civil court?   **YES   NO**
3 Are you aware of any adverse findings by a judge, magistrate or coroner about your
   professional competence or credibility as a witness?   **YES   NO**
4 Have you ever been the subject of any adverse findings by a professional or
   regulatory body?   **YES   NO**
5 Are there any proceedings, referrals or investigations pending against you that have
   been brought by a professional or regulatory body?   **YES   NO**
6 Are you aware of any other information that you think may severely affect your
   professional competence and credibility as an expert witness?   **YES   NO**

Should you have any queries in relation to your answers to any of the above, please contact the investigator.

Please note that the questions above apply to any proceedings, findings or other relevant information in this or any other jurisdiction.

If you have answered YES to any of the questions numbered 1–6, please give details below:

DECLARATION

All the information I have given in this certificate is true to the best of my knowledge and belief.

I will notify those instructing me of any change in this information.

I am aware that any false or misleading information I have given in this document, or any deliberate omission of relevant information may lead to disciplinary or criminal proceedings.

Signed

Name (in block capitals)

Date

INDEX

Figures are comprehensively referred to from the text. Therefore, significant material in figures have only been given a page reference in the absence of their concomitant mention in the text referring to that figure.